Handbook of Community and Home Health Nursing

Tools for Assessment, Intervention, and Education

D0154653

Handbook of Community and Home Health Nursing

Tools for Assessment, Intervention, and Education

MARCIA STANHOPE, RN, DSN, FAAN
Professor and Director
Division of Community Health Nursing and Administration
College of Nursing
University of Kentucky
Lexington, Kentucky

RUTH N. KNOLLMUELLER, RN, PhD
Visiting Professor
Division of Community Health Nursing and Administration
College of Nursing
University of Kentucky
Lexington, Kentucky

SECOND EDITION

illustrated

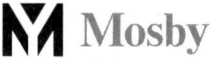

St. Louis Baltimore Boston Carlsbad Chicago Naples New York Philadelphia Portland
London Madrid Mexico City Singapore Sydney Tokyo Toronto Wiesbaden

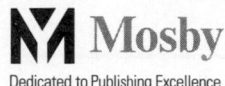
Mosby

Dedicated to Publishing Excellence

A Times Mirror
Company

Publisher: Nancy L. Coon
Editor: Loren Wilson
Associate Developmental Editor: Brian Dennison
Project Manager: Patricia Tannian
Production: Graphic World Publishing Services
Book Design Manager: Gail Morey Hudson
Manufacturing Manager: David Graybill
Cover Designer: Teresa Breckwoldt

SECOND EDITION

Printed in the United States of America
Composition by Graphic World, Inc.
Printing/binding by R.R. Donnelley & Sons Company

Mosby–Year Book, Inc.
11830 Westline Industrial Drive
St. Louis, Missouri 63146

Library of Congress Cataloging in Publication Data

Stanhope, Marcia.
    Handbook of community and home health nursing : tools for
  assessment, intervention, and education / Marcia Stanhope, Ruth N.
  Knollmueller. — 2nd ed.
      p. cm.
  Includes bibliographical references and index.
  ISBN 0-8151-8150-7
  1. Community health nursing. 2. Public health nursing. 3. Home
nursing.   I. Knollmueller, Ruth N. II. Title.
  [DNLM: 1. Community Health Nursing—handbooks. 2. Home Care
Services—handbooks.   WY 49 S786h 1996]
RT98.S782   1996
610.73′43—dc20
DNLM/DLC
for Library of Congress   95-44620
                                                        CIP

95 96 97 98 99 / 9 8 7 6 5 4 3 2 1

PREFACE

This work is a compilation of practical instruments, guidelines, hints, and charts that can be used to aid public health, community health, community-based, and home health nurses in implementing care plans and intervening with clients, whether families or individuals. Use of these tools will also aid the nurse in collecting information that can be used to evaluate health care outcomes. The tools herein are not exhaustive in identifying problems or strategies that may be useful in community and home settings. However, they do offer practical guidance for dealing with many of the problems community and home health nurses typically face.

The guidelines presented are general. Agency policies and procedures and client mix will dictate the specific strategies used for applying the nursing process to client care in the community. This handbook provides the nurse with a ready reference for reviewing pertinent nursing knowledge at the time of providing care. The information contained herein will also assist faculty and students by providing structure for the students' synthesis of knowledge related to all parameters of practice in community health nursing. In addition, researchers may apply these tools to the study of problems encountered in the community.

We wish to thank those who have permitted their work to be shared and acknowledge their expertise and the contributions they have made to promoting the health of communities, families, and individuals.

Marcia Stanhope   **Ruth N. Knollmueller**

CONTENTS

PART THREE: SCREENING TOOLS

PART FIVE: INTERVENTION GUIDES

PART ONE
RESOURCE DATA

 Quick Reference Information

The context of the home visit and safety guidelines are elements of the nurse's daily life in the field. Proper bag technique, essential supplies and equipment, and tips for improvising care in the home are all necessary to provide safe, quality care in an efficient manner.

Safety Guidelines

1. Do not take your purse with you on visits. Lock it in your desk or file cabinet before leaving the office.
2. Keep the interior of the car free of personal belongings. If you must keep personal items in your car, lock them in the trunk before leaving the office parking lot.
3. Alert the family (when possible) that you are coming and have them watch for you.
4. Have accurate directions to the street, building, and apartment.
5. If the area is unfamiliar to you, check with your supervisor for more detailed information.
6. If you are driving alone, drive with the windows closed and all car doors locked.
7. As you approach your destination, carefully observe your surroundings. Note location and activity of people; types and locations of cars; condition of buildings (abandoned or heavily congested buildings).
8. Park in a well-lighted and heavily traveled area.
9. Before getting out of the car, once again thoroughly check the surroundings. If you feel uneasy, do not get out of your car. Return to the office or call from a safe location.
10. Be alert at all times, from the moment you leave the office until you return.

Courtesy Visiting Nurse and Home Care, Inc, Waterbury, Conn.

Phases and Activities of a Home Visit

Phase	Activity
I Initiation phase	Clarify source of referral for visit Clarify purpose for home visit Share information on reason and purpose of home visit with family
II Previsit phase	Initiate contact with family Establish shared perception of purpose with family Determine family's willingness for home visit Schedule home visit Review referral and family record
III In-home phase	Introduction of self and professional identity Social interaction to establish rapport Establish nurse-client relationship Implement nursing process
IV Termination phase	Review visit with family Plan for future visits
V Postvisit phase	Record visit Plan for next visit

From Stanhope M, Lancaster J: *Community health nursing,* ed 4, St Louis, 1996, Mosby.

Essential Supplies and Equipment

The following checklists contain suggested supplies and equipment needed for the home visit.

Home visit bag

1. Sphygmomanometer   _____
2. Stethoscope   _____
3. Thermometer   _____
   a. Oral   _____
   b. Rectal   _____
4. Scissors   _____
5. Forceps   _____
6. Epinephrine   _____
7. TB syringe/needle   _____
8. Soap   _____
9. Towels   _____
10. Apron   _____
11. Antiseptic wipes   _____
12. Tape measure   _____

13. Penlight _____
14. Oto/Ophthalmoscope (optional) _____
15. Gloves/mask/eyeshield _____

Additional supplies/equipment for home visit

1. Wound care supplies _____
   a. 4 × 4 _____
   b. 2 × 2 _____
   c. Kling _____
   d. Antiseptic solution _____
   e. Irrigation solution _____
   f. Other _____ _____
2. Asepto syringe _____
3. Intravenous therapy setup _____
4. Catheter equipment _____
5. Suction catheter _____
6. Irrigation setup _____
7. Enema _____
8. Ace bandages _____
9. Slings _____
10. Splints _____
11. CPR mask _____
12. Other _____ _____

Bag Technique

- Follow agency policy and procedure for appropriate bag technique.
- Review plan of care and physician's orders.
- Check your bag for essential supplies and equipment to conduct home visit.
- To prevent nurse-to-client, client-to-nurse, or client-to-client contamination, place bag on paper towels or newspaper.
- Explain your actions to the client.
- Wash hands before removing contents of bag.
- Use good hand washing technique and turn off faucets with paper towels (see p. 385).
- Prepare a clean field with paper towels to lay out your equipment/ supplies.
- Follow universal precaution guidelines when providing home care.
- Discard used supplies, syringes, and needles according to agency policy.
- AFTER care is given, wash hands and clean equipment before repacking the bag.
- Organize the bag for efficient use.

Tips on Documentation

Basic Considerations

1. When appropriate, documentation should indicate that client is homebound with specific notation of physical limitations or restrictions that would not allow leaving home. Notes should indicate only activities done outside the home related to the client's health care. Example: physician or laboratory appointments. Some situations indicating homebound treatment follow:
   a. Fractures or disabilities that prevent ambulation without assistance or use of assistive aids, or that prevent weight bearing or the use of arms to open doors, etc.
   b. Shortness of breath with slight exertion as in chronic obstructive pulmonary disease (COPD) or chronic heart failure
   c. Weakness as result of surgery or illness or client being easily fatigued
   d. Dizziness, weakness, poor balance, or unsteady gait
   e. Incision, draining wound, or dressing changes
   f. Indwelling catheter
   g. Wheelchair or bedbound
   h. Sensory deficiencies such as visual or auditory impairment or aphasia
   i. Paraplegia, quadriplegia, hemiplegia, numbness of extremities, paresis, or impaired peripheral circulation
   j. Mental confusion, extreme anxiety, or paranoia
   k. Obesity
   l. Severe pain
2. List all medical diagnoses on care plan because care may be needed for more than one condition; document the most acute diagnosis as the principal diagnosis, using onset date.
3. Indicate a date for each problem or nursing diagnosis in care plan.
4. Documentation should be succinct, descriptive, and relevant. Omit items or words that do not relate or contribute to the necessary information.
5. Omit words describing care given, such as:
   a. Use of *chronic* for *acute exacerbation*
   b. Use of *monitor* for *assess* or *evaluate* if condition has stabilized
   c. Use of *reinforce* instead of *reinstruct* for instruction
   d. Use of *discussed* instead of *instructed*
   e. Use of *check* instead of *perform*
   f. Use of *observe* instead of *assess*

g. Use of words such as *stabilized* or *reviewed* instead of *responding to treatment*

6. Document what is wrong with client, not only client's progress or what is right with him or her. Indicate need for care, not that care is no longer needed, for example:
   Incorrect: respirations improving in rate, depth, and ease
   Correct: respirations remaining at 28 per minute with use of accessory muscles and presence of dyspnea

7. Document information in a factual, objective manner. Avoid injecting subjective information, for example:
   Incorrect: general weakness
   Correct: able to ambulate only 10 feet without fatigue and dizziness
   Incorrect: reddened area on right heel
   Correct: reddened area on right heel, measuring 1 cm in diameter

8. Document all care that relates to medical diagnoses and orders. Be specific and include all care and skills performed, for example, instruct client to draw insulin into syringe, using sterile technique.

9. Document unstable states that require interventions such as medication or catheter changes, sterile irrigations, pulmonary physiotherapy, and others that need skilled nursing care. Make sure skilled care matches the diagnoses and physician orders.

10. Document exercise or other regimens that are performed to restore function lost because of condition being treated and described by medical diagnoses.

11. Document in the care plan the exact services being provided that require skilled, professional nursing care.

12. Indicate in the care plan the time frames in which care will be provided such as two to three times per week or less, depending on condition and insurance parameters.

13. Document goal achievement with dates at least weekly on plan.

14. Each note should contain why the visit was needed; use specific information from assessment to affirm medical necessity and specific care given.

Additional Considerations*

Do not document the following:

• Private sitter or companion
• Client trips

---

*Modified from Jaffe M, Skidmore-Roth L: *Home health nursing care plans,* St Louis, 1988, Mosby.

- Medications reviewed
- Repetitive teaching
- Lack of progress when progress should be seen; instead document inability to participate in therapy

Do document the following:

- Why client or family cannot be taught a procedure
- Poor comprehension of client or family
- Specific signs and symptoms of disease taught to client
- Therapeutic diet taught with sample menus
- Return demonstrations by client to evaluate level of competence
- Medications taught; teach one each visit

PART TWO
ASSESSMENT TOOLS

◉ Environmental Assessment: Home

Healthy populations are active and reach out to various community groups. Individuals and families who function in a healthy way think of themselves as being part of a larger community. Part of successful coping is the ability to seek, receive, or accept appropriate resources to meet the need for a safe environment in which to live. The following assessment tools provide the structure for gathering valuable data related to the home.

Environmental Assessment for Children

Pediatric Review of Children's Environmental Support and Stimulation (PROCESS)

I. Preparation of clinical observation
II. Clinical observation
III. Clinical observation guide
IV. Parent questionnaire
V. Scoring procedures
VI. PROCESS recording form

Preparation of the clinical observation

Not all visits to the health clinic or pediatric office provide the appropriate conditions for making the kinds of observations needed to score items on the Clinical observation section of PROCESS. Generally, a 15- to 20-minute routine health maintenance visit is best suited for making the observation. The parent/child relationship is initially observed by the clinician while taking a medical history. During this portion of the visit, the child should be placed on the

Prepared by Patrick Casey, M.D., University of Arkansas for Medical Sciences and Robert Bradley, Ph.D., 1994, University of Arkansas at Little Rock.

parent's lap. The child should remain on the parent's lap during the less intrusive parts of the physical examination. The child should be separated from the parent and placed on the examination table only for the more invasive aspects of the physical examination. This semistructured format, which is typical for a health maintenance visit, allows observation of the parent/child relationship in increasingly stressful situations. However, it is not as constraining as a briefer clinic visit or a visit scheduled because of a child's illness. The 15 to 20 minutes used for such a visit provides an opportunity for a wide array of parenting behaviors to occur and, hopefully, provides the conditions for many parents to exhibit the kinds of behaviors typical of their behavior at home.

Clinical observation

Child's name _____   Observation date _____

Child's age _____   Sex _____   Race _____   Height _____

Child's weight _____   Observer _____

_____   1. Mother asks questions that are relevant and appropriate about the child.

     _____ irrelevant or no   _____ few questions asked
          questions asked   are relevant
     _____ most questions   _____ all questions are rel-
          asked are relevant   evant

_____   2. Mother shows interest in baby's behavior.

     _____ little or no interest   _____ only somewhat in-
     _____ moderately   terested
          interested   _____ very interested

_____   3. Mother reports how smart or how good baby is.

     _____ never   _____ once
     _____ 2 or 3 times   _____ many times

_____   4. Mother talks, sings, or otherwise vocalizes to baby.

     _____ never   _____ once
     _____ 2 or 3 times   _____ many times

_____   5. Mother is comfortable in caring for baby.

     _____ very uncomfortable/   _____ somewhat uncom-
          awkward   fortable
     _____ comfortable   _____ very comfortable

_____   6. Mother responds to child's social initiations with social response (smile, eye contact, laugh, etc.).

     _____ never   _____ once
     _____ 2 or 3 times   _____ many times

_____ 7. Mother initiates verbal interchanges with observer (asks questions, makes spontaneous comments, etc.).

_____ never   _____ once

_____ 2 or 3 times   _____ many times

_____ 8. Mother expresses ideas freely and easily; uses statements of appropriate length for conversation (more than brief answers).

_____ very poor expres-   _____ poor expressive
sive skills: one or   skills
two word answers   _____ very expressive

_____ appropriate expres-
sive skills

_____ 9. Mother eager to pat or pick up crying baby to quiet or comfort.

_____ ignores child, needs   _____ slow responding
prompting   _____ monitors child dur-

_____ adequate response   ing distress and eager to respond

_____ 10. Mother attends to baby's responses during the examination.

_____ never   _____ once

_____ usually   _____ almost all the time

_____ 11. Mother is detached and/or inwardly absorbed.

_____ not interested in   _____ not interested but
visit or communica-   neutral in emotion
tion, may be hos-   and communication
tile.   _____ extremely interested

_____ shows moderate   and involved
interest and
communication

_____ 12. Mother has eye-to-eye contact with the baby.

_____ never   _____ once

_____ 2 or 3 times   _____ many times

_____ 13. Mother stays within reach of the child.

_____ never   _____ only in distress

_____ most of the time   _____ always physically
available

_____ 14. Mother responds to child's vocalization with verbal responses.

_____ never   _____ once

_____ 2 or 3 times   _____ many times

_____ 15. Mother demonstrates negative responses or feelings toward child.

    _____ many times   _____ 2 or 3 times

    _____ once   _____ never

_____ 16. Mother caresses or strokes baby gently.

    _____ never   _____ once

    _____ 2 or 3 times   _____ many times

_____ 17. Mother looks at baby with warmth and tenderness.

    _____ never   _____ once

    _____ 2 or 3 times   _____ many times

_____ 18. Mother shows positive emotional response to praise of child offered by examiner.

    _____ no response   _____ little or poor response

    _____ some response

                          _____ very positive response

_____ 19. Mother smiles at baby.

    _____ never   _____ once

    _____ 2 or 3 times   _____ many times

_____ 20. Baby is clean. (Not every item necessary to score on a given level.)

    _____ smells bad, diaper area not clean, fingernails dirty, hair oily and matted, scalp dirty and crusty looking

    _____ body and hair clean

    _____ diaper area not clean, fingernails dirty, body dirty, hair dirty

    _____ hair is fixed and clean, smells of recent bath, powdered and "perfumed"

Observation total: _____

Clinical observation guide

Note: Throughout the Clinical Observation Guide the items have been stated for the mother, but this may be any person who is the prime caregiver (foster mother, grandmother, father, etc.).

1. Mother asks questions that are relevant and appropriate about the child or situation.

The key word is *relevant*. Credit is given for the quality of questions asked, not the quantity. "Most questions relevant" means most of the questions themselves were relevant in nature, not that there were many in number. If only one question is asked, but it is relevant, then credit is given for "most questions relevant."

2. Mother shows interest in baby's behavior.

Mother shows interest by close observation and may talk to the child in response to behavior. She may sit forward in the chair or stand to observe the exam more closely.

3. Mother reports how smart or how good baby is.

The mother will make a *spontaneous* comment about the "good things" the baby does. It will be more than a flat response to "what has he/she learned" or other questions.

4. Mother talks, sings, or otherwise vocalizes to baby.

Credit for this will include the soft humming, comforting sounds as well as the more audible vocalizations that may occur.

5. Mother is comfortable in caring for baby.

The mother seems at ease and relaxed with the child and her ability to meet the child's needs. She appears to *enjoy* the child and what he/she is doing. Discomfort can be awkwardness in handling the child (holding, diapering) or difficulty organizing self and the baby.

6. Mother responds to child's social initiations with social response.

This is a response to an action initiated by the child. If the child makes no overtures to the parent, the answer will be "never." The mother must respond to the baby's attention-getting actions (look, vocalization, touch, or gesture) by responding directly to the child.

7. Mother initiates verbal interchanges with observer.

The mother converses with the examiner besides responding to questions. She talks about the child's progress, problems, behavior, concerns, etc.

8. Mother expresses ideas freely and easily; uses statements of appropriate length for conversation.

"Very expressive" indicates good language use, expressing thoughts or concerns spontaneously; appropriate language and ease of manner. "Appropriate expressive" indicates more a simpler speech pattern with shorter sentences, but the speaker is generally fluent. Poor ability involves hesitancy in conversing, short answers, little or no spontaneous communication, sometimes saying "I don't know how to say it," etc. "Very poor expressive skills" indicates much difficulty conversing. Responses consist of one-word answers or prompting and/or assistance is needed. There is no spontaneous speech.

9. Mother eager to pat or pick up crying baby to quiet or comfort.

   The mother who monitors during the exam stands close to the child, has some reaching or touching, speaks to the child to comfort, and picks up child immediately upon conclusion of the exam. She may appear anxious during the child's distress. "Adequate response" involves more passivity or remaining seated, but watching attentively and picking up the child when certain the exam is completed. A slow response involves a mother who remains seated or at a distance, waits to respond after the exam, and moves to the child slowly. The mother who ignores or needs prompting must be told to get the child or have the child handed to her upon completion of the exam.

10. Mother attends to baby's responses during the examination.

    The mother who *attends* monitors the child carefully and with interest throughout the exam. She is aware of the child's responses and may discuss them with the examiner. "Usually" involves attending during most of the exam and observing whether standing by the child or not. "Some" indicates attending only when the child is easily visible. The mother remains seated and makes no special effort to monitor child. "Never" indicates the mother pays little or no attention to the exam, seems preoccupied, looks around, or does something else.

11. Mother is detached and/or inwardly absorbed.

    This mother is noncommunicative, shows little interest or no interest, and may be hostile. The mother who is not interested but neutral shows little interest or involvement but is not hostile. A moderately interested mother may stand back or look away, but is communicative. The extremely interested and involved mother is "present" both physically and mentally during the exam, is verbal and attentive to the child's behavior, and stays nearby.

12. Mother has eye-to-eye contact with baby.

    The eye contact involves the child looking at mother and the mother returning the gaze. If the child does not look at the mother, record this as *"never"* even though the mother looks at the child.

13. Mother stays within reach of the child.

    Mother stays nearby and within reach of the child. The mother is easily accessible to the child unless a physician removes to observe walking or other motor skill, etc.

14. Mother responds to vocalization with verbal responses.

    The mother makes some vocalization (words or sounds) in response to sounds made by the child. These may be imitative of the child's sound or verbal interpretations of what the child "says." May hold a "conversation" with the child. Credit is also given for verbal responses by the mother to the child's crying.

15. Mother demonstrates negative responses or feelings toward child.

    "Negative" means angry looks, frowning or scowling at the child; sharp verbal reprimands or commands; abrupt and/or rough handling (i.e., jerky or rough picking up or moving of the child); pulling or pushing roughly, thumping, pinching, or grabbing. May also include giving the child to someone else to care for, especially if the child is being difficult to manage.

16. Mother caresses or strokes baby gently.

    This includes gentle hugs, pats, petting strokes, and any other soft touch.

17. Mother looks at baby with warmth and tenderness.

    This is more than "just watching" to be sure the child is safe. It includes a genuine show of interest and pleasure, often accomplished by a soft smile and/or lingering look.

18. Mother shows positive emotional response to praise.

    Very positive response involves a positive comment, proud smile, and a further expansion of praised action, a "thank you" with enthusiasm. "Some response" indicates a brief general comment of a "thank you" with little enthusiasm. "Little or poor response" on the part of the mother may include only a nod, "yes," "uh-uh," or some other generalized reaction, usually flat and expressionless in tone. "No response" is completely ignoring the praise.

19. Mother smiles at baby.

    Mother smiles at the child's actions, seemingly showing approval of behavior or appearance. It is not in response to the child's social contact.

20. Baby is clean.

    Very clean babies are really "fixed up." The hair is "done up," the child smells good, obviously has been bathed recently, and is "powdered and perfumed." The clean baby has been bathed and is not dirty, but is not especially "fixed up." The dirty baby in general has marginally clean hair and/or scalp, evidence of not having been bathed recently, diaper area *not* clean, or dirty fingernails. The really dirty baby in general smells bad, the diaper area is not clean, the body is dirty, hair matted and oily, scalp dirty and/or crusty looking. There is evidence of not having been bathed and smell of old urine.

Parent questionnaire

CHILD'S NAME _____   TODAY'S DATE _____

BIRTH DATE _____ SEX _____ RACE _____ AGE _____

CAREGIVER'S NAME _____

RELATIONSHIP TO CHILD:

Mother _____   Grandmother _____

Foster mother _____ Other _____

PARENT'S AGE:

Mother _____   Father _____

PARENT'S EDUCATION:

Mother _____   Father _____

PARENT'S OCCUPATION:

Mother _____   Income _____

Father _____   Income _____

NUMBER OF CHILDREN: _____

BIRTH ORDER OF THIS CHILD: _____

CHILD LIVES WITH (list everyone who lives in household): ___

_____

HOME ADDRESS: _____

_____

TELEPHONE:

Home: _____   Work: _____

PARENT QUESTIONNAIRE INSTRUCTIONS—
PLEASE READ

1. Please **answer ALL questions.** Your answers will remain confidential.
2. Be **HONEST**—there are no right or wrong answers.
3. Mark the answer that is **MOST** appropriate for your situation when two answers seem to be correct. If the question **DOES NOT** seem to fit your child because of his/her age, etc., mark the answer that is closest to what you would do in the situation given.
4. If you need help or have questions about any part of the questionnaire, **PLEASE ASK.**

THANK YOU FOR YOUR TIME AND ASSISTANCE.

_____ 1. How long do you spend talking with your child each day?
   _____ 10 to 20 minutes   _____ 20 to 60 minutes
   _____ 1 to 2 hours   _____ more than 2 hours
                             a day

_____ 2. How often do you ask your friends or family for their suggestions on how to raise your baby?
   _____ hardly ever   _____ occasionally
   _____ about once a month _____ about once a week
                             or more

_____ 3. How often do you read the articles from newspapers, magazines, or books on how to raise a baby?
   _____ very rarely   _____ only occasionally
   _____ about once a month _____ about once a week

_____ 4. How often does your child's father or other adult male do some care giving for your child (dress, feed, bathe, put to bed, babysit while you are away)?
   _____ not very often   _____ once a week
   _____ about three to four _____ nearly every day
         times a week

_____ 5. What do you do when your baby starts to cry?
   _____ try to ignore the   _____ go to the baby only
         crying until he/she   if the crying keeps
         stops   on for a while
   _____ see if there is any- _____ pick him/her up and
         thing wrong, and if   hold or play with
         he/she is OK, let   him/her for a while
         him/her cry

_____ 6. Where does your baby usually sleep at nap time?
   _____ wherever he/she   _____ in whatever room
         falls asleep   I'm in
   _____ in a room alone   _____ in a room alone,
         while I go on with   and I keep the rest
         my household   of the house quiet
         activity

_____ 7. How would you describe your child?
   _____ often fussy and hard _____ sometimes fussy,
         to care for   but can be com-
   _____ usually happy and   forted without too
         easy to care for   much trouble
                             _____ always happy and
                                   easy to care for

_____ 8. How much is the T.V. or radio on while your child is awake?

    _____ nearly all the time   _____ about 3 to 5 hours
    _____ about 1 to 2 hours   a day
                                     _____ never

_____ 9. How often do you feel uncomfortable caring for your baby?

    _____ frequently   _____ some of the time
    _____ hardly ever   _____ never

_____ 10. Where does your child sleep at night?

    _____ in bed with parents   _____ in bed with his/her
    _____ in his/her own bed   brother or sister
    in his/her own room   _____ in his/her bed—
                                        sharing a room

_____ 11. What do you usually do when your child keeps on acting bad or misbehaving?

    _____ shake or spank   _____ scold him/her
    him/her   _____ try to get him/her
    _____ leave him/her alone   interested in some-
                                        thing else

_____ 12. How regular is your child's sleeping schedule?

    _____ at different times   _____ at the same time
    most every day   only 2 or 3 days a
    _____ at the same time 5   week
    or 6 days a week   _____ at about the same
                                        time every day

_____ 13. Where does your child spend his/her awake or play time?

    _____ in a playpen so   _____ in his/her room
    I know where   _____ I keep my child
    he/she is   within sight and
    _____ my child can go   check on him/her
    where he/she wants   often
    as long as he/she
    does not get hurt.

_____ 14. In how many places have you and your child lived in the past 2 years?

    _____ four or more   _____ three
    _____ two   _____ only one

_____ 15. How often do you change decorations or objects in your child's room?

    _____ do not change them   _____ seldom change them
    _____ occasionally change   _____ change them often
    them

_____ 16. How many people live in the same house with you and your baby?

_____ more than six   _____ four to six others
_____ two or three others   _____ one other

_____ 17. About how much time do you spend helping your child learn new things (crawling, walking, talking, using a spoon, holding/playing with a toy)?

_____ hardly any   _____ 10 to 15 minutes a
_____ 15 to 30 minutes a   couple of times a
      day   week

                             _____ an hour or more
                                   a day

_____ 18. How do you think young babies learn new things?

_____ Babies usually will   _____ Babies need some
      learn new things as   help when they are
      they grow up.   learning a few
_____ Babies need help   things like feed-
      when they are *first*   ing or dressing
      learning to do   themselves, using
      something, just to   the potty, etc.
      show them how,   _____ Babies need help all
      then they will learn   the time when they
      by themselves.   are learning to do
                                    things.

_____ 19. How often do you play with your baby using toys that will help him/her learn a new skill?

_____ once or twice a   _____ several times a
      month   week
_____ almost every day   _____ several times
                                   every day

_____ 20. What do you do when you get a new toy for your child?

_____ I buy only toys I   _____ I let him/her figure
      know he/she can   out how to use it by
      play with without   him/herself.
      help.   _____ I play with him/her
_____ I show him/her   and the toy until
      once or twice what   he/she can use it
      to do, then let   easily.
      him/her play with it
      and figure it out.

_____ 21. When your child is fussy, what do you do? (This is at times other than when he/she is tired or hungry.)

_____ scold or spank him/her

_____ try to get him/her interested in a toy or something

_____ let him/her fuss

_____ play with or hold him/her

IF YOUR CHILD IS YOUNGER THAN 8 MONTHS OF AGE, PLEASE ANSWER THE QUESTIONS 22a-24a. THEN COMPLETE THE TOY CHECK LIST.

_____ 22a. Who feeds your baby?

_____ I usually let the baby feed him/herself or prop the bottle

_____ Myself or one other person (this *must* be the same "other person" each time)

_____ whoever is available to help

_____ I usually feed the baby myself

_____ 23a. How often do you have to get someone else to hold or play with your baby when he/she is fussy so you can finish your work?

_____ several times every day

_____ only once or twice a week

_____ every day

_____ hardly ever/never

_____ 24a. On what kind of feeding schedule is your baby?

_____ a very set schedule

_____ a regular schedule about 3 or 4 days a week

_____ no set schedule— whenever he/she cries

_____ a regular schedule, but it will change to meet his/her needs if necessary

IF YOUR CHILD IS **8 MONTHS OF AGE OR OLDER,** AN-
SWER THE QUESTIONS 22b-24b, THEN COMPLETE THE **TOY
CHECK LIST.**

_____ 22b. How are family meals handled?

_____ unplanned, every-
one gets his/her
own

_____ planned, with foods
cooked but not al-
ways served at
regular times

_____ unplanned, food
is fixed whenever
someone is hungry

_____ planned, with foods
cooked and served
at regular times
every day

_____ 23b. How often does your child have at least one meal with
you and his/her father or other adult male figures. (The
other adult male must be the same adult male each
time—grandfather, uncle, etc.)

_____ less than once a
week

_____ three or four times
a week

_____ about once a week

_____ every day

_____ 24b. When does your child usually eat?

_____ whenever he/she is
hungry, seems like
all the time

_____ two or three times
a day, but not on
a regular basis

_____ whenever he/she
is hungry, usually
about four or five
times a day

_____ three meals a day
on a regular sched-
ule, with one or
two snacks during
the day

TOY CHECK LIST

We are interested in finding out what kinds of toys children have in their homes. The items below are for children of different ages.

Please check any of the following that you have in your home and that your child is allowed to play with. Do not check the ones you do not have now or that are broken.

_____ doll
_____ stroller
_____ toy telephone
_____ children's books
_____ crib gym
_____ squeeze toys
_____ car, truck, or train
_____ teething ring
_____ stacking rings
_____ surprise box
_____ plastic keys on a ring
_____ children's records
_____ measuring cups
_____ stuffed animal
_____ push or pull toy
_____ mobile
_____ plastic snap together beads
_____ shape sorting ball or box
_____ musical toy or music box
_____ shovel or other digging toy

_____ homemade toys (doll, etc.)
_____ boxes or plastic containers to fill
_____ pots and pans he/she can play with
_____ jump seat or door swing
_____ record player
_____ toy dishes
_____ busy bath
_____ toy animals
_____ walker
_____ ball
_____ building toys
_____ blocks
_____ swing
_____ pounding toy
_____ mirror
_____ bathtub toys
_____ bucket or pail
_____ rattles
_____ busy box
_____ pacifier

Thank you for your responses and time

Scoring procedures

PROCESS consists of three major sections:

1. Clinical observation (20 items each with four choices)
2. Parent questionnaire (24 items each with four choices)
3. Toy check list (40 items)

All items in the Clinical observation and Parent questionnaire sections are arranged in the following way:

Description of item:

| response A | response B |
| response C | response D |

Scoring for each item is as follows:

response A = 1 point   response B = 2 points
response C = 3 points   response D = 4 points

PROCESS recording form

On the PROCESS recording form are places to record scores for each section of PROCESS. Complete this form as follows:

1. **Enter** the score for each Clinical Observation item in the appropriate numbered space.

   Then **add** the points for each item in the columns to obtain an **Observation Total.**
2. **Enter** the score for each Parent Questionnaire item in the appropriate numbered space.

   Then **add** the points for items in the column labeled *Developmental Stimulation* to get the **DS Total.**

   Then **add** the points for items in the column labeled *Organization* to get the **Org Total.**

   Then **add** the **DS Total** and the **Org Total** to get the **Parent Quest. Total.**
3. **Compute** the **Toy Score** using the *Toys Table.*

   Then **compute** the **Weighted Toys Total** as presented on the Process Recording Form.
4. **Enter** the **Total** for each section in the **Summary Table** of the Process Recording Form.

   Then **add** the three **Total** scores to obtain the **PROCESS Total.**

Child's Name _____

Date _____

Date of Birth _____

PROCESS Recording Form

Parent questionnaire	
Developmental Stimulation	Organization
Item 1:	Item 2:
Item 3:	Item 4:
Item 5:	Item 6:
Item 7:	Item 8:
Item 9:	Item 10:
Item 11:	Item 12:
Item 13:	Item 14:
Item 15:	Item 16:
Item 17:	
Item 18:	
Item 19:	
Item 20:	
Item 21:	Item 22:
Item 23:	Item 24:
DS Total =	**Org** Total =
PARENT QUEST. TOTAL =	

Summary table
Parent quest. total =
Weighted toys total =
Observation total =
PROCESS TOTAL =

Clinical observation	
Item 1:	Item 11:
Item 2:	Item 12:
Item 3:	Item 13:
Item 4:	Item 14:
Item 5:	Item 15:
Item 6:	Item 16:
Item 7:	Item 17:
Item 8:	Item 18:
Item 9:	Item 19:
Item 10:	Item 20:
OBSERVATION TOTAL =	

Toys Table	
# of Toys:	**Toy Score =**
0	0
1-5	1
6-10	2
11-15	3
16-20	4
21-25	5
26-30	6
31-35	7
36-40	8
Toy Score _____ × 6 = _____ **WEIGHTED TOYS TOTAL**	

Home Assessment Checklist

General Household

1. Is there good lighting available, especially around stairwells?
2. Are there handrails (which can be easily grasped) on both sides of the staircases, designed to indicate when top and bottom steps have been reached?
3. Are top and bottom steps painted in easily seen colors? Are nonskid treads used?
4. Are the edges of rugs tacked down? (Suggest the use of wall-to-wall carpeting.)
5. Is a telephone present? Does the telephone have a dial that is easily readable? Are emergency numbers written in large print and kept near the telephone?
6. Are electrical cords, footstools, and other low-lying objects kept out of walkways?
7. Are electrical cords in good condition?
8. Is furniture arranged to allow for free movement in heavily traveled areas?
9. Is furniture sturdy enough to give support?
10. Is furniture designed to accommodate easy transfers on and off?
11. Is the temperature of the home within a comfortable range?
12. If fireplaces or other heating devices are present, do they have protective screens?
13. Are smoke detectors present (especially in the kitchen and bedroom)?
14. Are rapidly closing doors eliminated?
15. Are there alternative exits from the house?
16. Are basements and attics easy to get to, well lighted, and well ventilated?
17. Are slippers and shoes in good repair? Do they fit properly and have nonskid soles?

Kitchen

18. Are there loose extension cords, small sliding rugs, slippery linoleum tiles present? (Suggest the use of rubber-backed, nonskid rugs and nonskid floor wax.)
19. Is the cooking stove gas or electric?

From Tideiksaar R: New York, 1983, Ritter Department of Geriatrics and Adult Development, The Mount Sinai Medical Center. In Ebersole P, Hess P, editors: *Toward healthy aging*, ed 4, St Louis, 1994, Mosby.

20. Are there large, easily readable dials present on the stove or other appliances, with the "on" and "off" positions clearly marked?
21. Are refrigerators in good working order? Are refrigerators placed on 18-inch platforms so the client will not have to bend over?
22. Are spaces for food storage adequate? Are shelves at eye level and easily reachable?
23. Is a sturdy stepladder present for reaching?
24. Are electrical circuits overloaded with too many appliances?
25. Are electrical appliances disconnected when not in use?
26. Are sharp objects (such as carving knives) kept in special holders?
27. Are cleaning fluids, polishes, bleaches, detergents, and all poisons stored separately and clearly marked?
28. Are kitchen chairs sturdy, with arm rests with high backs?
29. Is stove free from flammable objects?
30. Are pot holders available for removing pots and pans from the stove?
31. Is baking soda available in case of fire?

Bathroom

32. Are there grab bars in the bath, in the shower, and around the toilet?
33. Are toilet seats high enough to get on and off of without difficulty?
34. Can the bathroom door be easily closed to ensure privacy? (Avoid locks.)
35. Are bathroom doorways wide enough for easy wheelchair and walker access?
36. Are there nonskid rubber mats in the bath, in the shower, and on the floor?
37. Is there good lighting in the area of the medicine cabinet?
38. Are internal and external medications stored separately? And safely (especially important with young grandchildren present in the house)?
39. Do medication containers have childproof tops? Are they labeled in large print? Is a magnifying glass present for reading medication instructions?
40. Have all outdated medications been discarded?
41. Do you notice any medications (both prescription and over-the-counter) that could cause adverse side effects or drug-drug interactions that the client is unaware of?
42. Can the water temperature be easily regulated?
43. Are electrical cords, outlets, and appliances a safe distance from the tub?

44. Are razor blades kept in a safe place?
45. Is a first-aid kit available?

Bedroom

46. Is there adequate lighting from the bedside to the bathroom?
47. Are lights easily accessible? (If not, suggest keeping a flashlight by the bedside or using a flashlight for entry into dark rooms if light switch is not within easy reach.)
48. Are beds in good repair?
49. Are beds at the proper height to allow for easy transfer on and off without difficulty?
50. Do bedroom rugs have nonskid rubber backings?

Environmental Assessment for the Elderly

1. How many rooms are available to client?
   Own bedroom   _____   If shared, with whom? _____
   Bathroom   _____
   Kitchen   _____
   Living/sitting room _____
2. Must client climb stairs to enter or leave house?
   Yes _____   No _____
   If yes, are they well lit and in good repair?
   Yes _____   No _____
3. Is neighborhood dangerous?
   Yes _____   No _____
4. Is house clean?
   Yes _____   No _____
5. Does house seem adequately insulated and ventilated?
   Yes _____   No _____
6. Are there signs of neglect?
   Old food in refrigerator   _____
   Unwashed dishes   _____
   Accumulated dirty clothing   _____
   Other (describe):   _____
7. Is there a sufficient supply of food for at least several days?
   Yes _____   No _____

From Kane R, Ouslander J, Abrass I: *Essentials of clinical geriatrics,* ed 3, New York, 1994, McGraw-Hill.

8. Safety checklist
   a. Can the client: Yes   No

	Yes	No
Lock and unlock the door	____	____
Reach light switches	____	____
Call for help (telephone and numbers accessible)	____	____
Safely transfer from bed, chair, toilet, tub	____	____

   b. Are there obvious dangers:

	Yes	No
Overloaded electrical outlets	____	____
Frayed electrical wires	____	____
Poor lighting	____	____
Cluttered furniture	____	____
Unsafe furniture	____	____
Frayed carpets or broken floors	____	____
Missing or broken smoke alarm	____	____

9. Fall hazard checklist (after *Clinical Report on Aging,* Volume 1, Number 5, 1987)
   a. Throughout the household, check that the following are in order:

   _____ 1. Flooring and carpeting are in good condition without protruding obstacles that may cause tripping and falling.

   _____ 2. Lighting is bright and without glare.

   _____ 3. Nightlights are strategically placed throughout the house, especially on stairways and along routes between bedroom and bathroom. Iluminated light switches are used when possible in similar high-risk locations.

   _____ 4. Telephones are positioned so that persons do not have to hurry to answer a ringing telephone.

   _____ 5. Electric cords are not located in walkways. When possible, they are shortened and tacked down to baseboards.

   _____ 6. Clutter does not obstruct walkways.

   b. Bathroom

   _____ 7. Railings are installed in the bathtub and toilet areas and are easily accessible for use.

   _____ 8. A nonslip surface is on the floor of the tub and shower. If a bath mat is used, it is of substantial quality.

   _____ 9. If a throw rug is used, it has a nonskid rubber backing.

   _____ 10. Water drainage is appropriate to prevent the development of slippery floors after bathing.

c. Bedroom

_____ 11. Throw rugs do not represent a slip or trip hazard, particularly those en route to the bathroom.

_____ 12. Bedside table is present for placement of glasses and other items rather than cluttering the floor beside the bed.

d. Kitchen

_____ 13. The floor is made of a nonslip material.

_____ 14. Spills are cleaned up quickly to prevent slipping.

_____ 15. Cleaning and cooking supplies are stored in locations that are not too high (for shorter persons who would otherwise climb) or too low (for persons who develop lightheadedness after stooping).

_____ 16. A high chair is available for doing dishes.

_____ 17. A sturdy step stool is available for reaching high places.

e. Living room

_____ 18. Throw rugs are not present over a carpet or otherwise scattered about.

_____ 19. Furniture is placed in positions that allow for wide walkways.

_____ 20. Chairs and sofas are of a height sufficient to permit easy sitting and standing for elderly persons.

f. Stairways

_____ 21. Sturdy railings are provided along both sides of stairways, including the stairway to the basement.

_____ 22. Step surfaces are nonskid.

_____ 23. Materials are not stored on stair landings or thresholds.

_____ 24. When possible, bright nonskid tape is placed on the top and bottom steps to indicate where the steps begin and end.

g. Outside the house

_____ 25. Front and back steps are in good condition. During the winter, sand (or salt) is available for slippery surfaces to ensure safety.

_____ 26. Walkways are shoveled free of ice and snow in the winter to prevent slips and falls.

_____ 27. Stairways and railings are sturdy.

Cultural Assessment

The community health nurse will want to learn the culture before beginning any efforts at intervention or change. When assessing families, the community health nurse needs to be aware of the following factors.

Cultural Characteristics Related to Health Care of Children and Families

Cultural group	Health beliefs	Health practices
Asians		
Chinese	A healthy body viewed as gift from parents and ancestors and must be cared for Health is one of the results of balance between the forces of *yin* (cold) and *yang* (hot)—energy forces that rule the world Illness caused by imbalance Believe blood is source of life and is not regenerated *Chi* is innate energy Lack of chi and blood results in deficiency that produces fatigue, poor constitution, and long illness	Goal of therapy is to restore balance of yin and yang Acupuncturist applies needles to appropriate meridians identified in terms of yin and yang Acupressure and *tai chi* replacing acupuncture in some areas *Moxibustion* is application of heat to skin over specific meridians Wide use of medicinal herbs procured and applied in prescribed ways Folk healers are herbalist, spiritual healer, temple healer, fortune healer Meals may or may not be planned to balance hot and cold Milk intolerance relatively common Use of condiments (e.g., monosodium glutamate and soy sauce) may create difficulty with some diet regimens (e.g., low-salt diets)

Japanese	Three major belief systems:
	Shinto religious influence
	  Humans inherently good
	  Evil caused by outside spirits
	  Illness caused by contact with polluting agents (e.g., blood, corpses, skin diseases)
		Believe evil removed by purification
		Energy restored by means of acupuncture, acupressure, massage, and moxibustion along affected meridians
		Kampō medicine—use of natural herbs
		Believe in removal of diseased parts

Family relationships	Communication	Comments
Extended family pattern common Strong concept of loyalty of young to old Respect for elders taught at early age—acceptance without questioning or talking back Children's behavior a reflection on family Family and individual honor and "face" important Self-reliance and self-restraint highly valued; self-expression repressed Males valued more highly than females; women submissive to men in family	Open expression of emotions unacceptable Often smile when do not comprehend	Do not react well to painful diagnostic workup; are especially upset by drawing of blood Deep respect for their bodies and believe it best to die with bodies intact; therefore may refuse surgery Believe in reincarnation Older members fear hospitals; often believe hospital is a place to go to die Children sometimes breast-fed for up to 4 or 5 years*
Close intergenerational relationships Family provides anchor Family tends to keep problems to self Value self-control and self-sufficiency Concept of *haji* (shame) imposes strong control; unacceptable behavior of children reflects on family	Issei—born in Japan; usually speak Japanese only Nisei, Sansei, and Yonsei have few language difficulties New immigrants able to read and write English better than able to speak or understand it Make significant use	Generational categories: *Issei*—1st generation to live in U S. *Nisei*—2nd generation *Sansei*—3rd generation *Yonsei*—4th generation Issei and Nissei—tolerant and permissive childrearing until 5 or 6, then emphasis

*Most Asian cultures consider the child 1 year old at the time of birth. Traditional Chinese custom adds 1 year on January 1 regardless of the birthday—a child born in December is 2 years old the next January.

From Wong D: *Whaley & Wong's nursing care of infants and children*, ed 5, St Louis, 1995, Mosby.   *Continued.*

Cultural Characteristics Related to Health Care of Children and Families—cont'd

Cultural group	Health beliefs	Health practices
Japanese—cont'd	Chinese and Korean influence Health achieved through harmony and balance between self and society Disease caused by disharmony with society and not caring for body Portuguese influence Upholds germ theory of disease	Trend is to use both Western and Oriental healing methods Care for disabled viewed as family's responsibility Take pride in child's good health Seek preventive care, medical care for illness May avoid some food combinations (e.g., milk and cherries, watermelon and crab) and believe pickled plums to have special properties
Vietnamese	Good health considered to be balance between yin and yang Believe person's life has been predisposed toward certain phenomena by cosmic forces Health believed to be result of harmony with existing universal order; harmony attained by pleasing good spirits and avoiding evil ones Belief in *am duc,* the amount of good deeds accumulated by ancestors Many use rituals to prevent illness Practice some restrictions to prevent incurring wrath of evil spirits	Family uses all means possible before using outside agencies for health care Fortune-tellers determine event that caused disturbance May visit temple to procure divine instruction Use astrologer to calculate cyclical changes and forces Regard health as family responsibility; outside aid sought when resources run out Certain illnesses considered only temporary (such as pustules, open wounds) and ignored Seek generalist health healers May use special diets to prevent illness and promote health Lactose intolerance prevalent

Family relationships	Communication	Comments
Many adopt practices of contemporary middle class Concern for child missing school may result in sending to school before fully recovered from illness	of nonverbal communication with subtle gestures and facial expression Tend to suppress emotions Will often wait silently	on emotional reserve and control Cleanliness highly valued Time considered valuable and used wisely Tendency to practice emotional control may make assessment of pain more difficult
Family is revered institution Multigenerational families Family is chief social network Children highly valued Individual needs and interests are subordinate to those of family group Father is main decision maker Women taught submission to men Parents expect respect and obedience from children	Many immigrants are not proficient in speaking and understanding English May hesitate to ask questions Questioning authority is sign of disrespect; asking questions considered impolite Use indirectness rather than forthrightness in expressing disagreement May avoid eye contact with health professionals as a sign of respect	Consider status more important than money Children taught emotional control Time concept more relaxed—consider punctuality less significant than other values (i.e., propriety) Place high value on social harmony

Continued.

Cultural Characteristics Related to Health Care
of Children and Families—cont'd

Cultural group	Health beliefs	Health practices
Filipinos	Believe God's will and supernatural forces govern universe Illness, accidents, and other misfortunes are God's punishment for violations of His will Widely accept "hot" and "cold" balance and imbalance as cause of health and illness	Some use amulets as a shield from witchcraft or as good luck pieces Catholics substitute religious medals and other items
Blacks	Illness classified as: Natural—affected by forces of nature without adequate protection (e.g., cold air, pollution, food and water) Unnatural—evil influences (e.g., witchcraft, voodoo, hoodoo, hex, fix, rootwork); symptoms often associated with eating Believe serious illness sent by God as punishment (e.g., parents punished by illness or death of child) Believe serious illness can be avoided May resist health care because illness is "will of God"	Self-care and folk medicine very prevalent Folk therapies usually religious in origin Attempt home remedies first; poorer people do not seek help until illness serious Usually seek help from: "Old lady"—woman in community with a common knowledge of herbs; consulted regarding pediatric care Spiritualist—has received gift from God for healing incurable diseases or solving personal problems; strongly based in Christianity Priest (voodoo priest/priestess)—most powerful healer Root doctor—meets need for herbs, oils, candles, and ointments Prayer is common means for prevention and treatment

Family relationships	Communication	Comments
Family is highly valued, with strong family ties Multigenerational family structure common, often with collateral members as well Personal interests are subordinated to family interests and needs Members avoid any behavior that would bring shame on the family	Immigrants and older persons may not be able to speak or understand English	Tend to have a fatalistic outlook on life Believe time and providence will solve all
Strong kinship bonds in extended family; members come to aid of others in crisis Less likely to view illness as a burden Augmented families common (unrelated persons living in same household) Place strong emphasis on work and ambition Sex-role sharing among parents Elderly members respected Maternal grandparent strong influence	Alert to any evidence of discrimination Place importance on nonverbal behavior May use nonstandard English or "black English" Use "testing" behaviors to assess personnel in health care situations before seeking active care Best to use simple, direct, but caring approach	High level of caution and distrust of majority group Social anxiety related to tradition of humiliation, oppression, and loss of dignity Will elect to retain dignity rather than seek care if values are compromised Strong sense of peoplehood High incidence of poverty Black minister a strong influence in black community Visits by family minister are sought, expected, and valued in helping to cope with illness and suffering

Continued.

Cultural Characteristics Related to Health Care of Children and Families—cont'd

Cultural group	Health beliefs	Health practices
Haitians†	Illnesses have a supernatural or natural origin Supernatural illnesses are caused by angry voodoo spirits, enemies, or the dead, especially deceased ancestors Natural illnesses are based on conceptions of natural causation: Irregularities of blood volume, flow, purity, viscosity, color and/or temperature (hot/ cold) Gas *(gaz)* Movement and consistency of mother's milk Hot/cold imbalance in the body Bone displacement Movement of diseases Health is maintained by good dietary and hygienic habits	Health is a personal responsibility Foods have properties of "hot"/"cold" and "light"/ "heavy" and must be in harmony with one's life cycle and bodily states Natural illnesses are treated by home remedies first Supernatural illness treated by healers: voodoo priest *(houngan)* or priestess *(mambo)*, midwife *(fam saj)*, and herbalist or leaf doctor *(dokte fey)* Amulets and prayer used to protect against illness due to curses or willed by evil people
Hispanics ***Mexicans (Latinos, Chicanos, Raza-Latinos)***	Health beliefs have strong religious association Believe in body imbalance as a cause of illness, especially imbalance between *caliente* (hot) and *frio* (cold) or "wet" and "dry" Some maintain good health is a result of "good luck"—a reward for good behavior Illness prevented by performing properly, eating proper foods, and working proper amount of time; accomplished through prayer, wearing religious medals or amulets, and sleeping with relics at home	Seek help from *curandero* or *curandera,* especially in rural areas Curandero(a) receives his/her position by birth, apprenticeship, or a "calling" via dream or vision Treatments involve use of herbs, rituals, and religious artifacts Practice for severe illness— make promises, visit shrines, offer medals and candles, offer prayers Adhere to "hot" and "cold" food prescriptions and prohibitions for prevention and treatment of illness

†This section was written by Lydia DeSantis, RN, PhD.

Family relationships	Communication	Comments
Maintenance of family reputation is paramount Lineal authority supreme; children in a subordinate position in family hierarchy Children valued for parental social security in old age and expected to contribute to family welfare at an early age Children viewed as "gifts from god" and treated with indulgence and affection	Recent immigrants and older persons may speak only Haitian creole May prefer family/friends to act as translators and confidants Often smile and nod in agreement when do not understand Quiet and gentle communication style and lack of assertiveness lead health care providers to falsely believe they comprehend health teaching and are compliant Will not ask questions if health care provider is busy or rushed	Will use biomedical and ethnomedical (folk) systems simultaneously Resistant to dietary and work restrictions Adherence to prescribed treatments directly related to perceived severity of illness
Traditionally men considered breadwinners and key decision makers in matters outside the home; women considered homemakers Males considered big and strong (*macho*) Strong kinship; extended families include *compadres* (godparents) established by ritual kinship Children valued highly and desired, taken everywhere with family Many homes contain shrines with statues	May use nonstandard English Some bilingual; many speak only Spanish May have a strong preference for native language and revert to it in times of stress May shake hands or engage in introductory embrace Interpret prolonged eye contact as disrespectful	High degree of modesty—often a deterrent to seeking medical care and open discussions of sex Youngsters often reluctant to share communal showers in schools Relaxed concept of time—may be late for appointments More concerned with present than with future and therefore may focus on immediate solutions rather than long-term goals Magicoreligious practices common

Continued.

Cultural Characteristics Related to Health Care of Children and Families—cont'd

Cultural group	Health beliefs	Health practices
Hispanics—cont'd	Illness is a punishment from God for wrongdoing, forces of nature, and the supernatural	
Puerto Ricans	Subscribe to the "hot-cold" theory of causation of illness Believe some illness caused by evil spirits and forces	Infrequent use of health care systems Seek folk healers—use of herbs, rituals Consult spiritualist medium for mental disorders *Santeria* is system, and practitioners are called *santeros* Treatments classified as "hot" or "cold"
Cubans‡	Prevention and good nutrition are related to good health	Diligent users of the medical model Eclectic health-seeking practices, including preventive measures, and, in some instances, folk medicine of both religious and nonreligious origins; home remedies; in many instances seek assistance of santeros and spiritualists to complement medical treatment Nutrition is important; parents show overconcern with eating habits of their children and spend a considerable part of the budget on food; traditional Cuban diet is rich in meat and starch; consumption of fresh vegetables added in U.S.

‡This section was written by Mercedes Sandaval, PhD.

Family relationships	Communication	Comments
and pictures of saints Elderly treated with respect		May view hospital as place to go to die
Family usually large and home centered— the core of existence Father has complete authority in family— family provider and decision maker Wife and children subordinate to father Children valued—seen as a gift from God Children taught to obey and respect parents; corporal punishment to ensure obedience	May use nonstandard English Spanish speaking or bilingual Strong sense of family privacy—may view questions regarding family as impudent	Relaxed sense of time Pay little attention to *exact* time of day Suspicious and fearful of hospitals
Strong family ties with mother and father kinships Children supported and assisted by parents long after becoming adults Elderly cared for at home	Most are bilingual (English/Spanish) except for segments of the senior population	In less than 30 years Cubans have been able to obtain a higher standard of living than other Hispanic groups in U.S. Have been able to retain many of their former social institutions: bilingual and private schools, clinics, social clubs, the family as an extended network of support, etc. Many do not feel discriminated against nor harbor feelings of inferiority with respect to Anglo-Americans or "mainstream" population

Continued.

Cultural Characteristics Related to Health Care
of Children and Families—cont'd

Cultural group	Health beliefs	Health practices
Native Americans (numerous tribes)	Believe health is state of harmony with nature and universe Respect of bodies through proper management All disorders believed to have aspects of supernatural Violation of a restriction or prohibition thought to cause illness Fear of witchcraft May carry objects believed to guard against witchcraft Theology and medicine strongly interwoven	Medicine persons: Altruistic persons who must use powers in purely positive ways Persons capable of both good and evil—perform negative acts against enemies Diviner-diagnosticians—diagnose but do not have powers or skill to implement medical treatment Specialists—use herbs and curative but non-sacred medical procedures Medicine persons—use herbs and ritual Singers—cure by the power of their song obtained from supernatural beings; effect cures by laying on of hands

Family relationships	Communication	Comments
Extended family structure—usually includes relatives from both sides of family Elder members assume leadership roles	Most continue to speak their Indian language, as well as English Nonverbal communication	Time orientation—present Respect for age Going to hospital associated with illness or disease; therefore may not seek prenatal care, since pregnancy viewed as natural process Tend to take time to form an opinion of professionals Sexual matters not openly discussed with members of opposite sex

Family or Individual
Sociocultural Factors

When assessing families or individuals, the community health nurse needs to be aware of the following:

1. Typical family households, roles played by family members and kinship groups, and patterns of residence
2. Events, rituals, and ceremonies considered important within the life cycle, such as birth, baptism, puberty, marriage, and death
3. The health beliefs and values of the family members and the social meaning attached to wellness and illness
   a. Beliefs concerning body organs and systems and how they function
   b. Particular methods used to help maintain health, such as hygienic and self-care practices
   c. Attitudes toward immunizations, screening tests, and other preventive health measures
   d. Beliefs and practices surrounding conception, pregnancy, childbirth, lactation, and rearing of children
   e. Attitudes toward mental illness, deformities, and death and dying
4. The person(s) in a family responsible for various health-related decisions, such as what to do when ill, where to go, who to see, and what advice to follow
5. Health topics that may be sensitive or taboo to the client
6. Possible conflicts between family health beliefs and practices and the teachings and practices of an established health program
7. Beliefs, rules, and preferences or prejudices concerning food, such as those believed to cause or cure illness
8. Culturally appropriate ways to enter and leave situations, including greetings, farewells, and convenient hours to make a home visit

Brownlee AT: *Community, culture, and care,* St Louis, 1978, Mosby. In Stanhope M, Lancaster J, editors: *Community health nursing: process and practice for promoting health,* ed 3, St Louis, 1992, Mosby.

Eleven Functional Health Patterns
Assessment Guidelines for Communities

Communities develop health patterns. In some practice settings the community is the primary client. In other cases an individual client or a family may have, or be predisposed to certain problems that require an assessment of certain community patterns. The following are guidelines for a comprehensive community assessment, but selected patterns can also be assessed, depending on the focus of care delivery:

1. *Health-perception–health-management pattern*
   History (community representatives):
   a. In general, what is the health/wellness level of the population on a scale of 1 to 5, with 5 being high? Any major health problems?
   b. Any strong cultural patterns influencing health practices?
   c. Do people feel that they have access to health services?
   d. Is there demand for any particular health services or prevention programs?
   e. Do people feel that fire, police, safety programs are sufficient?
   Examination (community records):
   a. Morbidity, mortality, disability rates (by age group, if appropriate)?
   b. Accident rates (by district, if appropriate)?
   c. Currently operating health facilities (types)?
   d. Ongoing health promotion–prevention programs; utilization rates?
   e. Ratios of health professionals to population?
   f. Laws regarding drinking age?
   g. Arrest statistics for drug use/drunk driving by age group?

2. *Nutritional-metabolic pattern*
   History (community representatives):
   a. In general, do most people seem well nourished? Children? Elderly?
   b. Food supplement programs? Food stamps: rate of use?
   c. Is cost of foods reasonable in this area relative to income?
   d. Are stores accessible for most? "Meals on Wheels" available?
   e. Water supply and quality? Testing services (if most have own wells)? (If appropriate: water usage cost? Any drought restrictions?)

From Gordon M: *Manual of nursing diagnosis: 1993-1994,* St Louis, 1993, Mosby.

    f. Any concern that community growth will exceed good water supply?

    g. Are heating/cooling costs manageable for most? Programs?

Examination:

    a. General appearance (nutrition, teeth, clothing appropriate for climate)? Children? Adults? Elderly?

    b. Food purchases (observations at food store checkout counters)?

    c. "Junk" food (machines in schools, etc.)?

3. *Elimination pattern*

History (community representatives):

    a. Major kinds of wastes (industrial, sewage, etc.)? Disposal systems? Recycling programs? Any problems perceived by community?

    b. Pest control? Food service inspection (restaurants, street vendors, etc.)?

Examination:

    a. Communicable-disease statistics?

    b. Air pollution statistics?

4. *Activity-exercise pattern*

History (community representatives):

    a. How do people find the transportation here? To work? For recreation? To health care?

    b. Do people (senior, others) have/use community centers? Recreation facilities for children? Adults? Seniors?

    c. Is housing adequate (availability, cost)? Public housing?

Examination:

    a. Recreation/cultural programs?

    b. Aids for the disabled?

    c. Residential centers, nursing homes, rehabilitation facilities relative to population needs?

    d. External maintenance of homes, yards, apartment houses?

    e. General activity level (e.g., bustling, quiet)?

5. *Sleep-rest pattern*

History (community representatives):

    a. Generally quiet at night in most neighborhoods?

    b. Usual business hours? Are industries round-the-clock?

Examination:

    a. Activity/noise levels in business district? Residential?

6. *Cognitive-perceptual pattern*

History (community representatives):

    a. Do most groups speak English? Bilingual?

    b. Educational level of population?

   c. Schools seen as good/need improving? Adult education desired/available?

   d. Types of problems that require community decisions? Decision-making process? What is best way to get things done/changed here?

Examination:

   a. School facilities? Dropout rate?

   b. Community government structure; decision-making lines?

7. *Self-perception–self-concept pattern*

History (community representatives):

   a. Good community to live in? Going up in status, down, or about the same?

   b. Old community? Fairly new?

   c. Does any age group predominate?

   d. People's mood, in general: enjoying life, stressed, feeling "down"?

   e. People generally have the kinds of abilities needed in this community?

   f. Community/neighborhood functions? Parades?

Examination:

   a. Racial, ethnic mix (if appropriate)?

   b. Socioeconomic level?

   c. General observations of mood?

8. *Role-relationship pattern*

History (community representatives):

   a. Do people seem to get along well together here? Places where people tend to go to socialize?

   b. Do people feel that they are heard by the government? High/low participation in meetings?

   c. Enough work/jobs for everybody? Are wages good/fair? Do people seem to like the kind of work available (happy in their jobs/job stress)?

   d. Any problems with riots, violence in the neighborhoods? Family violence? Problems with child/spouse/elder abuse?

   e. Does community get along with adjacent communities? Do people collaborate on any community projects?

   f. Do neighbors seem to support each other?

   g. Community get-togethers?

Examination:

   a. Observation of interactions (generally or at specific meetings)?

   b. Statistics on interpersonal violence?

   c. Statistics on employment, income/poverty?

   d. Divorce rate?

9. *Sexuality-reproductive pattern*

History (community representatives):
a. Average family size?
b. Do people feel there are any problems with pornography, prostitution, or other?
c. Do people want/support sex education in schools/community?

Examination:
a. Family sizes and types of households?
b. Male/female ratio?
c. Average maternal age? Maternal mortality rate? Infant mortality rate?
d. Teen pregnancy rate?
e. Abortion rate?
f. Sexual violence statistics?
g. Laws/regulations regarding information on birth control?

10. *Coping–stress-tolerance pattern*

History (community representatives):
a. Any groups that seem to be under stress?
b. Need/availability of phone help lines? Support groups (health-related, other)?

Examination:
a. Statistics on delinquency, drug abuse, alcoholism, suicide, psychiatric illness?
b. Unemployment rate by race/ethnic group/sex?

11. *Value-belief pattern*

History (community representatives):
a. Community values: what seem to be the top four things that people living here see as important in their lives? (Note health-related values, priorities.)
b. Do people tend to get involved in causes/local fund-raising campaigns? (Note if any are health related.)
c. Are there religious groups in the community? Churches available?
d. Do people tend to tolerate/not tolerate differences or socially deviant behavior?

Examination:
a. Zoning/conservation laws?
b. Scan of community government health committee reports (goals, priorities)?
c. Health budget relative to total budget?

Sociocultural Factors in Community Assessment

The following is a list of sociocultural factors to be considered when collecting community data, to give additional insight in the analysis of the data.

1. Existing influences that divide people into groups within the community, such as ethnicity, religion, social class, occupation, place of residence, language, education, sex, race, and age
2. Conditions that lead to social conflict or social cohesion
3. Attitudes toward minority groups, youth and the elderly, males and females, and age and gender groups
4. Division of the community into neighborhoods or districts and the characteristics of these
5. Formal and informal channels of communication between health programs and the community
6. Barriers that may be the result of differences in cultural beliefs and practices
7. Political orientation in the community (attitudes toward authority and its use in health problems)
8. Patterns of migration either in or out of a community and their effect on health care services
9. Relation of religion and medicine within the community (who and what causes various illnesses and how they can be prevented)
10. Types of diseases or illnesses thought by various members of the community to exist (culture-specific conditions, such as illnesses caused by hot and cold imbalances or diseases of magical origin)

Modified from Bauwens E, Anderson S: Social and cultural influences on health care. In Stanhope M, Lancaster J, editors: *Community health nursing: process and practice for promoting health,* ed 3, St Louis, 1992, Mosby.

Cross-Cultural Examples of Cultural Phenomena That Affect Nursing Care

Nations of origin	Communication	Space	Time orientation	Social organization	Environmental control	Biological variations
Asian China Hawaii Philippines Korea Japan Southeast Asia (Laos, Cambodia, Vietnam)	National language preference Dialects, written characters Use of silence Nonverbal and contextual cuing	Noncontact people	Present	Family: hierarchial structure, loyalty Devotion to tradition Many religions, including Taoism, Buddhism, Islam, and Christianity Community social organizations	Traditional health and illness beliefs Use of traditional medicines Traditional practitioners: Chinese doctors and herbalists	Liver cancer Stomach cancer Coccidioidomycosis Hypertension Lactose intolerance
African West Coast (as slaves) Many African countries West Indian Islands Dominican Republic Haiti Jamaica	National languages Dialect: Pidgin, Creole, Spanish, and French	Close personal space	Present over future	Family: many female, single parent Large, extended family networks Strong church affiliation within community Community social organizations	Traditional health and illness beliefs Folk medicine tradition Traditional healer: root-worker	Sickle cell anemia Hypertension Cancer of the esophagus Stomach cancer Coccidioidomycosis Lactose intolerance

Nations of Origin	Communication	Space	Time Orientation	Social Organization	Environmental Control	Biological Variations
Europe Germany England Italy Ireland Other European countries	National languages Many learn English immediately	Noncontact people Aloof Distant Southern countries: closer contact and touch	Future over present	Nuclear families Extended families Judeo-Christian religions Community social organizations	Primary reliance on modern health care system Traditional health and illness beliefs Some remaining folk medicine traditions	Breast cancer Heart disease Diabetes mellitus Thalassemia
Native American 170 Native American tribes Aleuts Eskimos	Tribal languages Use of silence and body language	Space very important and has no boundaries	Present	Extremely family oriented Biological and extended families Children taught to respect traditions Community social organizations	Traditional health and illness beliefs Folk medicine tradition Traditional healer: medicine man	Accidents Heart disease Cirrhosis of the liver Diabetes mellitus

Continued.

From Specter R: Culture, ethnicity, and nursing. In Potter PA, Perry AG, editors: *Fundamentals of nursing: concepts, process, and practice*, ed 3, St Louis, 1993, Mosby.

Cross-Cultural Examples of Cultural Phenomena That Affect Nursing Care—cont'd

Nations of origin	Communication	Space	Time orientation	Social organization	Environmental control	Biological variations
Hispanic countries Spain Cuba Mexico Central and South America	Spanish or Portuguese primary language	Tactile relationships Touch Handshakes Embracing Value physical presence	Present	Nuclear family Extended families *Compadrazzo:* godparents Community social organizations	Traditional health and illness beliefs Folk medicine tradition Traditional healers: *Curandero,* *Espiritista,* *Partera,* *Senora*	Diabetes mellitus Parasites Coccidioidomycosis Lactose intolerance

Characteristic Food Choices for Six Groups

	Vegetables	Fruits	Meats and alternatives	Grain products	Others
Black	Broccoli, corn, greens (mustard, collard, kale turnips, beet, etc.), lima beans, okra, peas, pumpkin	Grapefruit, grapes, nectarine, plums, watermelon	Sausage, pig's feet, ears, etc., bacon, luncheon meat, organ meats, turkey, catfish, perch, red snapper, tuna, salmon, sardines, shrimp, kidney beans, red beans, black-eyed peas, peanuts, and peanut butter	Corn bread, hominy grits, biscuits, muffins, cooked cereal, crackers	Chitterlings, salt pork, gravies, buttermilk
Hispanic	Avocado, chilies, corn, lettuce, peas, potato, prickly pear (cactus leaf called *nopales*), zucchini	Guava, lemon, mango, melons, prickly pear (cactus fruit called *tuna*), zapote (or sapote)	Lamb, tripe, sausage (*chorizo*), bologna, bacon, pinto beans, pink beans, garbanzo beans, lentils, peanuts, and peanut butter	Tortillas, corn flour, oatmeal, sweet bread (*pan dulce*)	Salsa (tomato-pepper, onion relish), chili sauce, guacamole, lard (*manteca*), pork cracklings

From Endres JB, Rockwell RE: *Food nutrition, and the young child*, ed 2, St Louis, 1985, Mosby. Modified from *Nutrition during pregnancy and lactation*, California Department of Public Health, revised 1975.

NOTE: Foods common to all ethnic groups have been omitted.

Continued.

Characteristic Food Choices for Six Groups—cont'd

Vegetables	Fruits	Meats and alternatives	Grain products	Others
Japanese				
Bamboo shoots, broccoli, burdock root, cauliflower, celery, cucumbers, eggplant, gourd (*Kampyo*), mushrooms, napa cabbage, peas, peppers, radishes (daikon or pickles called *takuwan*), snow peas, squash, sweet potato, turnips, water chestnuts, yamaimo	Apricot, cherries, grapefruit, grapes, lemon, lime, melons, persimmon, pineapple, pomegranate, plums (dried pickled *umeboshi*), strawberries	Turkey, raw tuna or sea bass (*sashimi*), mackerel, sardines (*mezashi*), shrimp, abalone, squid, octopus, soybean curd (tofu), soybean paste (*miso*), soybeans, red beans (*azuki*), lima beans, peanuts, almonds, cashews	Rice, rice crackers, noodles (whole-wheat noodle called *soba* or *udon*), oatmeal	Soy sauce, Nori paste (used to season rice), bean thread (*konyaku*), ginger (*shoga*; dried form called *denishoga*)

Chinese

Vegetables	Fruits	Protein Foods	Grains	Seasonings
Bamboo shoots, bean sprouts, bok choy, broccoli, celery, Chinese cabbage, corn, cucumbers, eggplant, greens (collard, Chinese, broccoli, mustard, kale), leeks, lettuce, mushrooms, peppers, scallions, snow peas, taro, water chestnuts, white radishes, winter melon	Figs, grapes, kumquats, locuats, mango, melons, persimmon, pineapple, plums, pomegranate	Organ meats, duck, white fish, shrimp, lobster, oyster, sardines, soybeans, tofu, black beans, chestnuts (*kuri*)	Rice, barley, millet	Soy sauce, sweet and sour sauce, mustard sauce, ginger root, plum sauce, red bean paste

Vietnamese*

Vegetables	Fruits	Protein Foods	Grains	Seasonings
Bamboo shoots, bean sprouts, cabbage, carrots, cucumbers, greens, lettuce, mushrooms, onions, peas, spinach, yams	Apple, banana, eggfruit (*o-ma*), grapefruit, jackfruit, lychee, mandarin, mango, orange, papaya, pineapple, tangerine, watermelon	Beef, blood, brain, chicken, duck, eggs, fish, goat, kidney, lamb, liver, pork, shellfish, soybeans	French bread, rice, rice noodles, wheat noodles	Fish sauce, fresh herbs, garlic, ginger, lard, MSG, peanut oil, sesame seeds, sesame seed oil, vegetable oil

Continued.

*Information supplied by Hanh-Trarg Tran-Viet, Carbondale, Ill.

Characteristic Food Choices for Six Groups—cont'd

Vegetables	Fruits	Meats and alternatives	Grain products	Others
Indian (East)				
Cauliflower, carrots, cucumber, corn gourds, leeks, eggplant, beets, radishes, hot pepper, bell pepper, peas, French beans, okra, pumpkin, red and white cabbage, mung sprouts, bean sprouts, potatoes, tapioca root, sweet potatoes	Oranges, limes, grapes, watermelon, mango, guava, honeydew, chiku, cantaloupe, pineapple, green, yellow, and red bananas, berries, custard apples	Lamb, beef, duck, chicken, shrimp, catfish, buffalo, sunfish, sardines, fresh crab, lobster, peanuts, cashews, almonds, chick-peas, split peas, black-eyed peas, dry mung beans	Rice pancakes, wheat chapati, puri, mixed grain flour bread	Fresh coconut juice, curries, tomato sauce; tamarind sauce, dried grain curries (*pulses*), yogurt-curry garnished with coriander (fresh leaves)

Foods Common to Most Ethnic Food Patterns

Meat and alternatives	Milk and milk products	Grain products	Vegetables	Fruits	Others
Pork*	Milk, fluid	Rice	Carrots	Apples	Fruit juices
Beef	Ice cream	White bread	Cabbage	Bananas	
Chicken		Noodles, macaroni, spaghetti	Green beans	Oranges	
Eggs		Dry cereal	Greens (especially spinach)	Peaches	
			Sweet potatoes or yams	Pears	
			Tomatoes	Tangerines	

From Endres JB, Rockwell RE: *Food nutrition, and the young child*, ed 2, St Louis, 1985, Mosby.
*May be restricted because of religious custom.

Cultural and Regional Foods

Name of food	Culture/region	Type of food	Description
Adobo	Filipino	Meat	Meat with soy sauce
Ajinomoto	Japanese	Grain	Wheat germ
Anadama	New England	Grain	Cornmeal-molasses yeast bread
Arroz blanco	Puerto Rican	Grain	Enriched white rice
Bacalao	Puerto Rican	Meat	Salted codfish
Bagels	Jewish	Grain	Bread dough, doughnut-shaped, boiled in water and baked
Baklava	Greek	Dessert	Layered pastry made with honey
Bok choy	Oriental	Vegetable	Green leafy, stalklike vegetable
Brioche	French	Grain	Egg-rich cake bread, used as sweet roll or shell for entrees
Bulgur	Middle Eastern	Grain	Granular wheat product with nutlike flavor
Burrito	Mexican	Combination	Sandwich; tortilla filled with beef-bean mixture and fried or baked
Café con leche	Latin American	Beverage	Coffee with milk
Cape Cod turkey	New England	Meat	Codfish balls
Challah	Jewish	Grain	Sabbath or holiday twisted eggbread
Chayote	Mexican	Vegetable	Squashlike vegetable
Chitterlings	Southern U.S.	Meat	Intestine of young pigs, soaked, boiled, and fried
Chorizo	Mexican	Meat	Sausage
Cilantro	Mexican	Seasoning	Coriander, similar to parsley
Crackling	Southern U.S.	Snack	Crispy pieces of fried pork fat
Croissants	French	Grain	Buttery, flaky, crescent-shaped rolls
Crumpets	English	Grain	Muffinlike produce cooked on griddle and then toasted

Cush	Montana	Grain	Cornbread mixed with butter and water and fried
Dandelion greens	Southern U.S.	Vegetable	Leaves from dandelion plant
Dolmathes	Greek	Combination	Grape leaves stuffed with beef
Enchiladas	Mexican	Combination	Tortilla filled with meat and cheese
Escargots	French	Meat	Snails
Falafel	Jewish	Meat	Mashed chick-peas mixed with spices and fried
Fatback	Southern U.S.	Fat	Fat from loin of pig
Feijoada	Brazilian	Meat	Black beans with meat
Feta	Greek	Milk	Soft, salty white cheese from sheep's or goat's milk
Finnan haddie	Scottish	Milk	Salted, smoked haddock
Frijoles fritos	Mexican	Meat	Refried pinto beans
Gazpacho	Spanish	Soup	Cold soup with chopped tomatoes, green peppers, and cucumbers
Gefilte fish	Jewish	Meat	Seasoned fish ground and shaped into balls
Goulash	Hungarian	Meat	Stew seasoned with paprika
Grits	Southern U.S.	Grain	Hulled and coarsely ground corn
Guava	Cuban	Fruit	Small, yellow or red sweet tropical fruit
Gumbo	Creole	Combination	Well-seasoned okra stew with meat or seafood
Hangtown fry	California	Meat	Fried oysters and eggs
Hoecake	Southeast U.S.	Grain	Thin corn cake
Mog maw	Southern U.S.	Meat	Stomach of pig
Hoppin' John	Southern U.S.	Combination	Blackeyed peas and rice
Hush puppies	Southern U.S.	Grain	Fried cornbread
Jalapeños	Latin American	Vegetable	Hot peppers

Continued.

From Burtis G, Davis J, Martin S: *Applied nutrition and diet therapy,* Philadelphia, 1988, Saunders.

Cultural and Regional Foods—cont'd

Name of food	Culture/region	Type of food	Description
Jambalaya	Creole	Combination	Well-seasoned combination of seafoods, tomatoes, and rice
Kale	Southern U.S.	Vegetable	Dark green leafy vegetable, similar to spinach
Kasha	Jewish	Grain	Coarsely ground buckwheat, toasted before cooking in liquid
Kelp	Oriental	Vegetable	Seaweed
Kibbeh	Middle East	Meat	Fresh raw lamb, ground and seasoned, similar to meat loaf
Kielbasa	Polish	Meat	Sausage
Kimchi	Korean	Vegetable	Peppery fermented combination of pickled cabbage, turnips, radishes, and other vegetables
Kuchen	German	Dessert	Yeast cake
Latkas	Jewish	Grain	Pancakes, sometimes from potatoes
Lard	—	Fat	Shortening-like product from pork
Limpa	Swedish	Grain	Rye bread
Lox	Jewish	Meat	Smoked salmon
Matzoh	Jewish	Grain	Unleavened bread
Menudo	Mexican	Meat	Stew made with tripe (cow's stomach)
Minestrone	Italian	Soup	Vegetable soup
Miso	Oriental	Meat	Fermented soybean paste
Moussaka	Greek	Combination	Meat and eggplant casserole
Mush	Southwest U.S.	Grain	Cooked cereal, usually cornmeal
Pandowdy	New England	Dessert	Dumplings and fruit
Papaya	—	Fruit	Large, yellow, melon-like tropical fruit

Pasta	Italian	Grain	Macaroni, spaghetti, and noodles in various shapes made from wheat
Pepperoni	Italian	Meat	Hot sausage
Phyllo	Greek	Grain	Paper-thin pastry for making meat, vegetables, cheese and egg dishes, and sweet pastries
Pilaf	Middle Eastern	Grain	Rice enriched with fat and sometimes vegetables, bits of meat, and spices
Poi	Polynesian	Vegetable	Root vegetable, especially taro, cooked and pounded, mixed with water, and sometimes fermented
Polenta	Italian	Grain	Cornmeal or cornmeal mush
Polk	Southern U.S.	Vegetable	Dark green leafy vegetable
Potato knishes	Jewish	Vegetable	Potato pancakes
Pot liquor (likker)	Southern U.S.	Vegetable	Liquid from cooking green vegetables or bones
Prosciutto	Italian	Meat	Ready-to-eat, cured, smoked ham
Prickly pear	Native American	Fruit	Fruit of cactus
Pumpernickel	—	Grain	Yeast bread with wheat, corn, rye, and potatoes
Ratatouille	French	Vegetable	Well-seasoned casserole of eggplant, zucchini, tomato, and green pepper
Redeye gravy	Southern U.S.	Gravy	Fried ham gravy
Sake	Oriental	Beverage	Rice wine
Salt pork	Southern U.S.	Fat	Salted port fat from the belly
Sancocho	Puerto Rican	Combination	Soup with meat and viandas
Sashimi	Japanese	Meat	Raw fish
Sauerbraten	German	Meat	Pot roast in spicy, aromatic, sweet-and sour marinade

Continued.

Cultural and Regional Foods—cont'd

Name of food	Culture/region	Type of food	Description
Scones	English	Grain	Round, flat, unleavened sweetened bread
Scrapple	Pennsylvania Dutch	Combination	Solid mush from cornmeal and the by-products of hog butchering
Shoofly pie	Pennsylvania Dutch	Dessert	Molasses pie
Shoyu	Japanese	Seasoning	Soy sauce
Sofrito	Puerto Rican	Seasoning	Specially seasoned tomato sauce
Sopapillas	Mexican	Grain	Rich fried bread
Spatzle	German	Grain	Small dumplings
Spoonbread	Virginia	Grain	Baked dish with cornmeal
Spumoni	Italian	Dessert	Fruited ice cream
Stollen	German	Dessert	Christmas fruitcake
Stricle sheets	Pennsylvania Dutch	Dessert	Coffee cake
Strudel	German	Dessert	Light pastry, filled with fruit or cheese
Tacos	Mexican	Combination	Fried tortillas, filled with meat, vegetables, and hot sauce
Tamales	Mexican	Grain	Pancakelike leathery bread
Tempura	Japanese	Combination	Deep-fried seafood or vegetables
Teriyaki sauce	Hawaiian	Accessory	Sweetened soy sauce
Tofu	Oriental	Meat	Soybean curd
Trotters	Southern U.S.	Meat	Pig's feet
Viandas	Puerto Rican	Vegetable	Starchy tropical vegetables, including plantain, green bananas, and sweet potatoes

Cultural Behaviors Relevant to Health Assessment

Cultural group	Cultural variations (Common belief/practice)	Nursing implications
African Americans	Dialect and slang terms require careful communication to prevent error (i.e., "bad" may mean "good").	Question the client's meaning or intent.
Mexican Americans	Eye behavior is important. An individual who looks at and admires a child without touching the child has given the child the "evil eye."	Always touch the child you are examining or admiring.
Native Americans	Eye contact is considered a sign of disrespect and is thus avoided.	Recognize that the client may be attentive and interested even though eye contact is avoided.
Appalachians	Eye contact is considered impolite or a sign of hostility. Verbal patter may be confusing.	Avoid excessive eye contact. Clarify statements.
American Eskimos	Body language is very important. The individual seldom disagrees publicly with others. Client may nod yes to be polite, even if not in agreement.	Monitor own body language closely as well as client's to detect meaning.
Jewish Americans	Orthodox Jews consider excess touching, particularly from members of the opposite sex, offensive.	Establish whether client is an Orthodox Jew and avoid excessive touch.
Chinese Americans	Individual may nod head to indicate yes or shake head to indicate no. Excessive eye contact indicates rudeness. Excessive touch is offensive.	Ask questions carefully and clarify responses. Avoid excessive eye contact and touch.

Continued.

From Kozier B et al: *Techniques in clinical nursing*, ed 2, Menlo Park, Calif, 1993, Addison-Wesley.

Cultural Behaviors Relevant to Health Assessment—cont'd

Cultural group	Cultural variations (Common belief/practice)	Nursing implications
Filipino Americans	Offending people is to be avoided at all cost. Nonverbal behavior is very important.	Monitor nonverbal behaviors of self and client, being sensitive to physical and emotional discomfort or concerns of the client.
Haitian Americans	Touch is used in conversation. Direct eye contact is used to gain attention and respect during communication.	Use direct eye contact when communicating.
East Indian Hindu Americans	Women avoid eye contact as a sign of respect.	Be aware that men may view eye contact by women as offensive. Avoid eye contact.
Vietnamese Americans	Avoidance of eye contact is a sign of respect. The head is considered sacred; it is not polite to pat the head. An upturned palm is offensive in communication.	Limit eye contact. Touch the head only when mandated and explain clearly before proceeding to do so. Avoid hand gesturing.

Family Assessment

Family Coping Index

The family coping index was developed in 1964 as a tool for practice, as an approach to identifying the family need for nursing care and assessing the potential for behavioral changes, and as a method of determining in a more systematic way how the nurse can help the family to manage.

Scaling Cues

The following descriptive statements are "cues" to help you as you rate family coping. They are limited to three points: *1*, or no competence; *3*, moderate competence; and *5*, complete competence. You will find, however, that most families will fall somewhere in between these points. Mark the point you feel most nearly describes the level of competence they have. The descriptions are not complete but suggestive. In the long run it is your own professional judgment that will be needed to make a decision. When there is no problem or the area is not relevant, check the "no problem" column.

1. Physical independence

This category is concerned with ability to move about, to get in and out of bed, to take care of daily grooming, walking, etc. Note that it is the *family* competence that is measured—even though an individual is dependent, if the family is able to compensate for this the family may be independent. However, the quality as well as quantity of ability is important; hence, if the *focus* of care is poor—if a mother is giving care to a handicapped child that the child could give himself/herself, or if one person is giving care that should be shared with other members—the independence might be considered incomplete. The *causes* of dependence may vary—lack of physical independence in the family may be due to actual physical incapacity, to lack of "know-how," to unwillingness or fear of doing the necessary tasks.

1 = Family failing entirely to provide required personal care to one or more of its members. *Example:* arthritic client unable to get out of bed alone, no one available to help; client "cannot" give his/her hypodermic medication because of fear.

Developed jointly by the Richmond IVNA City Nursing Service and the Johns Hopkins School of Hygiene and Public Health, 1964. From Freeman R, Heinrich J: *Community health nursing practice,* ed 2, Philadelphia, 1981, Saunders.

3 = Family providing partially for needs of its members, or providing care for some members but not for others. *Example:* mother may be doing well with own and husband's care, but failing to give daily care efficiently to newborn baby; daughter may be giving excellent physical care to aged mother but at cost of neglecting children somewhat, or with poor body mechanics that place undue strain upon herself.

5 = All family members, whether or not there is infirmity or disability in one or more members, are receiving the necessary care to maintain cleanliness, including skin care, are able to get about as far as possible within their physical abilities; are receiving assistance when needed without interruption or undue delay.

2. Therapeutic competence

This category includes all of the procecdures or treatment prescribed for the care of illness such as giving medications, using appliances (including crutches), dressings, exercises and relaxation, special diets, etc.

1 = Family either not carrying out procedures prescribed or doing it unsafely. For example, giving several medications without being able to distinguish one from the other, or taking them inappropriately, applying braces so they throw the limb out of line, measuring insulin incorrectly. Family resents, rejects, or refuses to give necessary care.

3 = Family carrying out some but not all of the treatments—for example, giving insulin but not adhering strictly to diet; carrying out procedures awkwardly, ineffectively, or with resentment or unnecessary anxiety. For example, crutch walking may be done, but with the helper using poor body mechanics, or not giving the client enough security and confidence; client may give own hypodermic, but say "I dread it every time." May be giving medications correctly, but not understanding purposes of the drug, or symptoms to be observed.

5 = Family able to demonstrate that they can carry out the prescribed procedures safely and efficiently, with the understanding of the principles involved and with a confident and willing attitude.

3. Knowledge of health condition

This category is concerned with the particular health condition that is the occasion for care. For example, knowledge of the disease or disability, understanding of communicability of disease and modes of transmission, understanding of general pattern of development of a newborn baby and the basic needs of infants for physical care and tender loving care (TLC).

1 = Totally uninformed or misinformed about the condition. For example, believes tuberculosis is caused by sin, or syphilis cured when symptoms subside; believes stroke patient must be bedridden, and that it is cruel to make them do for themselves; that overweight in the school-age child is "healthy."

3 = Has some general knowledge of the disease or condition, but has not grasped the underlying principles, or is only partially informed. For instance, may recognize need for TLC but not relate this to placing the baby's crib near people when the baby is awake or holding the baby when feeding; may accept fact that client is dying but not see need to prepare family for this event; may understand dietary and insulin control of diabetes, but not need for special care of feet, etc.

5 = Knows the salient facts about the disease well enough to take necessary action at the proper time, understands the rationale of care, able to observe and report significant symptoms.

4. Application of principles of personal and general hygiene

This is concerned with family action in relation to maintaining family nutrition, securing adequate rest and relaxation for family members, carrying out accepted preventive measures such as immunizations, medical appraisal, and safe homemaking habits in relation to storing and preparing food.

1 = Family diet grossly inadequate or unbalanced, necessary immunizations not secured for children; house dirty, food handled in unsanitary way; members of family working beyond reasonable limits; children and adults getting too little sleep; family members unkempt, dirty, inadequately clothed in relation to weather.

3 = Failing to apply some general principles of hygiene—for instance, keeping house in excellent condition but expending too much energy and becoming overfatigued as a result; secured initial immunizations but not boosters, or some but not all available immunizations; general diet and homemaking skills good, but father carrying two full-time jobs.

5 = Household runs smoothly, family meals well selected; habits of sleep and rest adequate to needs.

5. Health care attitudes

This category is concerned with the way the family feels about health care in general, including preventive services, care of illness, and public health measures.

1 = Family resents and resists all health care; has no confidence in doctors, uses patent medicines and quack nostrums, feels illness is unavoidable and to be borne rather than treated; feels community health agencies shouldn't interfere or bother them; practices folk medicine or superstitious rites in illness.

3 = Accepts health care in some degree, but with reservations. For example, may accept need for medical care for illness, but not general preventive measures; may have confidence in doctors generally, but not in the clinic or "free" doctors; may feel certain illnesses are hopeless (such as cancer), or care unnecessary—for instance, dental care for the young child.

5 = Understands and recognizes need for medical care in illness and for the usual preventive services, arranges for periodic physical appraisals and follows through with recommendations, accepts illness calmly and recognizes the limits it imposes while doing all possible to effect recovery and rehabilitation.

6. Emotional competence

This category has to do with the maturity and integrity with which the members of the family are able to meet the usual stresses and problems of life, and to plan for happy and fruitful living. The degree to which individuals accept the necessary disciplines imposed by one's family and culture; the development and maintenance of individual responsibility and decision; willingness to meet reasonable obligations, to accept adversity with fortitude, to consider the needs of others as well as one's own.

1 = Family does not face realities—assumes moribund client will get well, that they can eventually pay a hospital bill far beyond their means, that an unwanted pregnancy isn't so; one or more members lacking in any emotional control—uncontrollable rages, irresponsible sexual activities; one or more members alcoholic, family torn, suspicious of one another; evidences of great insecurity, guilt, or anxiety.

3 = Family members usually do fairly well, but one or more members evidence lack of security or maturity. For example, thumb sucking in late childhood; unusual concern with what the neighbors will think; failure to plan ahead for foreseeable emergencies; leaving children unattended, "fighting" in the family on occasion.

5 = All members of the family are able to maintain a reasonable degree of emotional calm, face up to illness realistically and hopefully; able to discuss problems and differences with objectivity and reasonable emotional control; do not worry unduly about trivial matters, consider the needs and wishes of other family members, of neighbors and those with whom they work and live in making decisions or deciding upon action.

7. Family living patterns

This category is concerned largely with the interpersonal or group aspects of family life—how well the members of the family get along with one another, the ways in which they make decisions affecting the family as a whole, the degree to which they support one another and do things as a family, the degree of respect and affection they show for one another, the ways in which they manage the family budget, the kind of discipline that prevails.

1 = Family consists of a group of individuals indifferent or hostile to one another, or strongly dominated and controlled by a single family member; no control of children, or family so totally dependent on one another that they are being stifled—for example, mother developing habits of dependence in sons so as to threaten future capacity for independence in own family life, no rational plan for managing available money; "battered" child.

3 = Family gets along but has habits or customs that interfere with their effectiveness or coherence as a family. For example, a family fond of one another, have many home activities, but dominated by a father in a kindly way; recreational habits separate family much of the time; children somewhat over-protected; expectations of the children unrealistic—parents expecting children with low academic competence to enter professions, etc.

5 = Family cohesive, does things together, each member acts with regard for the good of the family as a whole; children respect parents and vice versa; family tasks shared; evidence of planning.

8. Physical environment

This category is concerned with the home and community or work environment as it affects family health. The conditions for housing, presence of accident hazards, screening, plumbing, facilities for cooking and for privacy; level of community—(deteriorated or modern, presence of social hazards such as bars, street gangs, delinquency, pests such as rats), availability and condition of schools, transportation.

1 = House in poor condition, unsafe, unscreened, poorly heated, neighborhood deteriorated, juvenile and adult delinquency among neighbors, no play space except streets.

3 = House needs some repair or painting but fundamentally sound; neighborhood poor but possible to protect children from social influence through school or other community activities; house crowded but adjustments to this fairly adequate.

5 = House in good repair, provides for privacy for members and is free of accidents and pest hazards; neighborhood respectable and provided with play space for children; free from undesirable social elements; opportunities for community activity.

9. Use of community facilities

This category has to do with the degree to which the family knows about and the wisdom with which they use available community resources for health, education, and welfare. This would include the ways in which they use services of private physicians, clinics, emergency rooms, hospitals, schools, welfare organizations, churches, and so forth. The *coping ability* does not indicate the level of the *need* for services, but rather the degree to which they can cope when they must seek such aid. Even though a family has a severe housing problem, if they have used all appropriate facilities for enforcing landlord's compliance with sanitary regulations to secure public housing, their coping capacity in relation to *use* of community facilities is high, even though the underlying condition is not corrected.

1 = Family has obvious and serious social needs, but has not sought or found any help for them. For example, a family may be borrowing unreasonable sums of money for medical care, while not using available free hospitals or clinics; or leaving children without any supervision while the mother works; or fail to take steps to register for public housing when it is indicated. Using resources inappropriately, for example, calling ambulance or using emergency services for minor ills.

3 = Family knows about or uses some, but not all of the available community resources that they need. For example, the family may be under welfare care, and know how to use the social worker responsible for their care, but not have recognized that the counselor in the school could help with educational planning, or that the church might provide recreational activities for the children as well as spiritual guidance.

5 = Family using the facilities they need appropriately and promptly. Know when to call for help and whom to call. Feel secure in their relationship with community workers, such as social workers, teachers, doctors, etc.

Family coping estimate

Family _____   Nurse _____   Date _____

Initial _____   Periodic _____   Discharge _____

	Rating	
Coping area	x-status 0-est. change Poor . . . . Exc.	**Justification**
Physical independence	1 2 3 4 5 Not applicable ☐	
Therapeutic independence	1 2 3 4 5 Not applicable ☐	
Knowledge of condition	1 2 3 4 5 Not applicable ☐	
Application of principles of hygiene	1 2 3 4 5 Not applicable ☐	
Attitude toward health care	1 2 3 4 5 Not applicable ☐	
Emotional competence	1 2 3 4 5 Not applicable ☐	
Family living patterns	1 2 3 4 5 Not applicable ☐	
Physical environment	1 2 3 4 5 Not applicable ☐	
Use of community resources	1 2 3 4 5 Not applicable ☐	
Comments		

Family Assessment: Disability and Chronic Disease

The family provides nurturing, growth, socialization, and caretaking functions. The onset of a disability or chronic illness places stress on the individual and the family. This stress can test the limits of the bonds that hold the family together. The purpose of a family history is to identify genetic problems, communicable diseases, environmental problems, and interpersonal data relevant to the rehabilitation process. The nurse uses this information to identify problems of family function and to develop interventions that promote healthy family function.

I. Family: interdependent group system consisting of the biological or adoptive family; may also include influential others.
  A. Family forms.
    1. Nuclear family: husband, wife, and their children.
    2. Extended family: a family extended to include parents and sometimes other relatives.
    3. Alternate family: single-parent families, married adults without children, unmarried adults (homosexual or heterosexual), communes, and other types of family structures.
  B. Family history.
    1. The history may be recorded in narrative form, genogram, or family tree.
      a. The family tree lists all family relationships, including deaths, illnesses, divorces, and subsequent marriages. Data should be collected on grandparents, parents, siblings, spouse, and children. Age, general state of health, and health problems should be listed.
      b. Schematic representation of genogram.
  C. Family constellation.
    1. Number of family members, current living situation, and family roles.
    2. Communication patterns within the family.
      a. Who is the family spokesperson?
      b. How do family members express emotions?
      c. What are the patterns of communication among family members?

From Mumma CM, editor: *Rehabilitation nursing: concepts and practice, a core curriculum,* ed 2, Skokie, Ill, 1987, Rehabilitation Nursing Foundation.

3. Developmental level of the family refers to level of growth of the family and its ability to accomplish essential family tasks.
   a. Infancy: chaotic family that barely functions, and provides inadequate physical and emotional supports; distinguished by alienation from community, deviant behavior, distortion and confusion of roles, immaturity, child neglect, and depression failure.
   b. Childhood: intermediate family that is slightly above survival level due to variation in economic provisions; alienation present but greater ability to trust exists. Child neglect is not as great; family is defensive but slightly more willing to accept help.
   c. Adolescence: normal family, but with many conflicts and problems, plus variation in economic levels; greater trust and ability to seek and use help. Parents more mature, but still have emotional conflicts. Family members have successes and achievements and are more willing to seek solutions to problems; future oriented.
   d. Adulthood: family has solutions, is stable, healthy, and has few conflicts or problems. Very capable providers of physical and emotional supports. Parents are mature and confident, have fewer difficulties training children, are able to seek help, and are future oriented while enjoying present.
   e. Maturity: ideal family where homeostatic balance exists between individual and group goals and activities. Family meets its tasks well and is able to seek appropriate help when needed.
D. Framework for assessing impact of disability within family. Based on work of Hill and Hansen. Information should be gathered from client/family.
   1. Characteristics of disability.
      a. Nature of pathology and body systems affected.
         (1) Gradual versus sudden onset.
         (2) Degree of pain.
         (3) Visability of disability.
         (4) Threat to life.
         (5) Potential for transmission to other family members.
      b. Type of disability.
         (1) Temporary.
         (2) Chronic.
      c. Prognosis.
         (1) Will function improve or remain static?

       (2) Is disease fatal?

       (3) Anticipated lifespan?

   d. Potential for rehabilitation or restoration of function.

   e. Family perception of illness/disability.

2. Perceived threat to family relationships, status, and goals.
   a. Past family roles, relations, and communication patterns.
   b. Real and perceived changes in the above roles, relations, patterns secondary to illness/disability.
   c. Decision-making patterns before and after onset of illness/disability.
   d. Individual/family "life goals" and changes in these goals related to the onset of illness/disability.
   e. Feelings of individual/family members about changes in relationships, status, and goals.

3. Resources available to the family.
   a. Demographic data (refer to family history).
   b. Persons.
      (1) Family members.
      (2) Friends.
      (3) Community.
      (4) Family visiting expectations.

4. Past experiences with same or similar situations.
   a. Past crises experienced by family and methods of coping.
   b. Decision-making patterns employed during crisis.
   c. Individuals identified by the family as ones who can be counted on in time of crisis.

E. Future expectations related to caregiving role.
   1. Assessing caregiving capacity.
      a. Availability of a primary caregiver within family.
         (1) Desire.
         (2) Learning capacity.
         (3) Health.
      b. Tentative discharge residence and accessibility.
      c. Financial resources for help in home.
      d. Role changes within family to accommodate caretaking functions.
      e. Family's ability to handle emotional strain of caretaking.
      f. Availability of respite services.
         (1) Within family.
         (2) Within community.
      g. Community self-help programs.
         (1) For individual.
         (2) For family.

Family APGAR Questionnaire

Part 1

The following questions have been designed to help us better understand you and your family. You should feel free to ask questions about any item in the questionnaire.

The space for comments should be used when you wish to give additional information or if you wish to discuss the way the question is applied to your family.

Please try to answer all questions.

Family is defined as the individual(s) with whom you usually live. If you live alone, your "family" consists of persons with whom you now have the strongest emotional ties.*

For each question, check only one box.

	Almost always	Some of the time	Hardly ever
I am satisfied that I can turn to my family for help when something is troubling me.	☐	☐	☐

Comments: _____

_____

I am satisfied that my family talks over things with me and shares problems with me.	☐	☐	☐

Comments: _____

_____

I am satisfied that my family accepts and suports my wishes to take on new activities or directions.	☐	☐	☐

Comments: _____

_____

I am satisfied that my family expresses affection and responds to my emotions, such as anger, sorrow, and love.	☐	☐	☐

Comments: _____

_____

Modified from Smilkstein G et al: Validity and reliability of the family by APGAR as a test of family function, *J Fam Prac* 15(2):303-311, 1982.

*According to which member of the family is being interviewed the nurse may substitute for the word "family" either spouse, significant other, parents, or children.

Continued.

Family APGAR Questionnaire—cont'd

	Almost always	Some of the time	Hardly ever
I am satisfied with the way my family and I share time together.	☐	☐	☐

Comments: _____

_____

Scoring. The client checks one of three choices which are scored as follows: "Almost always" (2 points), "Some of the time" (1 point), or "Hardly ever" (0 points). The scores for each of the five questions are then totaled. A score of 7 to 10 suggests a highly functional family. A score of 4 to 6 suggests a moderately dysfunctional family. A score of 0 to 3 suggests a severely dysfunctional family.

Part II

Who lives in your home?* List the persons according to their relationship to you (for example, spouse, significant other,† child, or friend).

Check the column that best describes how you now get along with each member of the family listed.

Relationship	Age	Sex

Well	Fairly	Poorly

If you don't live with your own family, list the persons to whom you turn for help most frequently. List according to relationship (for example, family member, friend, associate at work, or neighbor).

Check the column that best describes how you now get along with each person listed.

Relationship	Age	Sex

Well	Fairly	Poorly

*If you have established your own family, consider your "home" as the place where you live with your spouse, children, or "significant other" (see next footnote for definition). Otherwise, consider home as your place of origin, for example, the place where your parents or those who raised you live.

†Significant other is the partner you live with in a physically and emotionally nurturing relationship but to whom you are not married.

Child Assessment

Pediatric Health History

The outline below provides a systematic procedure for completing a child health history. It is especially useful before completing a physical assessment to give the nurse essential background for health care planning.

Identifying Information

1. Name
2. Address
3. Telephone number
4. Age and birthdate
5. Birthplace
6. Race
7. Sex
8. Religion
9. Nationality
10. Date of interview
11. Informant

Additional information appropriate to older adolescent may include occupation, marital status, and temporary and permanent address.

Under informant include subjective impression of reliability, general attitude, willingness to communicate, overall accuracy of data, and any special circumstances, such as use of an interpreter.

Informants should include parent and child, as well as others who may be primary caregivers, such as grandparent.

Chief complaint (CC)

To establish the major specific reason for the individual's seeking professional health attention.

Record in client's own words; include duration of symptoms.
If informant has difficulty isolating *one* problem, ask which problem or symptom led person to seek help *now*.
In case of routine physical examination, state CC as reason for visit.

Modified from Wong DL, Whaley LF: *Essentials of pediatric nursing,* ed 4, St Louis, 1993, Mosby.

Present illness (PI)

To obtain all details related to the chief complaint.

In its broadest sense, *illness* denotes any problem of a physical, emotional, or psychosocial nature.

1. Onset
   a. Date of onset
   b. Manner of onset (gradual or sudden)
   c. Precipitating and predisposing factors related to onset (emotional disturbance, physical exertion, fatigue, bodily function, pregnancy, environment, injury, infection, toxins and allergens, or therapeutic agents)
2. Characteristics
   a. Character (quality, quantity, consistency, or other)
   b. Location and radiation (i.e., pain)
   c. Intensity or severity
   d. Timing (continuous or intermittent, duration of each, temporal relationship to other events)
   e. Aggravating and relieving factors
   f. Associated symptoms

Present information in chronologic order; may be referenced according to one point in time, such as *prior to admission* (PTA).

3. Course since onset
   a. Incidence
      (1) Single acute attack
      (2) Recurrent acute attacks
      (3) Daily occurrences
      (4) Periodic occurrences
      (5) Continuous chronic episode
   b. Progress (better, worse, unchanged)
   c. Effect of therapy

Concentrate on reason for seeking help now, especially if problem has existed for some time.

Past history (PH)

To elicit a profile of the individual's previous illnesses, injuries, or operations.

1. Pregnancy (maternal)
   a. Number (gravida)
      (1) Dates of delivery

   b. Outcome (parity)
      (1) Gestation (full-term, premature, postmature)
      (2) Stillbirths, abortions
   c. Health during pregnancy
   d. Medications taken

Importance of perinatal history depends on child's age; the younger
   the child, the more important the perinatal history.
Explain relevance of obstetric history in revealing important factors
   relating to the child's health.
Assess parents' emotional attitudes toward the pregnancy and birth.

2. Labor and delivery
   a. Duration of labor
   b. Type of delivery
   c. Place of delivery
   d. Medications

Assess parent's feelings regarding delivery; investigate factors
   affecting bonding, such as if awake and able to hold infant or if
   asleep and separated from infant.

3. Birth
   a. Weight and length
   b. Time of regaining birth weight
   c. Condition of health
   d. Apgar score
   e. Presence of congenital anomalies
   f. Date of discharge from nursery

If birth problems are reported, inquire about treatment, such as use of
   oxygen, phototherapy, surgery, and so on, and parents' emotional
   response to the event.

4. Previous illnesses, operations, or injuries
   a. Onset, symptoms, course, termination
   b. Occurrence of complications
   c. Incidence of disease in other family members or in community

Make positive statements about diphtheria, scarlet fever, measles,
   chickenpox, mumps, tonsillitis, pertussis, and common illnesses,
   such as colds, earaches, or sore throats.
Elicit a description of disease to verify the diagnosis.

   d. Emotional response to previous hospitalization
   e. Circumstances and nature of injuries

Be alert to areas of injury prevention.

5. Allergies
    a. Hay fever, asthma, or eczema

Have parent describe the type of allergic reaction.

    b. Unusual reactions to foods, drugs, animals, plants, or household products

Note sensitivity to egg albumin and reactions to certain immunizations.

6. Current medications
    a. Name, dose, schedule, duration, and reason for administration

Assess parents' knowledge of correct dosage of common drugs, such as acetaminophen; note underusage or overusage.

7. Immunizations
    a. Name, number of doses, ages when given
    b. Occurrence of reaction
    c. Administration of horse or other foreign serum, gamma globulin, or blood transfusion

May refer to immunizations as "baby shots."
Whenever possible, confirm information by checking medical or school records.

8. Growth and development
    a. Weight at birth, 6 months, 1 year, and present
    b. Dentition
        (1) Age of eruption/shedding
        (2) Number
        (3) Problems with teething
    c. Age of head control, sitting unsupported, walking, first words
    d. Present grade in school, scholastic achievement
    e. Interaction with peers and adults
    f. Participation in organized activities, such as scouts, sports, and so on

Compare parents' responses with own observations of child's achievement and results from objective tests, such as DDST or DASE.
School and social history can be more thoroughly explored under Family Assessment.

9. Habits
    a. Behavior patterns
        (1) Nail biting
        (2) Thumb sucking

    (3) Pica
    (4) Rituals, such as "security blanket"
    (5) Unusual movements (headbanging, rocking)
    (6) Temper tantrums

Assess parents' attitudes toward habits and any remedies used to curtail them, such as punishment for bed-wetting.

  b. Activities of daily living
    (1) Hour of sleep and arising
    (2) Duration of nocturnal sleep/naps
    (3) Age of toilet training
    (4) Pattern of stools and urination; occurrence of enuresis

Record child's usual terms for defecation and urination.

    (5) Type of exercise

  c. Use/abuse of drugs, alcohol, coffee, or cigarettes

With adolescents, estimate the quantity of drugs used.

  d. Usual disposition; response to frustration

Review of systems (ROS)

To elicit information concerning any potential health problem.

1. **General**—overall state of health, fatigue, recent or unexplained weight gain or loss, period of time for either, contributing factors (change of diet, illness, altered appetite), exercise tolerance, fevers (time of day), chills, night sweats (unrelated to climatic conditions), frequent infections, general ability to carry out activities of daily living

Explain relevance of questioning to parents (similar to pregnancy section) in comprising total health history of child.
Make positive statements about each system, for example, "Mother denies headaches, bumping into objects, squinting, or excessive rubbing of eyes."
Use terms parents are likely to understand, such as "bruises" for ecchymoses.

2. **Integument**—pruritus, pigment or other color changes, acne, eruptions, rashes (location), tendency to bruising, petechiae, excessive dryness, general texture, disorders or deformities of nails, hair growth or loss, hair color change (for adolescent, use of hair dyes or other potentially toxic substances, such as hair straighteners)
3. **Head**—headaches, dizziness, injury (specific details)

4. **Eyes**—visual problems (ask about behaviors that indicate blurred vision, such as bumping into objects, clumsiness, sitting very close to television, holding a book close to the face, writing with head near desk, squinting, rubbing the eyes, bending the head in an awkward position), "cross-eye" (strabismus), eye infections, edema of lids, excessive tearing, use of glasses or contact lenses, date of last optic examination

5. **Nose**—nosebleeds (epistaxis), constant or frequent running or stuffy nose, nasal obstruction (difficulty in breathing), sense of smell

6. **Ears**—earaches, discharge, evidence of hearing loss (ask about behaviors such as need to repeat requests, loud speech, inattentive behavior), results of any previous auditory testing

7. **Mouth**—mouth breathing, gum bleeding, toothaches, tooth-brushing, use of fluoride, difficulty with teething (symptoms), last visit to dentist (especially if temporary dentition is complete), response to dentist

8. **Throat**—sore throats, difficulty in swallowing, choking (especially when chewing food, which may be caused by poor chewing habits), hoarseness or other voice irregularities

9. **Neck**—pain, limitation of movement, stiffness, difficulty in holding head straight (torticollis), thyroid enlargement, enlarged nodes or other masses

10. **Chest**—breast enlargement, discharge, masses, enlarged axillary nodes (for adolescent female, ask about breast self-examination)

11. **Respiratory**—chronic cough, frequent colds (number per year), wheezing, shortness of breath at rest or on exertion, difficulty in breathing, sputum production, infections (pneumonia, tuberculosis), date of last chest x-ray examination; date of last tuberculin test and type of reaction, if any

12. **Cardiovascular**—cyanosis or fatigue on exertion, history of heart murmur or rheumatic fever, anemia, date of last blood count, blood type, recent transfusion

13. **Gastrointestinal**—(much of this in regard to appetite, food tolerance, and elimination habits has been asked elsewhere) concentrate on nausea, vomiting (if not associated with eating, it may indicate brain tumor or increased intracranial pressure), jaundice or yellowing skin or sclera, belching, flatulence, recent change in bowel habits (blood in stools, change of color, diarrhea, or constipation)

14. **Genitourinary**—pain on urination, frequency, hesitancy, urgency, hematuria, nocturia, polyuria, unpleasant odor of urine, direction and force of stream, discharge, change in size of scrotum, date of last urinalysis (for adolescent, sexually trans-

mitted disease, type of treatment; for adolescent male, ask about testicular self-examination)

15. **Gynecologic**—menarche, date of last menstrual period, regularity or problems with menstruation, vaginal discharge, pruritus, date and result of last Pap test (include obstetric history as discussed under birth history when applicable), if sexually active, type of contraception
16. **Musculoskeletal**—weakness, clumsiness, lack of coordination, unusual movements, back or joint stiffness, muscle pains or cramps, abnormal gait, deformity, fractures, serious sprains, activity level
17. **Neurologic**—seizures, tremors, dizziness, loss of memory, general affect, fears, nightmares, speech problems, any unusual habits
18. **Endocrine**—intolerance to weather changes, excessive thirst, excessive sweating, salty taste to skin, signs of early puberty

Nutrition history

To elicit information about adequacy of child's dietary intake and eating patterns.

Family medical history

To identify the presence of genetic traits or diseases that have familial tendencies; to assess family habits and exposure to a communicable disease that may affect family members.

Choose terms wisely when asking about child's parentage, for example, inquire about paternal history by referring to the child's "father" rather than mother's husband; use term "partner" rather than spouse.

1. Family pedigree and guidelines for construction

A pedigree is a pictorial representation or diagram of a family tree to visualize patterns of disease transmission

2. Familial diseases and congenital anomalies, such as heart disease, hypertension, cancer, diabetes mellitus, obesity, congenital anomalies, allergy, asthma, tuberculosis, sickle cell disease, mental retardation, convulsions, insanity or other emotional problems, syphilis, or rheumatic fever; indicate symptoms, treatment, and sequelae
3. Family habits, such as smoking or chemical use
4. Geographic location, such as recent travel or contact with foreign visitors

Important for identification of endemic diseases.

Family personal/social history

To gain an understanding of the family's structure and function.

Sexual history

To elicit information concerning young person's concerns or activities and any pertinent data regarding adults' sexual activity that influences child.

1. Sexual concerns/activity of youngster
2. Sexual concerns/activity of adults if warranted

Sexual history is an essential component of preadolescents' and adolescents' health assessment.

Degree of investigation into parents' sexual history depends on its relevance to the child's health. It may be limited to family planning concerns or it may be more detailed if overt sexual activity or abuse is suspected.

Investigate toward end of history when rapport is greatest.

Respect sensitive and complex nature of questioning.

Give parents and youngster option of discussing sexual matters alone with nurse.

Assure confidentiality.

Clarify terms such as "sexually active" or "having sex?"

Refer to sexual contacts as "partners," not "girlfriends" or "boyfriends," to avoid biasing discussion of homosexual activity.

Discussion may flow easily after review of genitourinary tract, such as asking female about menstruation or male about urinary problems.

Suggestions for beginning discussion include the following:

"Tell me about your social life."

"Who are your closest friends?"

"Is there one very special friend?"

"Some teenagers have decided to have sex. What do you think about that?"

Take detailed history of all contacts if sexually transmitted disease is suspected or diagnosed.

Client profile (C/P)

To summarize the interviewer's overall impression of the child's and family physical, psychological, and socioeconomic background.

1. Health status
2. Psychological status
3. Socioeconomic status

A comprehensive summary often identifies nursing diagnoses based on subjective and objective findings.

Physical Assessment and
Examination of the Newborn

The following is a suggested guide for the physical examination of the newborn. In most instances this task is performed in the hospital, but there may be times when the nurse will want a copy of this assessment, or need to perform such an assessment in the home.

Provide a normothermic and nonstimulating examination area.

Undress only body area examined to prevent heat loss.

Proceed in an orderly sequence (usually head to toe) with the following exceptions:

Perform all procedures that require quiet first, such as auscultating the lungs, heart, and abdomen.

Perform disturbing procedures, such as testing reflexes, last.

Measure head, chest, and length at same time to compare results.

Proceed quickly to avoid stressing infant.

Check that equipment and supplies are working properly and are accessible.

Comfort infant during and after examination; involve parent in the following:

Talk softly.

Hold infant's hands against chest.

Swaddle and hold.

Give pacifier or gloved finger to suck.

From Wong D: *Whaley and Wong's nursing care of infants and children,* ed 5, St Louis, 1995, Mosby.

Summary of Physical Assessment of the Newborn

Usual findings	Common variations/minor abnormalities	Potential signs of distress/major abnormalities
General measurements		
Head circumference—33-35 cm (13-14 inches); about 2-3 cm (1 inch) larger than chest circumference	Molding after birth may decrease head circumference Head and chest circumferences may be equal for first 1-2 days after birth	Head circumference <10th or >90th percentile
Chest circumference—30.5-33 cm (12-13 inches)		
Crown-to-rump length—31-35 cm (12.5-14 inches); approximately equal to head circumference		
Head-to-heel length—48-53 cm (19-21 inches)		
Birth weight—2700-4000 g (6-9 pounds)	Loss of 10% of birth weight in first week; regained in 10-14 days	Birth weight <10th or >90th percentile
Vital signs		
Temperature		
Axillary—36.5°-37°C (97.7°-98.6°F)	Crying may increase body temperature slightly Radiant warmer will falsely increase axillary temperature	Hypothermia Hyperthermia

From Wong D: *Whaley and Wong's nursing care of infants and children,* ed 5, St Louis, 1995, Mosby.

Continued.

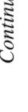

Summary of Physical Assessment of the Newborn—cont'd

Usual findings	Common variations/minor abnormalities	Potential signs of distress/major abnormalities
Heart Rate Apical—120-140 beats/min	Crying will increase heart rate; sleep will decrease heart rate During first period of reactivity (6 to 8 hours), rate can reach 180 beats/min	Bradycardia—resting rate below 80-100 beats/min Tachycardia—rate above 160-180 beats/min Irregular rhythm
Respirations 30-60 breaths/min	Crying will increase respiratory rate; sleep will decrease respiratory rate During first period of reactivity (6 to 8 hours), rate can reach 80 breaths/min	Tachypnea—rate above 60 breaths/min Apnea >15 seconds
Blood Pressure Oscillometric—65/41 mm Hg in arm and calf See inside back cover for auscultatory BP measurements	Crying and activity will increase BP Placing cuff on thigh may agitate infant; thigh BP may be higher than arm or calf BP by 4-8 mm Hg	Oscillometric systolic pressure in calf 6-9 mm Hg less than in upper extremity (sign of coarctation of aorta)
General appearance *Posture*—flexion of head and extremities, which rest on chest and abdomen	*Frank breech*—extended legs, abducted and fully rotated thighs, flattened occiput, extended neck	Limp posture, extension of extremities

Continued.

Skin

At birth, bright red, puffy, smooth

Second to third day, pink, flaky, dry

Vernix caseosa

Lanugo

Edema around eyes, face, legs, dorsa of hands, feet, and scrotum or labia

Acrocyanosis—cyanosis of hands and feet

Cutis marmorata—transient mottling when infant is exposed to decreased temperature

Neonatal jaundice after first 24 hours

Ecchymoses or petechiae caused by birth trauma

Milia—distended sebaceous glands that appear as tiny white papules on cheeks, chin, and nose

Miliaria or sudamina—distended sweat (eccrine) glands that appear as minute vesicles, especially on face

Erythema toxicum—pink papular rash with vesicles superimposed on thorax, back, buttocks, and abdomen; may appear in 24 to 48 hours and resolve after several days

Harlequin color change—clearly outlined color change as infant lies on side; lower half of body becomes pink, and upper half is pale

Mongolian spots—irregular areas of deep blue pigmentation, usually in sacral and gluteal regions; seen predominantly in newborns of African, Native American, Asian, or Hispanic descent

Telangiectatic nevi ("stork bites")—flat, deep pink localized areas usually seen in back of neck

Progressive jaundice, especially in first 24 hours

Cracked or peeling skin

Generalized cyanosis

Pallor

Mottling

Grayness

Plethora

Hemorrhage, ecchymoses, or petechiae that persist

Sclerema—hard and stiff skin

Poor skin turgor

Rashes, pustules, or blisters

Café-au-lait spots—Light brown spots

Nevus flammeus—Port-wine stain

Summary of Physical Assessment of the Newborn—cont'd

Usual findings	Common variations/minor abnormalities	Potential signs of distress/major abnormalities
Head		
Anterior fontanel—diamond shaped, 2.5-4.0 cm (1-1.75 inches)	Molding following vaginal delivery	Fused sutures
Posterior fontanel—triangular, 0.5-1 cm (0.2-0.4 inch)	Third sagittal (parietal) fontanel	Bulging or depressed fontanels when quiet
Fontanels should be flat, soft, and firm	Bulging fontanel because of crying or coughing	Widened sutures and fontanels
Widest part of fontanel measured from bone to bone, not suture to suture	*Caput succedaneum*—edema of soft scalp tissue	*Craniotabes*—snapping sensation along lambdoid suture that resembles indentation of Ping-Pong ball
	Cephalhematoma (uncomplicated)—hematoma between periosteum and skull bone	
Eyes		
Lids usually edematous	Epicanthal folds in Oriental infants	Pink color of iris
Color—slate gray, dark blue, brown	Searching nystagmus or strabismus	Purulent discharge
Absence of tears	*Subconjunctival (scleral) hemorrhages*—ruptured capillaries, usually at limbus	Upward slant in non-Orientals
Presence of red reflex		Hypertelorism (3 cm or greater)
Corneal reflex in response to touch		Hypotelorism
Pupillary reflex in response to light		Congenital cataracts
Blink reflex in response to light or touch		Constricted or dilated fixed pupil

Rudimentary fixation on objects and ability to follow to midline		Absence of red reflex Absence of pupillary or corneal reflex Inability to follow object or bright light to midline Blue sclera Yellow sclera
Ears		
Position—top of pinna on horizontal line with outer canthus of eye Startle reflex elicited by a loud, sudden noise Pinna flexible, cartilage present	Inability to visualize tympanic membrane because of filled aural canals Pinna flat against head Irregular shape or size Pits or skin tags	Low placement of ears Absence of startle reflex in response to loud noise Minor abnormalities may be signs of various syndromes, especially renal
Nose		
Nasal patency Nasal discharge—thin white mucus Sneezing	Flattened and bruised	Nonpatent canals Thick, bloody nasal discharge Flaring of nares (alae nasi) Copious nasal secretions or stuffiness (may be minor)

Continued.

Summary of Physical Assessment of the Newborn—cont'd

Usual findings	Common variations/minor abnormalities	Potential signs of distress/major abnormalities
Mouth and throat		
Intact, high-arched palate	*Natal teeth*—Teeth present at birth; benign but may be associated with congenital defects	Cleft lip
Uvula in midline		Cleft palate
Frenulum of tongue	*Epstein's pearls*—small, white epithelial cysts along midline of hard palate	Large, protruding tongue or posterior displacement of tongue
Frenum of upper lip		Profuse salivation or drooling
Sucking reflex—strong and coordinated		*Candidiasis (thrush)*—white, adherent patches on tongue, palate, and buccal surfaces
Rooting reflex		Inability to pass nasogastric tube
Gag reflex		Hoarse, high-pitched, weak, absent, or other abnormal cry
Extrusion reflex		
Absent or minimal salivation		
Vigorous cry		
Neck		
Short, thick, usually surrounded by skinfolds	*Torticollis* (wryneck)—head held to one side with chin pointing to opposite side	Excessive skinfolds
Tonic neck reflex		Resistance to flexion
		Absence of tonic neck reflex
		Fractured clavicle

Chest

Normal Findings	Common Variations/Deviations	Abnormal Findings
Anteroposterior and lateral diameters equal	Funnel chest (pectus excavatum)	Depressed sternum
Slight sternal retractions evident during inspiration	Pigeon chest (pectus carinatum)	Marked retractions of chest and intercostal spaces during respiration
Xiphoid process evident	Supernumerary nipples	Asymmetric chest expansion
Breast enlargement	Secretion of milky substance from breasts ("witch's milk")	Redness and firmness around nipples
		Wide-spaced nipples

Lungs

Normal Findings	Common Variations/Deviations	Abnormal Findings
Respirations chiefly abdominal	Rate and depth of respirations may be irregular, periodic breathing	Inspiratory stridor
Cough reflex absent at birth, present by 1-2 days	Crackles shortly after birth	Expiratory grunt
Bilateral equal bronchial breath sounds		Retractions
		Persistent irregular breathing
		Periodic breathing with repeated apneic spells
		Seesaw respirations (paradoxical)
		Unequal breath sounds
		Persistent fine crackles
		Wheezing
		Diminished breath sounds
		Peristaltic sounds on one side, with diminished breath sounds on same side

Continued.

Summary of Physical Assessment of the Newborn—cont'd

Usual findings	Common variations/minor abnormalities	Potential signs of distress/major abnormalities
Heart		
Apex—fourth to fifth intercostal space, lateral to left sternal border	*Sinus arrhythmia*—heart rate increases with inspiration and decreases with expiration	*Dextrocardia*—heart on right side
S_2 slightly sharper and higher in pitch than S_1	Transient cyanosis on crying or straining	Displacement of apex, muffled
		Cardiomegaly
		Abdominal shunts
		Murmurs
		Thrills
		Persistent cyanosis
		Hyperactive precordium
Abdomen		
Cylindric in shape	Umbilical hernia	Abdominal distention
Liver—palpable 2-3 cm below right costal margin	*Diastasis recti*—midline gap between recti muscles	Localized bulging
Spleen—tip palpable at end of first week of age	*Wharton's jelly*—unusually thick umbilical cord	Distended veins
Kidneys—palpable 1-2 cm above umbilical cord		Absent bowel sounds
Umbilical cord—bluish white at birth with two arteries and one vein		Enlarged liver and spleen
Femoral pulses—equal bilaterally		Ascites
		Visible peristaltic waves
		Scaphoid or concave abdomen
		Green umbilical cord
		Presence of only one artery in cord

		Urine or stool leaking from cord
		Palpable bladder distention following scanty voiding
		Absent femoral pulses
		Cord bleeding or hematoma

Female genitalia

Labia and clitoris usually edematous	*Pseudomenstruation*—blood-tinged or mucoid discharge	Enlarged clitoris with urethral meatus at tip
Urethral meatus behind clitoris	Hymenal tag	Fused labia
Vernix caseosa between labia		Absence of vaginal opening
Urination within 24 hours		Meconium from vaginal opening
		No urination within 24 hours
		Masses in labia
		Ambiguous genitalia

Male genitalia

Urethral opening at tip of glans penis	Urethral opening covered by prepuce	*Hypospadias*—urethral opening on ventral surface of penis
Testes palpable in each scrotum	Inability to retract foreskin	*Epispadias*—urethral opening on dorsal surface of penis
Scrotum usually large, edematous, pendulous, and covered with rugae; usually deeply pigmented in dark-skinned ethnic groups	*Epithelial pearls*—small, firm, white lesions at tip of prepuce	*Chordee*—ventral curvature of penis
	Erection or priapism	

Continued.

Summary of Physical Assessment of the Newborn—cont'd

Usual findings	Common variations/minor abnormalities	Potential signs of distress/major abnormalities
Male genitalia—cont'd		
Smegma	Testes palpable in inguinal canal	Testes not palpable in scrotum or inguinal canal
Urination within 24 hours	Scrotum small	No urination within 24 hours
		Inguinal hernia
		Hypoplastic scrotum
		Hydrocele—fluid in scrotum
		Masses in scrotum
		Meconium from scrotum
		Discoloration of testes
		Ambiguous genitalia
Back and rectum		
Spine intact, no openings, masses, or prominent curves	Green liquid stools in infant under phototherapy	Anal fissures or fistulas
Trunk incurvation reflex	Delayed passages of meconium in very-low-birth-weight neonates	Imperforate anus
Anal reflex		Absence of anal reflex
Patent anal opening		No meconium within 36 hours
Passage of meconium within 48 hours		Pilonidal cyst or sinus
		Tuft of hair along spine
		Spina bifida (any degree)

Extremities

Ten fingers and toes

Full range of motion

Nail beds pink, with transient cyanosis immediately after birth

Creases on anterior two thirds of sole

Sole usually flat

Symmetry of extremities

Equal muscle tone bilaterally, especially resistance to opposing flexion

Equal bilateral brachial pulses

Partial syndactyly between second and third toes

Second toe overlapping into third toe

Wide gap between first (hallux) and second toes

Deep crease on plantar surface of foot between first and second toes

Asymmetric length of toes

Dorsiflexion and shortness of hallux

Polydactyly—extra digits

Syndactyly—fused or webbed digits

Phocomelia—hands or feet attached close to trunk

Hemimelia—absence of distal part of extremity

Hyperflexibility of joints

Persistent cyanosis of nail beds

Yellowing of nail beds

Sole covered with creases

Transverse palmar (simian) crease

Fractures

Decreased or absent ROM

Dislocated or subluxated hip

  Limitation in hip abduction

  Unequal gluteal or leg folds

  Unequal knee height (Allis or Galeazzi sign)

  Audible click on abduction (Ortolani sign)

Asymmetry of extremities

Unequal muscle tone or range of motion

Continued.

Summary of Physical Assessment of the Newborn—cont'd

Usual findings	Common variations/minor abnormalities	Potential signs of distress/major abnormalities
Neuromuscular system		
Extremities usually maintain some degree of flexion	Quivering or momentary tremors	*Hypotonia*—floppy, poor head control, extremities limp
Extension of an extremity followed by previous position of flexion		*Hypertonia*—jittery, arms and hands tightly flexed, legs stiffly extended, startles easily
Head lag while sitting, but momentary ability to hold head erect		Asymmetric posturing (except tonic neck reflex)
Able to turn head from side to side when prone		*Opisthotonic posturing*—arched back
Able to hold head in horizontal line with back when held prone		Signs of paralysis
		Tremors, twitches, and myoclonic jerks
		Marked head lag in all positions

Pediatric Physical Assessment

The following is a suggested guide for the physical examination of the child. The nurse may adapt the examination based on the child's age.

1. General
   a. Frequent colds, infections, or illnesses
   b. Frequent fevers, sweats
   c. Fatigue patterns
   d. Energetic or overactive patterns
2. Nutritional
   a. Recent weight gain or loss (describe)
   b. Appetite
   c. Twenty-four-hour recall, including types, amount of food eaten (formula, breast milk, meat, fruits, vegetables, cereals, juices, eggs, sweets, milk, snacks), and frequency (e.g., how many times a day or week)
   d. Child feeding self?
   e. Where does child eat?
   f. Who does child eat with?
   g. Parent's perception of child's nutritional status (note problems)
   h. Vitamins?
   i. Junk food consumption (amount and kinds)
3. Integumentary
   a. Skin
      (1) Chronic rashes
      (2) Easy bruising or petechiae
      (3) Easy bleeding
      (4) Acne (treatment pattern)
      (5) Excessive sweating
      (6) Skin diseases, problems, or lesions
      (7) Itching
      (8) Pigmentation changes, discolorations, mottling
      (9) Excessive dryness
      (10) Skin growths or tumors
   b. Hair
      (1) Changes in amount, texture, characteristics
      (2) Infections, lice
      (3) Alopecia

From Bowers AC, Thompson JM: *Clinical manual of health assessment,* ed 4, St Louis, 1992, Mosby.

    c. Nails
       (1) Changes in appearance
       (2) Cyanosis
       (3) Texture

4. Head
    a. Headache (frequency, type, location, duration, care for)
    b. Past significant trauma
    c. Dizziness
    d. Syncope

5. Eyes
    a. Crossed eyes
    b. Strabismus
    c. Discharge
    d. Complaint of vision changes
    e. Reading difficulty
    f. Sitting close to television
    g. History of infections
    h. Pruritus
    i. Excessive tearing
    j. Pain in eyeball
    k. Swelling around eyes
    l. Cataracts
    m. Unusual sensations or twitching
    n. Excessive blinking
    o. Eye injury history
    p. Currently wears glasses
    q. Diplopia
    r. Blurring
    s. Gives history of inability to see distant images

6. Ears
    a. Multiple infections or earaches
    b. Myringotomy tubes in ears
    c. Discharge
    d. Cerumen
    e. Care habits
    f. Cracking or ringing
    g. Parent perceives problem in child's hearing

7. Nose, nasopharynx, and paranasal sinuses
    a. Discharge (character of)
    b. Epistaxis
    c. Allergies
    d. General olfactory ability
    e. Pain over sinuses

    f. Postnasal drip

    g. Sneezing

    h. Nasal stuffiness

8. Mouth and throat
   a. Sore throats (frequent)
   b. Tonsils present
   c. Mouth sores
   d. Toothaches, caries
   e. Voice changes
   f. Hoarseness
   g. Mouth breathing
   h. Chewing difficulties
   i. Swallowing difficulties
   j. Teeth brushing pattern

9. Neck
   a. Swollen glands
   b. Tenderness
   c. Limitations of movement
   d. Stiffness

10. Breast: applicable only with teenagers; refer to adult data base

11. Cardiovascular
    a. History of murmur
    b. History of heart problem
    c. Palpitations
    d. Hypertension
    e. Postural hypotension
    f. Cyanosis (what precipitates)
    g. Dyspnea on exertion
    h. Limitation of activities
    i. Frequent complaints of extremity coldness

12. Respiratory
    a. Breathing trouble
    b. Chronic cough
    c. Wheezing (precipitating factors)
    d. Croup history
    e. Noisy breathing
    f. Shortness of breath

13. Hematolymphatic
    a. Lymph node swelling (note frequency and location)
    b. Excessive bleeding or easy bruising
    c. Anemia
    d. Blood dyscrasias
    e. Lead exposures, deleading in past

14. Gastrointestinal
    a. Ulcer history
    b. Previously diagnosed problem
    c. Vomiting
    d. Diarrhea
    e. Constipation or stool-holding problems
    f. Rectal bleeding
    g. Stool color change
    h. Abdominal pains
    i. Pinworms by history
    j. Perianal pruritus
    k. Use of evacuation aids
    l. Toilet trained? If not, is it planned? Any problems?
15. Urinary
    a. Urinary tract infections during past year
    b. Previously diagnosed problems
    c. Characteristics of urine (cloudy, dark)
    d. Suprapubic pains
    e. Steadiness and force of urination stream
    f. Dysuria
    g. Nocturia
    h. Bed-wetting (Associated with emotional upsets? Family history of bed-wetting?)
    i. Urinary frequency
    j. Dribbling or incontinence
    k. Polyuria/oliguria
    l. Bubble bath used?
16. Genital
    a. Birth defects
    b. Discharges
    c. Odors
    d. Rashes, irritation
    e. Pruritus
    f. How is sexuality education handled in the home?
    g. Areas of concern
    h. If client is female and menstruating, refer to adult data base for appropriate questioning
17. Musculoskeletal
    a. Muscles
        (1) Twitching
        (2) Cramping
        (3) Pain
        (4) Weakness
        (5) Pain with use

   b. Extremities
- (1) General complaints of pain, weakness, deformity
- (2) Night pains in legs
- (3) Gait ability—strength and coordination

   c. Bones and joints
- (1) Joint swelling
- (2) Joint pain
- (3) Redness, stiffness
- (4) Joint deformity
- (5) Fracture or dislocation history

   d. Back
- (1) History of back injury
- (2) Curvature of spine
- (3) Characteristics of problems and corrective measures

18. Central nervous system
   a. General
- (1) Unusual episodic behaviors
- (2) History of central nervous system diseases
- (3) Birth injury

   b. Seizure: febrile versus afebrile

   c. Speech
- (1) Stuttering
- (2) Speech misarticulations
- (3) Language delay

   d. Cognitive changes
- (1) Hallucinations
- (2) Passing out episodes
- (3) Staring spells
- (4) Learning difficulties

   e. Motor-gait
- (1) Coordination
- (2) Developmental clumsiness
- (3) Balance problems
- (4) Tic
- (5) Tremor, spasms

   f. Sensory
- (1) Pain pattern
- (2) Tingling sensations

19. Endocrine
   a. Diagnosis of disease states (e.g., thyroid, diabetes)
   b. Changes in skin texture (e.g., increased or decreased dryness or perspiration)
   c. Pigmentation
   d. Abnormal hair distribution

    e. Sudden or unexplained changes in height and weight
    f. Intolerance to heat or cold
    g. Exophthalmos
    h. Goiter
    i. Polydipsia (increased thirst)
    j. Polyphagia (increased food intake)
    k. Polyuria (increased urination)
    l. Anorexia (decreased appetite)
    m. Weakness
    n. Precocious puberty
20. Allergic and immunological
    a. Dermatitis (inflammation or irritation of the skin)
    b. Eczema
    c. Pruritus (itching)
    d. Urticaria (hives)
    e. Sneezing
    f. Vasomotor rhinitis (inflammation and swelling of mucous membrane of nose, nasal discharge)
    g. Conjunctivitis (inflammation of conjunctiva)
    h. Interference with activities of daily living
    i. Environmental and seasonal causes
    j. Treatment techniques

Performing a Pediatric Physical Examination

Perform examination in appropriate, nonthreatening area.
    Have room well lit and decorated with neutral colors.
    Have room temperature comfortably warm.
    Place all strange and potentially frightening equipment out of sight.
    Have some toys, dolls, stuffed animals, and games available for child.
    If possible, have rooms decorated and equipped for children of different ages.
    Provide privacy, especially for school-age children and adolescents.
Provide time for play and becoming acquainted.
Observe behaviors that signal child's readiness to cooperate:
    Talking to nurse
    Making eye contact

From Wong D: *Whaley and Wong's nursing care of infants and children,* ed 5, St Louis, 1995, Mosby.

Accepting offered equipment

Allowing physical touching

Choosing to sit on examining table rather than parent's lap

If signs of readiness are not observed, use the following techniques:

Talk to parent while essentially "ignoring" child; gradually focus on child or a favorite object, such as a doll.

Make complimentary remarks about child, such as appearance, dress, or a favorite object.

Tell a funny story or play a simple magic trick.

Have a nonthreatening "friend" available, such as a hand puppet to "talk" to child for the nurse.

If child refuses to cooperate, use the following techniques:

Assess reason for uncooperative behavior; consider that a child who is unduly afraid may have had a previous traumatic experience.

Try to involve child and parent in process.

Avoid prolonged explanations about examining procedure.

Use a firm, direct approach regarding expected behavior.

Perform examination as quickly as possible.

Have attendant gently restrain child.

Minimize any disruptions or stimulation.

Limit number of people in room.

Use isolated room.

Use quiet, calm, confident voice.

Begin examination in a nonthreatening manner for young children or children who are fearful:

Use those activities that can be presented as games, such as test for cranial nerves or parts of developmental screening tests.

Use approaches such as "Simon says" to encourage child to make a face, squeeze a hand, stand on one foot, and so on.

Use "paper-doll" technique.

Lay child supine on an examining table or floor that is covered with a large sheet of paper.

Trace around child's body outline.

Use body outline to demonstrate what will be examined, such as drawing a heart and listening with the stethoscope before performing the activity on child.

If several children in the family will be examined, begin with the most cooperative child to provide modeling of desired behavior.

Involve child in examination process:

Provide choices, such as sitting on table or in parent's lap.

Allow child to handle or hold equipment.

Encourage child to use equipment on a doll, family member, or examiner.

Explain each step of the procedure in simple language.

Examine child in a comfortable and secure position:

Sitting in parent's lap

Sitting upright if in respiratory distress

Proceed to examine the body in an organized sequence (usually head to toe) with the following exceptions:

Alter sequence to accommodate needs of children of different ages.

Examine painful areas last.

In emergency situation, examine vital functions (airway, breathing, and circulation) and injured area first.

Reassure child throughout examination, especially about bodily concerns that arise during puberty.

Discuss findings with family at end of examination.

Praise child for cooperation during examination; give reward such as a small toy or sticker.

Age-Specific Approaches to Physical Examination During Childhood

Position	Sequence	Preparation
Infant		
Before sits alone: supine or prone, preferably in parent's lap; before 4 to 6 months: can place on examining table	If quiet, auscultate heart, lungs, abdomen	Completely undress if room temperature permits
After sits alone: use sitting in parent's lap whenever possible	Record heart and respiratory rates	Leave diaper on male
If on table, place with parent in full view	Palpate and percuss same areas	Gain cooperation with distraction, bright objects, rattles, talking
	Proceed in usual head-to-toe direction	Have older infants hold a small block in each hand; until voluntary release develops toward end of the first year, infants will be unable to grasp other objects
	Perform traumatic procedures last (eyes, ears, mouth [while crying])	(e.g., stethoscope, otoscope) (Farber, 1991)
	Elicit reflexes as body part examined	Smile at infant; use soft, gentle voice
	Elicit Moro reflex last	Pacify with bottle of sugar water or feeding
		Enlist parent's aid for restraining to examine ears, mouth
		Avoid abrupt, jerky movements
Toddler		
Sitting or standing on/by parent	Inspect body area through play: "count fingers," "tickle toes"	Have parent remove outer clothing
Prone or supine in parent's lap	Use minimal physical contact initially	Remove underwear as body part examined
	Introduce equipment slowly	Allow to inspect equipment; demonstrating use of equipment is usually ineffective

Continued.

From Wong DL: *Whaley and Wong's nursing care of infants and children*, ed 5, St Louis, 1995, Mosby.

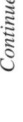

Age-Specific Approaches to Physical Examination During Childhood—cont'd

Position	Sequence	Preparation
Toddler—cont'd		
	Auscultate, percuss, palpate whenever quiet	If uncooperative, perform procedures quickly
	Perform traumatic procedures last (same as for infant)	Use restraint when appropriate; request parent's assistance
		Talk about examination if cooperative; use short phrases
		Praise for cooperative behavior
Preschool child		
Prefer standing or sitting	If cooperative, proceed in head-to-toe direction	Request self-undressing
Usually cooperative prone/supine	If uncooperative, proceed as with toddler	Allow to wear underpants if shy
Prefer parent's closeness		Offer equipment for inspection; briefly demonstrate use
		Make up "story" about procedure: "I'm seeing how strong your muscles are" (blood pressure)
		Use paper-doll technique
		Give choices when possible
		Expect cooperation; use positive statement: "Open your mouth"

School-age child

Prefer sitting	Proceed in head-to-toe direction	Request self-undressing
Cooperative in most positions	May examine genitalia last in older child	Allow to wear underpants
Younger child prefers parent's presence	Respect need for privacy	Give gown to wear
Older child may prefer privacy		Explain purpose of equipment and significance of procedure, such as otoscope to see eardrum, which is necessary for hearing
		Teach about body functioning and care

Adolescent

Same as for school-age child	Same as for older school-age child	Allow to undress in private
Offer option of parent's presence		Give gown
		Expose only area to be examined
		Respect need for privacy
		Explain findings during examination: "Your muscles are firm and strong"
		Matter-of-factly comment about sexual development: "Your breasts are developing as they should be"
		Emphasize normalcy of development
		Examine genitalia as any other body part; may leave to end

Adult Assessment

Adult Health History

The outline below suggests a systematic procedure for completing an adult health history. It is especially useful before a physical assessment to give the nurse background data for health care planning.

1. Biographical data
2. Reason for visit (chief complaint)
3. Present health status (general summary and symptom analysis; also known as history of present illness—HOPI)
4. Current health data
5. Past health status
6. Family history
7. Review of physiological systems
8. Psychosocial history

Biographical Data
- Name
- Age
- Race
- Culture
- Address and telephone number
- Marital status
- Children and family in home (if not family, significant others)
- Occupation
- Means of transportation to health care facility if pertinent
- Description of home and size and type of community

Reason for Visit
One statement that describes the reason for the client's visit or the chief complaint, stated in the client's own words.

Present Health Status
- Summary of client's current major health concerns
- If illness is present, record symptom analysis
  1. When client was last well
  2. Date of problem onset
  3. Character of complaint
  4. Nature of problem onset

From Bowers A, Thompson J: *Clinical manual of health assessment,* ed 4, St Louis, 1992, Mosby.

5. Course of problem
6. Client's hunch of precipating factors
7. Location of problem
8. Relation to other body symptoms, body positions, and activity
9. Patterns of problem
10. Efforts of client to treat
11. Coping ability

Current Health Data

- Current medications
    1. Type (prescription, over-the-counter drugs, vitamins, etc.)
    2. Prescribed by whom
    3. When first prescribed
    4. Amount per day
    5. Problems
- Allergies (description of agent and reactions)
    1. Drugs
    2. Foods
    3. Contact substances
    4. Environmental factors
- Last examinations (physician/clinic, findings, advice, instructions)
    1. Physical
    2. Dental
    3. Vision
    4. Hearing
    5. EKG
    6. Chest radiograph
    7. Pap smear (females)
    8. Tuberculosis tine test
- Immunization status (dates or year of last immunization)
    1. Tetanus, diphtheria, pertussis
    2. Mumps
    3. Rubella
    4. Polio
    5. Influenza

Past Health Status

Although each of the following is asked separately, the examiner must summarize and record the data *chronologically:*

- Childhood illnesses: rubeola, rubella, mumps, pertussis, scarlet fever, chickenpox, strep throat
- Serious or chronic illnesses: scarlet fever, diabetes, kidney problems, hypertension, sickle cell anemia, seizure disorders, blood infections

- Serious accidents or injuries: head injuries, fractures, burns, other trauma
- Hospitalizations: description of, including reason for, location, primary care providers, duration
- Operations: what, where, when, why, by whom
- Emotional health: past problems, help sought, support persons
- Obstetrical history
  1. Complete pregnancies: number, pregnancy course, postpartum course, and condition, weight, and sex of each child
  2. Incomplete pregnancies: duration, termination, circumstances (including abortions and stillbirths)
  3. Summary of complications

Family History

Family members include the client's blood relatives, spouse, and children. Specifically the interviewer should inquire about the client's maternal and paternal grandparents, parents, aunts, uncles, spouse, and children, as well as about the general health, stress factors, and illnesses of other family members. Questions should include a survey of the following:

Alzheimer's disease	Mental illnesses
Cancer	Developmental delay
Diabetes	Alcoholism
Heart disease	Endocrine diseases
Hypertension	Sickle cell anemia
Epilepsy (or seizure disorder)	Kidney disease
	Unusual limitations
Emotional stresses	Other chronic problems

The most concise method to record these data is by a family tree. Fig. 1 is an example.

Review of Physiological Systems

The purpose of this component of the data base is to collect information about the body regions or systems and their function.

- General—reflect from client's previous description of current health status
  1. Fatigue patterns
  2. Exercise and exercise tolerance
  3. History of weakness episodes, if any
  4. History of fever, sweats, if any
  5. Frequency of colds, infections, or illnesses
  6. Ability to carry out activities of daily living

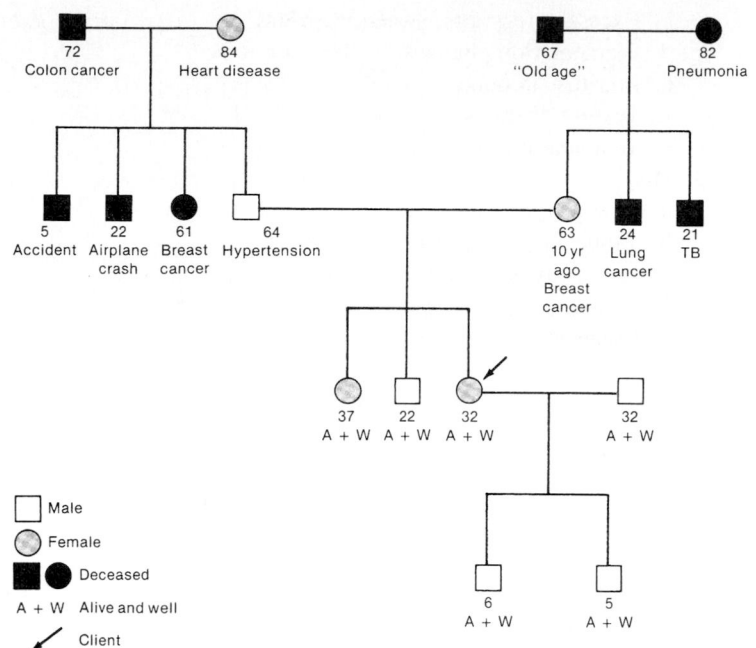

Fig. 1. Sample family tree (identifying grandparents, parents, aunts and uncles, siblings, spouse, and children).

- Nutritional
    1. Client's average, maximum, and minimum weights during past month; 1 year; 5 years
    2. History of weight gains or losses (time element); specific efforts to change weight
    3. Twenty-four-hour diet recall (helpful to mail the client a chart to fill in before visit)
    4. Cultural or religious practices regarding intake
    5. Current appetite
    6. Extreme deviations in physical activity that would affect appetite (e.g., athletic or immobilization influences)
    7. Person(s) who buys and prepares food
    8. Person(s) client normally eats with
    9. Availability of money to buy preferred food
    10. Status of ability to chew; condition of teeth or dentures
    11. Client's self-evaluation of nutritional status
- Integumentary
    1. Skin
        a. Skin disease, problems, lesions (wounds, sores, ulcers)
        b. Skin growths, tumors, masses

    c. Excessive dryness, sweating, odors
    d. Pigmentation changes or discolorations
    e. Pruritus (itching)
    f. Texture changes
    g. Temperature changes
  2. Hair
    a. Changes in amount, texture, character
    b. Alopecia (loss of hair)
    c. Use of dyes
  3. Nails
    a. Changes in appearance, texture

- Head
  1. Headache (characteristics, including frequency, type, location, duration, care for)
  2. Past significant trauma
  3. Dizziness
  4. Syncope
- Eyes
  1. Discharge (characteristics)
  2. History of infections, frequency, treatment
  3. Pruritus
  4. Lacrimation (excessive tearing)
  5. Pain in eyeball
  6. Spots (floaters)
  7. Swelling around eyes
  8. Cataracts, glaucoma
  9. Unusual sensations or twitching
  10. Vision changes (generalized or vision field)
  11. Use of corrective or prosthetic devices
  12. Diplopia (double vision)
  13. Blurring
  14. Photophobia
  15. Difficulty reading
  16. Interference with activities of daily living
- Ears
  1. Pain (characteristics)
  2. Cerumen (wax)
  3. Infection
  4. Hearing changes (describe)
  5. Use of prosthetic devices
  6. Increased sensitivity to environmental noise
  7. Vertigo
  8. Ringing and cracking
  9. Care habits
  10. Interference with activities of daily living

- Nose, nasopharynx, and paranasal sinuses
  1. Discharge (characteristics)
  2. Epistaxis
  3. Allergies
  4. Pain over sinuses
  5. Postnasal drip
  6. Sneezing
  7. General olfactory ability
- Mouth and throat
  1. Sore throats (characteristics)
  2. Tongue or mouth lesion (abscess, sore, ulcer)
  3. Bleeding gums
  4. Hoarseness
  5. Voice changes
  6. Use of prosthetic devices (dentures, bridges)
  7. Altered taste
  8. Chewing difficulty
  9. Swallowing difficulty
  10. Pattern of dental hygiene
- Neck
  1. Node enlargement
  2. Swellings, masses
  3. Tenderness
  4. Limitation of movement
  5. Stiffness
- Breasts
  1. Pain or tenderness
  2. Swelling
  3. Nipple discharge
  4. Changes in nipples
  5. Lumps, dimples
  6. Unusual characteristics
  7. Breast examination (pattern, frequency)
- Cardiovascular
  1. Cardiovascular
     a. Palpitations
     b. Heart murmur
     c. History of heart disease
     d. Hypertension
     e. Chest pain (character and frequency)
     f. Shortness of breath
     g. Orthopnea
     h. Paroxysmal nocturnal dyspnea

2. Peripheral vascular
   a. Coldness, numbness
   b. Discoloration
   c. Peripheral edema
   d. Varicose veins
   e. Intermittent claudication
- Respiratory
  1. History of asthma
  2. Other breathing problems (when, precipitating factors)
  3. Sputum production
  4. Hemoptysis
  5. Chronic cough (characteristics)
  6. Shortness of breath (precipitating factors)
  7. Night sweats
  8. Wheezing or noise with breathing
- Hematolymphatic
  1. Lymph node swelling
  2. Excessive bleeding or easy bruising
  3. Petechiae, ecchymoses
  4. Anemia
  5. Blood transfusions
  6. Excessive fatigue
  7. Radiation exposure
- Gastrointestinal
  1. Food idiosyncrasies
  2. Change in taste
  3. Aphagopraxia or dysphagia (inability to swallow or difficulty in swallowing)
  4. Indigestion or pain (associated with eating?)
  5. Pyrosis (burning sensation in esophagus and stomach with sour eructation)
  6. Ulcer history
  7. Nausea/vomiting (time, degree, precipitating or associated factors)
  8. Hematemesis
  9. Jaundice
  10. Ascites
  11. Bowel habits (diarrhea/constipation)
  12. Stool characteristics
  13. Change in bowel habits
  14. Hemorrhoids (pain, bleeding, amount)
  15. Dyschezia (constipation resulting from habitual neglect in responding to stimulus to defecate)
  16. Use of digestive or evacuation aids (what, how often)

- Urinary
  1. Characteristics of urine
  2. History of renal stones
  3. Hesitancy
  4. Urinary frequency (in 24-hour period)
  5. Change in stream of urination
  6. Nocturia (excessive urination at night)
  7. History of urinary tract infection, dysuria (painful urination), urgency, flank pain
  8. Suprapubic pain
  9. Dribbling or incontinence
  10. Stress incontinence
  11. Polyuria (excessive excretion of urine)
  12. Oliguria (decrease in urinary output)
  13. Pyuria
- Genital
  1. General
     a. Lesions
     b. Discharges
     c. Odors
     d. Pain, burning, pruritus
     e. Venereal disease history
     f. Satisfaction with sexual activity
     g. Birth control methods practiced
     h. Sterility
  2. Men
     a. Prostate problems
     b. Penis and scrotum self-examination practices
  3. Women
     a. Menstrual history (age of onset, last menstrual period [LMP], duration and amount of flow, problems)
     b. Amenorrhea (absence of menses)
     c. Menorrhagia (excessive menstruation)
     d. Dysmenorrhea (painful menses), treatment method
     e. Metrorrhagia (uterine bleeding at times other than during menses)
     f. Dyspareunia (pain with intercourse)
- Musculoskeletal
  1. Muscles
     a. Twitching
     b. Cramping
     c. Pain
     d. Weakness

2. Extremities
   a. Deformity
   b. Gait or coordination difficulties
   c. Interference with activities of daily living
   d. Walking (amount per day)
3. Bones and joints
   a. Joint swelling
   b. Joint pain
   c. Redness
   d. Stiffness (time-of-day related)
   e. Joint deformity
   f. Crepitus (noise with joint movement)
   g. Limitations of movement
   h. Interference with ADLs (activities of daily living)
4. Back
   a. History of back injury (characteristics of problems, corrective measures)
   b. Interference with ADLs
- Central nervous system
  1. History of central nervous system disease
  2. Fainting episodes
  3. Seizures
     a. Characteristics
     b. Medications
  4. Cognitive changes
     a. Inability to remember (recent versus distant)
     b. Disorientation
     c. Phobias
     d. Hallucinations
     e. Interference with ADLs
  5. Motor-gait
     a. Coordinated movement
     b. Ataxia, balance problems
     c. Paralysis (partial versus complete)
     d. Tic, tremor, spasm
     e. Interference with ADLs
  6. Sensory
     a. Paresthesia (patterns)
     b. Tingling sensations
     c. Other changes
- Endocrine
  1. Diagnosis of disease states (e.g., thyroid, diabetes)
  2. Changes in skin pigmentation or texture
  3. Changes in or abnormal hair distribution

4. Sudden or unexplained changes in height and weight
5. Intolerance of heat or cold
6. Exophthalmos
7. Goiter
8. Hormone therapy
9. Polydipsia (increased thirst)
10. Polyphagia (increased food intake)
11. Polyuria
12. Anorexia (decreased appetite)
13. Weakness

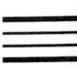

- Allergic and immunological (optional; use if client indicates allergy history; note precipitating factors in each case.)
    1. Dermatitis (inflammation or irritation of skin)
    2. Eczema
    3. Pruritus
    4. Urticaria (hives)
    5. Sneezing
    6. Vasomotor rhinitis (inflammation and swelling of mucous membrane of nose, nasal discharge)
    7. Conjunctivitis (inflammation of conjunctiva)
    8. Interference with ADLs
    9. Environmental and seasonal correlation
    10. Treatment techniques
- Any other physiological problems or disease states not specifically discussed. (If present, explore in detail [e.g., fatigue, insomnia, nervousness]).

Psychosocial History

- General statement of client's feelings about self
- Feelings of satisfaction or frustration in interpersonal relationships
    1. Home, occupants
    2. Client's position in home relationships
    3. Most significant relationship (in and out of home)
    4. Community activities
    5. Work or school relationships
    6. Family cohesiveness patterns
- Activities of daily living
    1. General description of work, leisure, and rest distribution
    2. Significant hobbies or methods of relaxation
    3. Family demands
    4. Community activities and involvement
    5. Ability to accomplish all that is desired during period of day/week

- General statement about client's ability to cope with ADLs
- Occupational history
  1. Jobs held in past
  2. Current employer
  3. Educational preparation
  4. Satisfaction with present and past employment
  5. Time spent at work versus time spent at play
- Recent changes or stresses in client's life-style (e.g., divorce, moving, new job, family illness, new baby, financial stresses)
- Patterns in which client copes with situations of stress
- Response to illness
  1. Client's ability to cope during own or others' illness
  2. Client's family and friends' response during periods of illness
- History of psychiatric care or counseling
- Feelings of anxiety or nervousness (characteristics and coping mechanisms)
- Feelings of depression (such symptoms as insomnia, crying, fearfulness, marked irritability, or anger)
- Changes in personality, behavior, or mood
- Use of medications or other techniques during times of anxiety, stress, or depression
- Habits
  1. Alcohol
     a. Kinds (beer, wine, mixed drinks)
     b. Frequency per week
     c. Pattern over past 5 years; 1 year
     d. Drinking companions
     e. Alcohol consumption variances (increase) when anxious or stressed
  2. Smoking
     a. Kind (pipe, cigarette, cigar)
     b. Amount per week; day
     c. Pattern over past 5 years; 1 year
     d. Enclosed with others who smoke
     e. Smoking amount variances (increase) when anxious or stressed
     f. Desire to quit smoking (methods, attempts)
  3. Coffee and tea
     a. Amount per day
     b. Pattern over past 5 years; 1 year
     c. Consumption variances (increase) when anxious or stressed
     d. Physiological effects

4. Other
   a. Overeating or sporadic eating (e.g., always in refrigerator, soft drink abuse, cookie jar syndrome)
   b. Nail biting
   c. "Street drug" usage
   d. Nervous noneating
- Financial status
1. Sources
2. Adequacy
3. Recent changes in resources and expenditures

Notes

Adult Nursing Assessment Data Base

Name _____   Age _____ Sex _____
Address _____   Race _____
City, state _____   Religion _____
Phone number _____   Occupation _____
Marital status _____   Place of employment _____
Private physician _____   Education _____

Health history

Check the problems that you presently have or have had that were diagnosed and treated by a physician.

Yes	No	Problem	Yes	No	Problem
___	___	Alcoholism	___	___	High blood pressure
___	___	Anemia			High blood fats
___	___	Bleeding trait	___	___	Cholesterol
___	___	Bronchitis	___	___	Triglycerides
		Cancer	___	___	Obesity (more than 20
___	___	Breast			pounds overweight)
___	___	Cervix	___	___	Pneumonia
___	___	Lung	___	___	Polyps in colon (over-
___	___	Uterus			growths in colon)
___	___	Other	___	___	Rheumatic fever
___	___	Cirrhosis	___	___	Stroke
___	___	Colitis	___	___	Suicide
___	___	Depression	___	___	Tuberculosis
___	___	Diabetes			
___	___	Emphysema			In the past year have you had:
___	___	Fibrocystic	**Yes**	**No**	
		breasts (lumps			
		in breast)	___	___	Chest pain on exertion
		Heart Problems			relieved by rest?
___	___	Heart attack	___	___	Shortness of breath
___	___	Coronary disease			lying down, relieved
___	___	Rheumatic heart			by sitting up?
___	___	Heart valve	___	___	Unexplained weight
		problem			loss of more than 10
___	___	Heart murmur			pounds?
___	___	Enlarged heart	___	___	Unexplained rectal
___	___	Heart rhythm			bleeding?
		problem	___	___	Unexplained vaginal
___	___	Other			bleeding?

From Koge NT, Bodnar BW: *The nursing process.* In Edelman CL, Mandle CL, editors: *Health promotion throughout the lifespan,* ed 3, St Louis, 1994, Mosby.

Family medical history
Check items that apply to your blood relatives (parents, grandparents, siblings, children):

Yes	No	Illness	Yes	No	Illness
___	___	Anemia	___	___	High blood pressure
___	___	Bleeding trait	___	___	Mental illness
___	___	Cancer	___	___	Stroke
___	___	Diabetes	___	___	Suicide
___	___	Heart disease	___	___	Tuberculosis

Check the items that apply:

Yes	No	Problem
___	___	Father died of heart attack before age 60
___	___	Mother died of heart attack before age 60
___	___	Mother or sister had breast cancer

Surgical history
List any operations and dates _____

_____

Females: describe obstetric history (if appropriate) _____

_____

_____

List childhood illnesses _____

_____

_____

Immunizations:	Yes	No		Yes	No
Tetanus	___	___	Rubella		
Pertussis	___	___	(German measles)	___	___
Diphtheria	___	___	Mumps	___	___
Polio	___	___	Flu	___	___
Measles	___	___			

List any allergies (food, drugs, other) _____

_____

List current medications (if appropriate) _____

_____

_____

Psychological history

Mark the frequency with which you have the feelings listed by placing a check mark in the appropriate column, (*M*—Most of the time; *S*—some of the time; *R*—rarely or none)

M	S	R	
___	___	___	Feel sad, depressed?
___	___	___	Wish to end it all?
___	___	___	Feel tense and anxious?
___	___	___	Worry about things generally?
___	___	___	More aggressive and hard driving than friends?
___	___	___	Have an intense desire to achieve?
___	___	___	Feel optimistic about the future?

Continued.

Adult Nursing Assessment Data Base—cont'd

Social history

Family members (parents, siblings, spouse, children, grandparents)
List family members, their ages, and health status or cause of
death _____
_____
_____

Educational history (schools attended, diplomas or degrees earned)
_____
_____
_____

Marital history (how many years; any past or present difficulties)
_____
_____

Work history (types and places of employment) _____
_____
_____

Leisure time activities _____
_____
_____

Financial status (plans for retirement, insurance, medical coverage)
_____
_____

Environmental background

Place of residence: apartment __ home __ Do you own? Yes __ No __
Travel time to work or school _____
Means of transportation _____
Environmental pollutants in area of residence _____
Place of residence in past and travel history _____
_____
_____

Describe present neighborhood (noisy or quiet; location to shopping, social, cultural, and religious centers) _____
_____
_____

Review of systems

Head and neck _____
Skin _____
Respiratory _____
Cardiovascular _____
Gastrointestinal _____
Genitourinary _____
Reproductive _____
Musculoskeletal _____
Central nervous _____

Endocrine _____

Circulatory _____

Physical examination

Height _____   Weight _____

Blood pressure ____ Pulse ____ Respirations ____ Temperature __

Functional health pattern assessment

The nurse should use these questions as a basis to explore the
health patterns listed.

1. Health perception and health management pattern.
   How has your general health been?
   Describe the most important things you do to stay healthy.
   Which statement is more like you?
      "If it's meant to be, I will stay healthy."
         or
      "If I take care of myself, I will stay healthy."
   Regularly use dental floss?
   Has had dental examination in past 2 years?
   Has had eyes checked in past 2 years?
   Seeks professional advice for unusual physical or mental
      changes?
   Has smoke detector in house?
   Has emergency phone numbers posted?
   (If responsible for children) Keeps medicines and cleaning
      products in locked cabinet?
   Women
      Have had Pap test within a year?   Conduct monthly breast
         self-examinations?
   Men
      Conduct monthly testicular examinations?

   Any concerns about current health practices?
   Behaviors you think you should change? Would like to change?
Strengths and areas for improvement _____
_____
_____

Weaknesses and problem areas _____
_____
_____

2. Nutritional and metabolic pattern
   Describe typical daily food and fluid intake.
   Any supplements? Appetite? Discomfort? Diet restrictions?
   Heals well or poorly?
   Skin problems?
   Dental problems?
   Drinks less than three alcoholic beverages (including beer) per
      week?
   Drinks less than five soft drinks per week?

Continued.

Adult Nursing Assessment Data Base—cont'd

Drinks less than three cups of coffee or tea per day?
Any foods avoided? Why?
Snacks between meals? What kind?
Limits intake of refined sugars (junk foods, desserts)?
Adds salt to food? Cooking? At the table?
Checks ingredients in prepackaged food?
Describe cooking facilities.
Limits intake of high-cholesterol foods?
Uses foods containing polyunsaturated fats?
Adds brans to diet to provide roughage?
Eats at least one uncooked fruit or vegetable a day?
Knows ideal weight? Current weight? Recent changes?
Considers self overweight? Underweight? Ideal weight?
Any concerns in this area?
Behaviors you think you should change? Would like to change?
Strengths and areas for improvement _____
_____
_____

Weaknesses and problem areas _____
_____
_____

3. Elimination pattern
    Describe bowel elimination pattern.
    Frequency? Character? Discomfort? Laxatives?
    Describe urinary elimination pattern.
    Frequency? Problems with control?
    Excess perspiration?
    Odor problem?
    Do you have to get up during the night to go to the bathroom?
    If so, how often?
    Any concerns?
    Behaviors you think you should change? Would like to change?
Strengths and areas for improvement _____
_____
_____

Weaknesses and problem areas _____
_____
_____

4. Activity and exercise pattern
    Describe daily pattern of activity.
    Has sufficient energy for desired and required activities?
    Exercise? Type? How often?
    Spare time activities?
    Climbs stairs rather than rides elevator?
    Participates in any strenuous exercise or sports?
    Engages in warm-up exercises?
    Participates in sports for competition or enjoyment?
    Any concerns?
    Behaviors you think you should change? Would like to change?

Strengths and areas of improvement _____

_____

_____

Weaknesses and problem areas _____

_____

_____

5. Sleep and rest pattern.
   Describe sleep pattern.
   Generally rested and ready for daily activities after sleeping?
   Any onset problem? Aids? Dreams? Nightmares? Early
     awakening?
   Takes time to relax each day? How?
   Enjoys spending time without planned activities?
   Any concerns?
   Behaviors you think you should change? Would like to change?
Strengths and areas for improvement _____

_____

_____

Weaknesses and problem areas _____

_____

_____

6. Cognitive and perception pattern
   Has hearing difficulties? Aids?
   Has difficulties with vision? Wears glasses or contact lenses?
     Any pain? Discomfort?
   Changes in memory? Describe.
   New interest areas?
   Easiest way to learn things?
   Any difficulty learning?
   Estimate of reading ability
   Likes to read?
   Any concerns?
   Behaviors you think you should change? Would like to change?
Strengths and areas for improvement _____

_____

_____

Weaknesses and problem areas _____

_____

_____

7. Self-perception and self-concept pattern
   How would you describe yourself?
   Most of the time, do you feel good or not so good about
     yourself?
   Perceives self as being well accepted by others?
   Any recent body changes? Changes in the things you do? Is
     this a problem for you?
   Any changes in the way you feel about your body? Yourself?

Continued.

Adult Nursing Assessment Data Base—cont'd

Has an enthusiastic and optimistic outlook?
Enjoys expressing self through arts, hobbies, or sports?
Continues to grow and change? Describe.
Enjoys work or school?
Member of community group? How active?
Proud of self?
Respects own accomplishments?
Finds it easy to express concern, love, and warmth to others?
Enjoys meeting and getting to know new people?
Can accept constructive criticism easily and not react
   defensively?
Looks forward to the future?
Any concerns?
Behaviors you think should change? Would like to change?
Strengths and areas for improvement _____
_____
_____
Weaknesses and problem areas _____
_____
_____

8. Role and relationship pattern
   Any family problems? Difficulty handling? Describe.
   Problems with children (if appropriate)? Difficulty handling?
      Describe.
   Finds it easy or difficult to communicate with others?
   If difficult, with whom? Actions taken to resolve?
   Belongs to social groups?
   Enjoys family? Friends?
   Has at least three close friends?
   Things generally go well for you at work or school?
   Enjoys touching other people? Being touched by others?
   Finds it easy or difficult to express love, warmth, and concern
      to those you care about?
   Any concerns?
   Behaviors that you think you should change? Would like to
      change?
Strengths and areas for improvement _____
_____
_____
Weaknesses and problem areas _____
_____
_____

9. Sexuality and reproductive pattern
   Any problems or changes in sexual relations? Describe.
   (If appropriate) Use of contraceptives? Any problems?
   Any concerns?
   Behaviors you think you should change? Would like to change?
   Number of sexual partners?
   Use of safe sex practice? Describe.

Number of pregnancies? Of living children?
Menstrual cycles? Describe (regular, experience discomfort,
   bloating).
Practice BSE? Regularly? When?
Strengths and areas for improvement _____

_____

_____

Weaknesses and problem areas _____

_____

_____

10. Coping and stress tolerance pattern
    Tense a lot of time? Causes? What helps?
    Who's most helpful when you're distressed? Available now?
    Any big change in your life recently?
    Practices any methods of relaxation? Meditation? Yoga?
    Considers it acceptable to cry, feel sad, angry, or afraid?
    Can laugh at self?
    Able to say no without feeling guilty?
    Any concerns?
    Behaviors you think you should change? Would like to change?
Strengths and areas for improvement _____

_____

_____

Weaknesses and problem areas _____

_____

_____

11. Value and belief pattern
    How important is "health" to you?
    Generally get things out of life that you want?
    Is religion important? Is it a help when difficulties arise?
    Are you satisfied with how you spend a typical work day?
       School day? Leisure day?
    Any concerns?
    Behaviors you think you should change? Would like to change?
Strengths and areas for improvement _____

_____

_____

Weaknesses and problem areas _____

_____

_____

Adult Physical Examination

There is no one right way to put together the parts of the physical examination so that the end product is an easily flowing process that minimizes the number of times the client has to change position and that conserves energy. The following is a suggested approach. In reality, this or any other approach may need to be adapted for a particular setting, client condition, or client disability.

General Inspection

Begin the inspection as you greet the client on entering the room, and look for signs of distress or disease. You can perform parts of your physical examination at any time as long as the client is within your view. There are no blank moments when you are with the client. On your first greeting, you can judge the alacrity with which you are met; the moistness of the palm when you shake hands; the gait as you walk back to the room; and the eyes, their luster, and their expression of emotion. All of this contributes to your examination, along with assessments of the following:

1. Skin color
2. Facial expression
3. Mobility
   a. Use of assistive devices
   b. Gait
   c. Sitting, rising from chair
   d. Taking off coat
4. Dress and posture
5. Speech pattern, disorders, foreign language
6. Difficulty hearing, assistive devices
7. Stature and build
8. Musculoskeletal deformities
9. Vision problems, assistive devices
10. Eye contact with examiner
11. Orientation, mental alertness
12. Nutritional state
13. Respiratory problems
14. Significant others accompanying client

Client Instructions

Instruct the client to empty bladder, remove clothing, and put on gown. Then begin the examination. A suggested sequence follows.

Modified from Seidel H et al: *Mosby's guide to physical examination,* ed 3, St Louis, 1995, Mosby.

Measurements

1. Measure height.
2. Measure weight.
3. Assess distance vision: Snellen chart.
4. Document vital signs: temperature, pulse, respiration, and blood pressure in both arms.

Client Seated, Wearing Gown

Client is seated on examining table; examiner stands in front of client.

Head and face

1. Inspect skin characteristics
2. Inspect symmetry and external characteristics of eyes and ears.
3. Inspect configuration of skull.
4. Inspect and palpate scalp and hair for texture, distribution, and quantity of hair.
5. Palpate facial bones.
6. Palpate temporomandibular joint while client opens and closes mouth.
7. Palpate sinus regions; if tender, transilluminate.
8. Inspect ability to clench teeth, squeeze eyes tightly shut, wrinkle forehead, smile, stick out tongue, puff out cheeks (CN V, VII).
9. Test light sensation of forehead, cheeks, chin (CN V).

Eyes

1. External examination
   a. Inspect eyelids, eyelashes, palpebral folds.
   b. Determine alignment of eyebrows.
   c. Inspect sclera, conjunctiva, iris.
   d. Palpate lacrimal apparatus.
2. Near vision screening: Rosenbaum chart (CN II)
3. Eye function
   a. Test pupillary response to light and accommodation.
   b. Perform cover-uncover test and light reflex.
   c. Test extraocular eye movements (CN III, IV, VI).
   d. Assess visual fields (CN II).
   e. Test corneal reflex (CN V).
4. Ophthalmoscopic examination
   a. Test red reflex.
   b. Inspect lens.
   c. Inspect disc, cup margins, vessels, retinal surface, vitreous humor.

Ears

1. Inspect alignment.
2. Inspect surface characteristics.
3. Palpate auricle.
4. Assess hearing with whisper test or ticking watch (CN VIII).
5. Perform otoscopic examination.
   a. Inspect canals.
   b. Inspect tympanic membranes for landmarks, deformities, inflammation.
6. Perform Rinne and Weber tests.

Nose

1. Note structure, position of septum.
2. Determine patency of each nostril.
3. Inspect mucosa, septum, and turbinates with nasal speculum.
4. Assess olfactory function: test sense of smell (CN I).

Mouth and pharynx

1. Inspect lips, buccal mucosa, gums, hard and soft palates, floor of mouth for color and surface characteristics.
2. Inspect oropharynx: note anteroposterior pillars, uvula, tonsils, posterior pharynx, mouth odor.
3. Inspect teeth for color, number, surface characteristics.
4. Inspect tongue for color, characteristics, symmetry, movement (CN XII).
5. Test gag reflex and "ah" reflex (CN IX, X).
6. Perform taste test (CN VII).

Neck

1. Inspect for symmetry and smoothness of neck and thyroid.
2. Inspect for jugular venous distention.
3. Inspect and palpate range of motion; test resistance against examiner's hand.
4. Test shoulder shrug (CN IX).
5. Palpate carotid pulses.
6. Palpate tracheal position.
7. Palpate thyroid.
8. Palpate lymph nodes: preauricular and postauricular, occipital, tonsillar, submaxillary, submental, superficial cervical chain, posterior cervical, deep cervical, supraclavicular.
9. Auscultate carotid arteries and thyroid.

Upper extremities

1. Observe and palpate hands, arms, and shoulders.
   a. Skin and nail characteristics
   b. Muscle mass
   c. Musculoskeletal deformities
   d. Joint range of motion: fingers, wrists, elbows, shoulders
2. Assess pulses: radial, brachial.
3. Palpate epitrochlear nodes.

Client Seated, Back Exposed

Client is still seated on examining table. Gown is pulled down to the waist for males so the entire chest and back are exposed; back is exposed, but breasts are covered for females. Examiner stands behind the client.

Back and posterior chest

1. Inspect skin and thoracic configuration.
2. Inspect symmetry of shoulders, musculoskeletal development.
3. Inspect and palpate scapula and spine.
4. Palpate and percuss costovertebral angle.

Lungs

1. Inspect respiration: excursion, depth, rhythm, pattern.
2. Palpate for expansion and tactile fremitus.
3. Palpate scapular and subscapular nodes.
4. Percuss posterior chest and lateral walls systematically for resonance.
5. Percuss for diaphragmatic excursion.
6. Auscultate systematically for breath sounds: note characteristics and adventitious sounds.

Client Seated, Chest Exposed

Examiner moves around to front of the client. The gown is lowered in females to expose anterior chest.

Anterior chest, lungs, and heart

1. Inspect skin, musculoskeletal development, symmetry.
2. Inspect respirations: client posture, respiratory effort.
3. Inspect for pulsations or heaving.
4. Palpate chest wall for stability, crepitation, tenderness.
5. Palpate precordium for thrills, heaves, pulsations.
6. Palpate left chest to locate apical impulse.
7. Palpate for tactile fremitus.

8. Palpate nodes: infraclavicular, axillary.
9. Percuss systematically for resonance.
10. Auscultate systematically for breath sounds.
11. Auscultate systematically for heart sounds: aortic area, pulmonic area, second pulmonic area, apical area.

Female breasts

1. Inspect in the following positions: client's arms extended over head, pushing hands on hips, hands pushed together in front of chest, client leaning forward.
2. Palpate breasts in all four quadrants, tail of Spence, over areolae; if breasts are large, perform bimanual palpation.
3. Palpate nipple; compress breasts to observe for discharge.

Male breasts

1. Inspect breasts and nipples for symmetry, enlargement, surface characteristics.
2. Palpate breast tissue.

Client Reclining 45 Degrees

Assist the client to a reclining position at a 45-degree angle. Examiner stands to the right side of the client.

1. Inspect chest in recumbent position.
2. Inspect jugular venous pulsations and measure jugular venous pressure.

Client Supine, Chest Exposed

Assist the client into a supine position. If the client cannot tolerate lying flat, maintain head elevation at 30-degree angle. Uncover the chest while keeping abdomen and lower extremities draped.

Female breasts

1. Inspect in recumbent position.
2. Palpate systematically with client's arm over head and arm at side.

Heart

1. Palpate chest wall for thrills, heaves, pulsations.
2. Auscultate systematically; you can turn client slightly to left side and repeat auscultation.

Client Supine, Abdomen Exposed

Client remains supine. Cover the chest with the client's gown. Arrange draping to expose the abdomen from pubis to epigastrium.

Abdomen

1. Inspect skin characteristics, contour, pulsations, movement.
2. Auscultate all quadrants for bowel sounds.
3. Auscultate aorta, renal arteries, femoral arteries for bruits, venous hums.

4. Percuss all quadrants for tone.
5. Percuss liver borders and estimate span.
6. Percuss left midaxillary line for splenic dullness.
7. Lightly palpate all quadrants.
8. Deeply palpate all quadrants.
9. Palpate right costal margin for liver border.
10. Palpate left costal margin for spleen.
11. Palpate for right and left kidneys.
12. Palpate midline for aortic pulsation.
13. Test abdominal reflexes.
14. Have client raise head as you inspect abdominal muscles.

Inguinal area

Palpate for lymph nodes, pulses, hernias.

External genitalia, males

1. Inspect penis, urethral meatus, scrotum, pubic hair.
2. Palpate scrotal contents.

Client Supine, Legs Exposed

Client remains supine. Arrange drapes to cover abdomen and pubis and to expose lower extremities.

Feet and legs

1. Inspect for skin characteristics, hair distribution, muscle mass, musculoskeletal configuration.
2. Palpate for temperature, texture, edema, pulses (dorsal pedis, posterior tibial, popliteal).
3. Test range of motion and strength of toes, feet, ankles, knees.

Hips

1. Palpate hips for stability.
2. Test range of motion and strength of hips.

Client Sitting, Lap Draped

Assist the client to a sitting position. Client should have gown on with drape across lap.

Musculoskeletal

1. Observe client moving from lying to sitting position.
2. Note coordination, use of muscles, ease of movement.

Neurological

1. Test sensory function: dull and sharp sensation of forehead, paranasal sinus area, lower arms, hands, lower legs, feet.
2. Test vibratory sensation of wrists, ankles.
3. Test two-point discrimination of palms, thighs, back.
4. Test stereognosis, graphesthesia.
5. Test fine motor function, coordination, and position sense of upper extremities.
   a. Touch nose with alternating index fingers.
   b. Rapidly alternate fingers to thumb.
   c. Rapidly move index finger between own nose and examiner's finger.
6. Test fine motor function, coordination, and position sense of lower extremities.
   a. Run heel down tibia of opposite leg.
   b. Alternately and rapidly cross leg over knee.
7. Test deep tendon reflexes and compare bilaterally: biceps, triceps, brachioradial, patellar, Achilles.
8. Test Babinski reflex bilaterally.

Client Standing

Assist client to a standing position. Examiner stands next to client.

Spine

1. Inspect and palpate spine as client bends over at waist.
2. Test range of motion: hyperextension, lateral bending, rotation of upper trunk.

Neurological

1. Observe gait.
2. Test proprioception and cerebellar function.
   a. Assess Romberg test.
   b. Ask the client to walk heel to toe.
   c. Ask the client to stand on one foot then the other with eyes closed.

d. Ask the client to hop in place on one foot then the other.
e. Ask the client to do deep knee bends.

Abdominal/genital

Test for inguinal and femoral hernias.

Female Client, Lithotomy Position

Assist female clients into lithotomy position and drape appropriately.
Examiner is seated.

External genitalia

1. Inspect pubic hair, labia, clitoris, urethral opening, vaginal opening, perineal and perianal area, anus.
2. Palpate labia and Bartholin's glands; milk Skene's glands.

Internal genitalia

1. Perform speculum examination.
   a. Inspect vagina and cervix.
   b. Collect Pap smear and other necessary specimens.
2. Perform bimanual palpation to assess for characteristics of vagina, cervix, uterus, adnexae.
3. Perform rectovaginal examination to assess rectovaginal septum, broad ligaments.
4. Perform rectal examination.
   a. Assess anal sphincter tone and surface characteristics.
   b. Obtain rectal culture if needed.
   c. Note characteristics of stool when gloved finger is removed.

Male Client, Bending Forward

Assist male clients in leaning over examining table or into knee-chest position. Examiner is behind client.

1. Inspect sacrococcygeal and perianal areas.
2. Perform rectal examination.
   a. Palpate sphincter tone and surface characteristics.
   b. Obtain rectal culture if needed.
   c. Palpate prostate gland and seminal vesicles.
   d. Note characteristics of stool when gloved finger is removed.

Elderly Assessment

Important Aspects of the History in the Elderly

Social History
Living arrangements
Relationships with family and friends
Economic status
Abilities to perform activities of daily living
Social activities and hobbies
Mode of transportation

Past Medical History
Previous surgical procedures
Major illnesses and hospitalizations
Immunization status
   Influenza, pneumococcal, tetanus
Tuberculosis history and testing
Medications (use the "brown bag" technique; see text)
   Previous allergies
   Knowledge of current medication regimen
   Compliance
Perceived beneficial or adverse drug effects

Systems Review
Ask questions about general symptoms that may indicate treatable underlying disease such as fatigue, anorexia, weight loss, and insomnia.
Attempt to elicit key symptoms in each organ system, including:

System	Key symptoms
Respiratory	Increasing dyspnea
	Persistent cough
Cardiovascular	Orthopnea
	Edema
	Angina
	Claudication

From Kane R, Ouslander J, Abrass I: *Essentials of clinical geriatrics,* ed 3, New York, 1994, McGraw-Hill.

System	Key symptoms
Cardiovascular—cont'd	Palpitations Dizziness Syncope
Gastrointestinal	Difficulty chewing Dysphagia Abdominal pain Change in bowel habit
Genitourinary	Frequency Urgency Nocturia Hesitancy, intermittent stream, straining 　to void Incontinence Hematuria Vaginal bleeding
Musculoskeletal	Focal or diffuse pain Focal or diffuse weakness
Neurological	Visual disturbances (transient or progressive) Progressive hearing loss Unsteadiness or falls Transient focal symptoms
Psychological	Depression Anxiety or agitation Paranoia Forgetfulness or confusion

Normal Physical Assessment Findings for Elderly Clients

Cardiovascular Changes

Cardiac output	Heart loses elasticity; therefore decreased heart contractility in response to increased demands
Arterial circulation	Decreased vessel compliance with increased peripheral resistance to blood flow resulting from general or localized arteriosclerosis
Venous circulation	Does not exhibit change with aging in the absence of disease
Blood pressure	Significant increase in the systolic, slight increase in the diastolic, increase in peripheral resistance and pulse pressure

From Ebersole P, Hess P: *Toward healthy aging,* ed 4, St Louis, 1994, Mosby. Data from Malasanos L et al: *Health assessment,* ed 3, St Louis, 1985, Mosby; Blake D: *Physiology and aging seminar for nurses,* Napa, Calif, May, 1979; and Wardell S, editor: *Acute interventions: nursing process throughout the life span,* Reston, Va, 1979, Reston.

Continued.

Normal Physical Assessment
Findings for Elderly Clients—cont'd

Cardiovascular Changes—cont'd

Heart	Dislocation of the apex because of kyphoscoliosis; therefore diagnostic significance of location is lost
	Increased premature beats, rarely clinically important
Murmurs	Diastolic murmurs in over half the aged; the most common heard at the base of the heart because of sclerotic changes on the aortic valves
Peripheral pulses	Easily palpated because of increased arterial wall narrowing and loss of connective tissue; feeling of tortuous and rigid vessels
	Possibility that pedal pulses may be weaker as a result of arteriosclerotic changes; colder lower extremities, especially at night; possibility of cold feet and hands with mottled color
Heart rate	No changes with age at normal rest

Respiratory Changes

Pulmonary blood flow and diffusion	Decreased blood flow to the pulmonary circulation; decreased diffusion
Anatomic structure	Increased anterior-posterior diameter
Respiratory accessory muscles	Degeneration and decreased strength; increased rigidity of chest wall
	Muscle atrophy of phayrnx and larynx
Internal pulmonic structure	Decreased pulmonary elasticity creates senile emphysema
	Shorter breaths taken with decreased maximum breathing capacity, vital capacity, residual volume, and functional capacity
	Airway resistance increases; less ventilation at the base of the lung and more at the apex

Integumentary Changes

Texture	Skin loses elasticity; wrinkles, folding, sagging, dryness
Color	Spotty pigmentation in areas exposed to sun; face paler, even in the absence of anemia
Temperature	Extremities cooler; decreased perspiration
Fat distribution	Less on extremities; more on trunk
Hair color	Dull gray, white, yellow, or yellow-green
Hair distribution	Thins on scalp, axilla, pubic area, upper and lower extremities; decreased facial hair in men, women may develop chin and upper lip hair
Nails	Decreased growth rate

Genitourinary and Reproductive Changes

Renal blood flow	Because of decreased cardiac output, reduced filtration rate and renal efficiency; possibility of subsequent loss of protein from kidneys
Micturition	In men possibility of increased frequency as a result of prostatic enlargement
	In women decreased perineal muscle tone; therefore urgency and stress incontinence
	Increased nocturia for both men and women
	Possibility that polyuria may be diabetes related
	Decreased volume of urine may relate to decrease in intake but evaluation needed
Incontinence	Increased occurrence with age, specifically in those with dementia
Male reproduction	
Testosterone production	Decreases; phases of intercourse slower, lengthened refractory time
Frequency of intercourse	No changes in libido and sexual satisfaction; decreased frequency to one or two times weekly
Testes	Decreased size; decreased sperm count; diminished viscosity of seminal fluid
Female reproduction	
Estrogen	Decreased production with menopause
Breasts	Diminished breast tissue
Uterus	Decreased size; mucous secretions cease; possibility that uterine prolapse may occur as a result of muscle weakness
Vagina	Epithelial lining atrophies; narrow and shortened canal
Vaginal secretions	Become more alkaline as glycogen content increases and acidity declines

Gastrointestinal Changes

Mastication	Impaired because of partial or total loss of teeth, malocclusive bite, and ill-fitting dentures
Swallowing and carbohydrate digestion	Swallowing more difficult as salivary secretions diminish
Esophagus	Decreased esophageal peristalsis
	Increased incidence of hiatus hernia with accompanying gaseous distention
Digestive enzymes	Decreased production of hydrochloric acid, pepsin, and pancreatic enzymes
Fat absorption	Delayed, affecting the absorption rate of fat-soluble vitamins A, D, E, and K
Intestinal peristalsis	Reduced gastrointestinal motility
	Constipation because of decreased motility and roughage

Continued.

Normal Physical Assessment
Findings for Elderly Clients—cont'd

Musculoskeletal Changes

Muscle strength and function	Decrease with loss of muscle mass; bony prominences normal in aged, since muscle mass decreased
Bone structure	Normal demineralization, more porous
	Shortening of the trunk as a result of intervertebral space narrowing
Joints	Become less mobile; tightening and fixation occur
	Activity may maintain function longer
	Normal posture changes; some kyphosis
	Range of motion limited
Anatomic size and height	Total decrease in size as loss of body protein and body water occurs in proportion to decrease in basal metabolic rate
	Increased body fat; diminished in arms and legs, increased in trunk
	Decreased height from 2.5 to 10 cm from young adulthood

Nervous System Changes

Response to stimuli	All voluntary or automatic reflexes slower
	Decreased ability to respond to multiple stimuli
Sleep patterns	Stage IV sleep reduced in comparison to younger adulthood; increased frequency of spontaneous awakening
	Stay in bed longer but get less sleep; insomnia a problem, which should be evaluated
Reflexes	Deep tendon reflexes responsive in the healthy aged
Ambulation	Kinesthetic sense less efficient; may demonstrate an extrapyramidal Parkinson-like gait
	Basal ganglions of the nervous system influenced by the vascular changes and decreased oxygen supply
Voice	Decreased range, duration, and intensity of voice; may become higher pitched and monotonous

Sensory Changes

Vision	
Peripheral vision	Decreases
Lens accommodation	Decreases, requires corrective lenses

Ciliary body	Atrophy around disc
Iris	Development of arcus senilis
Choroid	Atrophy around disc
Lens	May develop opacity, cataract formation; more light necessary to see
Color	Fades or disappears
Macula	Degenerates
Conjunctiva	Thins and looks yellow
Tearing	Decreases; increased irritation and infection
Pupil	May differ in size
Cornea	Presence of arcus senilis
Retina	Observable vascular changes
Stimuli threshold	Increased threshold for light touch and pain
	Ischemic paresthesias common in the extremities
Hearing	Less perceptible high-frequency tones; hence greatly impaired language understanding; promotes confusion and seems to create increased rigidity in thought processes
Gustatory	Decreased acuity as taste buds atrophy; may increase the amount of seasoning on food

Situational Assessment

The community health nurse encounters a variety of situational interruptions when caring for clients. Assessment of selected and common events will assist the nurse to develop an appropriate plan of care. The following tools are examples to help the nurse working with clients in the community.

Activities of Daily Living

The assessment of the client's ability to perform the activities of daily living provides the nurse with data to indicate the client's self-care ability. The following tools may be used to plan the assistance given to the client to regain a maximum level of independence, and to plan for support services. Basic activities of daily living and instrumental activities of daily living are both given.

Index of Independence in Basic Activities of Daily Living

The Index of Independence in Activities of Daily Living is based on an evaluation of the functional independence or dependence of clients in bathing, dressing, going to toilet, transferring, continence, and feeding. Specific definitions of functional independence and dependence appear below the index.

A — Independent in feeding, continence, transferring, going to toilet, dressing, and bathing.
B — Independent in all but one of these functions.
C — Independent in all but bathing and one additional function.
D — Independent in all but bathing, dressing, and one additional function.
E — Independent in all but bathing, dressing, going to toilet, and one additional function.
F — Independent in all but bathing, dressing, going to toilet, transferring, and one additional function.
G — Dependent in all six functions.
Other — Dependent in at least two functions but not classifiable as C, D, E, or F.

Independence means without supervision, direction, or active personal assistance, except as specifically noted on p. 143. This is based on actual status and not on ability. A client who refuses to perform a function is considered as not performing the function, even though the client is deemed able.

Bathing (sponge, shower, or tub)
Independent: assistance only in bathing a single part (as back or disabled extremity) or bathes self completely
Dependent: assistance in bathing more than one part of body; assistance in getting in or out of tub or does not bathe self

Dressing
Independent: gets clothes from closets and drawers; puts on clothes, outer garments, braces; manages fasteners; act of tying shoes is excluded
Dependent: does not dress self or remains partly undressed

Going to toilet
Independent: gets to toilet; gets on and off toilet; arranges clothes; cleans organs of excretion (may manage own bedpan used at night only and may or may not be using mechanical supports)
Dependent: uses bedpan or commode or receives assistance in getting to and using toilet

Transfer
Independent: moves in and out of bed independently and moves in and out of chair independently (may or may not be using mechanical supports)
Dependent: assistance in moving in or out of bed or chair; does not perform one or more transfers

Continence
Independent: urination and defecation entirely self-controlled
Dependent: partial or total incontinence in urination or defecation; partial or total control by enemas, catheters, or regulated use of urinals or bedpans

Feeding
Independent: gets food from plate or its equivalent into mouth (precutting of meat and preparation of food, as buttering bread, are excluded from evaluation)
Dependent: assistance in act of feeding (see above); does not eat at all or parenteral feeding

---

Evaluation form

Name _____ Date of evaluation _____

For each area of functioning listed below, check description that applies. (The word "assistance" means supervision, direction of personal assistance.)

Bathing—either sponge bath, tub bath, or shower

☐ Receives no assistance (gets in and out of tub by self if tub is usual means of bathing)

☐ Receives assistance in bathing only one part of the body (such as back or a leg)

☐ Receives assistance in bathing more than one part of the body (or not bathed)

From Katz S et al: Studies of illness in the aged, *JAMA* 185:914-919, September 21, 1963. Copyright 1963, American Medical Association. *Continued.*

Evaluation form—cont'd

Dressing—gets clothes from closets and drawers—including underclothes, outer garments, and using fasteners (including braces if worn)

☐	☐	☐
Gets clothes and gets completely dressed without assistance	Gets clothes and gets dressed without assistance except for assistance in tying shoes	Receives assistance in getting clothes or in getting dressed, or stays partly or completely undressed

Toileting—going to the "toilet room" for bowel and urine elimination; cleaning self after elimination, and arranging clothes

☐	☐	☐
Goes to "toilet room," cleans self, and arranges clothes without assistance (may use object for support such as cane, walker, or wheelchair and may manage night bedpan or commode, emptying same in morning)	Receives assistance in going to "toilet room," in cleansing self, or in arranging clothes after elimination or in use of night bedpan or commode	Doesn't go to room termed "toilet" for the elimination process

Transfer—

☐	☐	☐
Moves in and out of bed as well as in and out of chair without assistance (may be using object for support such as cane or walker)	Moves in or out of bed or chair with assistance	Doesn't get out of bed

Continence—

☐	☐	☐
Controls urination and bowel movement completely by self	Has occasional "accidents"	Supervision helps keep urine or bowel control; catheter is used, or is incontinent

Feeding—

☐	☐	☐
Feeds self without assistance	Feeds self except for getting assistance in cutting meat or buttering bread	Receives assistance in feeding or is fed partly or completely by using tubes or intravenous fluids

Activities of Daily Living Assessment

I. Introduction
  A. Definition: Activities of daily living (ADL) are those activities a person performs on his or her own behalf in maintaining life, health, and well-being.
  B. Nursing assessment of client needs and functional abilities.
    1. Determine ability to communicate verbally and nonverbally.
    2. Assess desire to engage in self-assessment and self-care.
    3. Medical history relevant to disability and preexisting health status.
    4. Social history.
    5. Home responsibilities.
    6. Home accessibility.
    7. Education.
    8. Vocational status.
    9. Avocational testing.
    10. Transportation issues.
    11. Endurance and level of fatigue.
II. Evaluation of activities of daily living
  A. Assess client's status using predetermined indicators and project discharge goals with evaluation of ADL.
    1. Use of assistive devices.
    2. Ability to secure own equipment.
    3. Toileting/cleansing.
    4. Bathing (washing and drying).
    5. Care of teeth (brushing; denture care, including oral placement/removal and storage).
    6. Hair care (shampooing, brushing, and combing).
    7. Skin care.
    8. Grooming (social/psychological additions to general appearance/self-image enhancement).
    9. Dressing/undressing, upper and lower extremities.
    10. Eating (preparing meals and feeding self).
    11. Personal care clean-up activities.
    12. Social/psychological activities.
    13. Kitchen tasks.
    14. Homemaking tasks.

From Mumma CM, editor: *Rehabilitation nursing concepts and practice: a core curriculum,* ed 2, Skokie, Ill, 1987, Rehabilitation Nursing Foundation.

        15. Child care.
        16. Community skills.
        17. Communication skills.
        18. Recreational activities.
        19. Sexual activity/function.
   B. Review findings of other team members.
III.   Designed program to increase self-care abilities
   A. Program should include the following:
      1. Evaluation of client's current functional status, actual and potential problems.
      2. Precautions to be exercised in view of medical status.
      3. Client and family interactions and determination of primary caregiver.
      4. Discharge plans and particular needs of client.
      5. Treatment plan established with physician, therapist, client, family, nurse, and other team members.
   B. Evaluate factors contributing to inability to perform activities of daily living.
      1. Situational or environmental factors (inaccessibility, sensory overload, etc.).
      2. Complexity of task and sequencing.
      3. Impaired ability to focus attention on task.
      4. Primary or secondary illnesses, disabilities, or deficits.
      5. Visual neglect.
      6. Impaired balance.
      7. Impaired endurance; low activity tolerance caused by fatigue.
      8. Sensation deficit.
      9. Coordination deficit.
    10. Perceptual deficit.
    11. Impaired judgment.
    12. Impaired memory.
    13. Communication deficit.
    14. Apraxia.
    15. Spasticity.
    16. Contracture.
    17. Pain.
    18. Paralysis.
    19. Paresis.
    20. Lack of one or more extremity(ies).
    21. Visual impairment.
    22. Auditory impairment.
    23. Mobility deficit.
    24. Learning impairments.

25. Psychological impairment.
    a. Loss, grief, or depression.
    b. Self-image deficit.
    c. Motivation (role in self-initiation of care tasks).
C. Specific elements to consider in activities of daily living training.
    1. Feeding.
       a. Utensil, cup, plate management, and napkin use.
       b. Tidiness/organization.
       c. Awareness of swallowing, chewing, or pocketing problems.
       d. Ability to handle different food consistencies, e.g., finger foods versus soups.
       e. Mouth care after eating.
    2. Bathing.
       a. Assembling of items and appropriate equipment.
       b. Management of caps, lids, sprays, etc.
       c. Facial cleansers and cosmetic application.
       d. Shaving foam or soap application versus electric razor.
       e. Shaving face, underarms, or legs.
       f. Hair care.
       g. Deodorant application.
       h. Tooth/denture care.
       i. Nail care.
       j. Replacement of care items.
       k. Location of bath facilities in hospital and home.
       l. Transfer ability to bathtub or shower.
    3. Dressing.
       a. Selection of clothing.
       b. Assembling of clothing.
       c. Application of underwear.
       d. Management of fasteners.
       e. Application of trousers/slacks, belt, or suspenders.
       f. Management of buckles and zippers.
       g. Application of pullover tops.
       h. Application of shirt, jacket, dress (front opening), or tie.
       i. Management of buttons.
       j. Application of socks or stockings.
       k. Application of shoes and tying laces.
       l. Location of dressing activities; bed, sitting, or standing.
       m. Ability to care for and apply glasses, contact lenses, or hearing aid.

4. Toileting and elimination management.
   a. Transfer ability.
   b. Clothing management.
   c. Cognitive function.
   d. Bowel and bladder control.
   e. External devices: assembly, application, removal, and care of equipment.
   f. Suppository insertion (include preparation of suppository and cleaning of insertion device if used).
   g. Post-toileting hygiene.
   h. Timing of bowel program (morning or evening).
   i. Employment/school/home/environmental considerations.
   j. Colostomy or ileal conduit care.
   k. Performance of bladder management programs.
   l. Accident management.

Instrumental Activities of Daily Living

Evaluation of autonomy of the older adult helps in making decisions with family and clients about client care. This scale can be an effective therapeutic tool in planning care and in identifying strengths and limitations of the older adult.

Instructions

The instrumental activities of daily living (IADL) has eight categories of activities that help the nurse determine the client's level of functioning beyond simple physical tasks of self-care. The highest possible score for both males and females is *eight*. For males, the possible score for each item in a category appears in the first column at the right of the category items. For females, the possible score for each item in a category appears in the second column at the right of the category items. The highest possible score for a category is one and the lowest possible score is zero.

Give a score for each category, choosing the category item that best reflects the client's level of functioning. For example, A: Ability to Use Telephone = 1. Item chosen: #2—Dials a few well-known numbers.

Modified from Lawton M, Brody E: Assessment of older people: self-maintaining and instrumental activities of daily living, *The Gerontologist* 9:179-186, 1969. Copyright © The Gerontological Society of America.

Sum the score.

a score of 7-8 = high level independence

5-6 = moderate level independence

3-4 = moderate level dependence

1-2 = dependence

Although a summed score will give an overall picture of the level of independence in IADL, each category should be considered separately to determine the rehabilitative needs of clients.

Category	Male score	Female score
A. Ability to use telephone		
1. Operates telephone on own initiative— looks up and dials numbers, etc.	1	1
2. Dials a few well-known numbers.	1	1
3. Answers telephone but does not dial.	1	1
4. Does not use telephone at all.	0	0
B. Shopping		
1. Takes care of all shopping needs independently.	1	1
2. Shops independently for small purchases.	0	0
3. Needs to be accompanied on any shopping trip.	0	0
4. Completely unable to shop.	0	0
C. Food preparation	(if applicable)	
1. Plans, prepares, and serves adequate meals independently.	1	1
2. Prepares adequate meals if supplied with ingredients.	0	0
3. Heats and serves prepared meals, or prepares meals but does not maintain adequate diet.	0	0
4. Needs to have meals prepared and served.	0	0
D. Housekeeping	(if applicable)	
1. Maintains house alone or with occasional assistance (e.g., "heavy work–domestic help").	1	1
2. Performs light daily tasks such as dish washing, bed making.	1	1
3. Performs light daily tasks but cannot maintain acceptable level of cleanliness.	1	1
4. Needs help with all home maintenance tasks.	1	1
5. Does not participate in any housekeeping tasks.	0	0
E. Laundry	(if applicable)	
1. Does personal laundry completely.	1	1
2. Launders small items—rinses socks, stockings, etc.	1	1
3. All laundry must be done by others.	0	0

Continued.

Category	Male score	Female score
F. Mode of transportation		
1. Travels independently on public transportation or drives own car.	1	1
2. Arranges own travel via taxi, but does not otherwise use public transportation.	1	1
3. Travels on public transportation when assisted or accompanied by another.	0	1
4. Travel limited to taxi or automobile with assistance of another.	0	0
5. Does not travel at all.	0	0
G. Responsibility for own medications		
1. Is responsible for taking medication in correct dosages at correct time.	1	1
2. Takes responsibility if medication is prepared in advance in separate dosages.	0	0
3. Is not capable of dispensing own medication.	0	0
H. Ability to handle finances.		
1. Manages financial matters, independently budgets, writes checks, pays rent, bills, goes to bank, collects and keeps track of income.	1	1
2. Manages own finances with assistance for banking.	1	1
3. Is not capable of managing finances.	0	0

Dementia Assessment

Dementia involves loss of intellectual functioning and memory over time, which results in dysfunction in daily living. It is important for the nurse to compute the results of an assessment of dementia to provide anticipatory guidance needed for education and support of clients and family.

A. History

1. Active medical conditions

_____

_____

_____

From Kane R, Ouslander J, Abrass I: *Essentials of clinical geriatrics,* New York, 1994, McGraw-Hill.

2. Medications

_____

_____

_____

3. History of (describe):
_____ Hypertension
_____ Stroke
_____ Transient ischemic attack
_____ Depression
_____ Other psychiatric disorder

4. Current symptoms (complaints of client or family)
_____ Memory loss
_____ Forgets recent events
_____ Forgets things just said
_____ Forgets names of people
_____ Forgets words
_____ Gets lost
_____ Asks questions or tells stories repeatedly
_____ Confused about date or place
_____ Can't do simple calculations
_____ Can't understand what is read or said
_____ Impairment of other cognitive functions
_____ Anxiety/agitation
_____ Paranoia
_____ Delusions/hallucinations
_____ Wandering
_____ Disruptive behavior
_____ Incontinence

5. Onset of symptoms
_____ Recent (days to few weeks)
_____ Longer duration (months)
_____ Uncertain

6. Progression of symptoms
_____ Rapid
_____ Gradual
_____ Stepwise (irregular, stuttering deteriorations)
_____ Uncertain

7. Activities of daily living (ADL)
Does the impairment of cognitive function interfere with instrumental ADL?
_____ Yes _____ No
If yes, which ones? _____
Basic ADL? _____ Yes _____ No
If yes, which ones? _____

B. Physical Examination

1. General appearance
_____ Normal
_____ Abnormal (Describe: _____)

2. Blood pressure
Right arm   _____ / _____
Left arm_____ / _____

3. Hearing

	Normal	Abnormal
Normal voice		
1024-Hz tuning fork		

4. Orientation

	No	Yes
Person		
Place		
Time		
Situation		

5. Memory function

	Normal	Impaired
Remote		
Recent (object recall after 5 minutes)		
Immediate (digit repetition)		

6. Short Portable Status Questionnaire
(Many other standardized tests are also available.)

Right	Wrong	
_____	_____	What is the date today (month/day/year)?
_____	_____	What day of the week is it?
_____	_____	What is the name of this place?
		What is your telephone number? (If no telephone,
_____	_____	what is your street address?)
_____	_____	How old are you?
_____	_____	When were you born (month/day/year)?
_____	_____	Who is the current president of the United States?
_____	_____	Who was the president just before him?
_____	_____	What was your mother's maiden name?
		Subtract 3 from 20 and keep subtracting 3 from each
_____	_____	new number you get, all the way down.

Number of errors _____
0-2 errors—intact
3-4 errors—mild intellectual impairment
5-7 errors—moderate intellectual impairment
8-10 errors—severe intellectual impairment

7. Other cognitive functions

	Normal	Impaired
Remote	_____	_____
General fund of knowledge	_____	_____
Simple calculations	_____	_____
Ability to write name	_____	_____
Ability to copy diagrams	_____	_____
Interpretations of proverbs	_____	_____
Naming common objects	_____	_____
Insight	_____	_____
Judgment	_____	_____
Ability to follow simple written commands (e.g., "Close your eyes")	_____	_____
Ability to follow simple verbal commands (e.g., "Touch your left ear with your right hand")	_____	_____

8. Thought content

_____ Normal

_____ Delusions

_____ Paranoid ideation

_____ Other (Describe: _____)

9. Mood/affect

_____ Appropriate _____ Depressed _____ Labile _____ Agitated

_____ Other (Describe: _____)

10. Behavior during examinations

	Yes	No
Good attention and concentration	_____	_____
Good effort to answer questions and perform tasks	_____	_____
Many "don't know" answers	_____	_____

11. Remainder of neurological examination

_____ Focal neurological signs (Describe: _____

_____)

_____ Signs of parkinsonism (Describe: _____

_____)

Pathological reflexes:

_____ Babinski

_____ Hoffman

_____ Grasp

_____ Palmomental

Gait:

_____ Normal

_____ Abnormal (Describe: _____)

_____ Other abnormality (Describe: _____)

Sensory examination:

_____ Normal

_____ Abnormal (Describe: _____)

12. Hachinski ischemia score

Characteristic	Point score
Abrupt onset	2
Stepwise deterioration	1
Somatic complaints	1
Emotional incontinence	1
History or presence of hypertension	1
History of strokes	2
Focal neurological symptoms	2
Focal neurological signs	2

Total score: _____

(Score of 4 or more suggests multi-infarct dementia.)

C. Diagnostic Studies

	Normal	Abnormal
Blood:		
CBC	_____	_____
Sedimentation rate	_____	_____
Glucose	_____	_____
BUN	_____	_____
Electrolytes	_____	_____
Calcium	_____	_____
Liver function tests	_____	_____
Free thyroxine index	_____	_____
TSH	_____	_____
VDRL	_____	_____
Vitamin B_{12}	_____	_____
Folate	_____	_____
Radiographic:		
Chest film	_____	_____
CT scan	_____	_____
Other:		
Urinalysis	_____	_____
EKG	_____	_____
EEG	_____	_____
Lumbar puncture	_____	_____
Audiology	_____	_____

D. Diagnosis

_____ Probable primary degenerative dementia (Alzheimer's type)
_____ Multi-infarct dementia
_____ Mixed
_____ Other (describe)
_____ Depression
_____ Other potentially reversible cause of dementia (describe)

Incontinence Assessment

The control of urine is said to be a requirement for social acceptability. There are a number of underlying causes of incontinence. Assessment of incontinence is essential for referral and establishment of appropriate physiological management.

I. Assessment of Acute Incontinence

If incontinence is of recent onset (within a few days) or associated with an acute illness, check for any of the following:

_____ Acute urinary tract infection

_____ Fecal impaction

_____ Acute confusion (delirium)*

_____ Immobility*

_____ Drug effects (e.g., excessive sedation, polyuria caused by diuretics, urinary retention, other autonomic effects)

_____ Metabolic abnormality with polyuria (e.g., hyperglycemia, hypercalcemia)

*Such that ability to get to a toilet (or toilet substitute) is impaired. If incontinence persists despite management of any of these conditions or resolution of an acute illness, further assessment (as shown in Part II) should be pursued.

II. Assessment of Persistent Incontinence

A. History

1. Do you ever leak urine when you don't want to?
   _____ No, never   _____ Yes
2. Do you ever have trouble getting to the toilet on time or have accidents getting your clothes or bed wet?
   _____ No, never   _____ Yes
3. How long have you had a problem with urinary leakage?
   _____ Less than 1 week
   _____ 1 to 4 weeks
   _____ 1 to 3 months
   _____ 4 to 12 months
   _____ 1 to 5 years
   _____ Longer than 5 years

From Kane R, Ouslander J, Abrass I: *Essentials of clinical geriatrics,* New York, 1994, McGraw-Hill.

4. How often do you leak urine?

_____ Less than once per week

_____ More than once per week, but less than once per day

_____ About once per day

_____ More than once per day

_____ Continual leakage

_____ Variable

5. When does the leakage occur?

_____ Mainly during the day

_____ Mainly at night

_____ Both night and day

6. When you leak urine, how much leaks?

_____ Just a few drops

_____ More than a few drops, but less than a cupful

_____ More than a cupful (enough to wet clothes or bed linens)

_____ Variable

_____ Unknown

7. Do any of the following cause you to leak urine?

_____ Coughing

_____ Laughing

_____ Exercise or other forms of straining

_____ Inability to get to the toilet in time

8. How often do you normally urinate?

_____ Every 6 to 8 hours or less often

_____ About every 3 to 5 hours

_____ About every 1 or 2 hours

_____ At least every hour or more often

_____ Frequency varies

_____ Unknown

9. Do you wake up at night to urinate?

_____ Never or rarely

_____ Yes, usually between one and three times

_____ Yes, four or more times per night

_____ Yes, but frequency varies

10. Once your bladder feels full, how long can you hold your urine?

_____ As long as you want (several minutes at least)

_____ Just a few minutes

_____ Less than a minute or two

_____ Not at all

_____ Cannot tell when bladder is full

11. Do you have any of the following when you urinate?

_____ Difficulty in getting the urine started

_____ Very slow stream or dribbling

_____ Straining to finish

_____ Discomfort or pain

_____ Burning

_____ Blood in the urine

12. Are you using any of the following to help with the urinary leakage?

_____ Bed or furniture pads

_____ Sanitary napkins

_____ Other types of pads in your underwear

_____ Special undergarments

_____ Medication

_____ Bedside commode

_____ Urinal

_____ Other (Describe: _____)

13. Is the urinary leakage enough of a problem that you would like further evaluation and treatment?

_____ Yes _____ No

14. Do you ever have uncontrolled loss of stool?

_____ No, never _____ Yes

15. Relevant medical history

_____ Stroke

_____ Dementia

_____ Parkinson's disease

_____ Prior CNS trauma/surgery

_____ Other neurological disorder

_____ Diabetes

_____ Congestive heart failure

_____ Other (Specify: _____)

16. Prior genitourinary history

_____ Multiple vaginal deliveries

_____ Cesarean section(s)

_____ Abdominal hysterectomy

_____ Vaginal hysterectomy

_____ Bladder suspension

_____ TURP (transurethral prostate resection)

_____ Suprapubic prostatectomy

_____ Urethral stricture/dilatation

_____ Bladder tumor

_____ Pelvic irradiation

_____ Recurrent urinary tract infections

17. Medications

Diuretic   _____

                              _____

Antihypertensive   _____

                              _____

Other drugs that   _____

affect the autonomic   _____

nervous system   _____

B. Physical examination

1. Mental status
   _____ Normal
   _____ Mild/moderate cognitive impairment
   _____ Severe cognitive impairment (unaware of toileting needs)
2. Mobility
   _____ Ambulates independently, with adequate speed
   _____ Ambulates independently, but slowly (so that ability to get to a toilet is impaired)
   _____ Not independently ambulatory, but able to use urinal, bedpan, or bedside commode independently
   _____ Chair- or bed-bound, but able to use urinal or bedpan independently
   _____ Dependent on others for toileting
3. Abdominal examination
   _____ Bladder enlarged and palpable
   _____ Bladder not palpable
4. Neurological examination of lower extremities
   _____ Normal
   _____ Evidence of upper motor neuron lesion
   _____ Evidence of lower motor neuron lesion
   _____ Peripheral neuropathy
5. Rectal examination
   _____ Decreased rectal sphincter tone
   _____ Decreased perianal sensation
   _____ Absent bulbocavernosus reflex
   _____ Prostate enlarged
   _____ Prostate cancer suspected
6. External genitalia
   _____ Skin irritation
   _____ Diminished sensation
   _____ Abnormal (Describe: _____)
7. Vaginal examination
   _____ Atrophic vaginitis
   _____ Mild prolapse
   _____ Moderate/severe prolapse
   _____ Rectocele
   _____ Adnexal or uterine mass

C. Diagnostic studies

1. Pad test with full bladder
   _____ No leakage
   _____ Leakage, small amount
   _____ Leakage, large amount
   _____ Delayed leakage
2. Voided volume
   _____ Unable _____ ml

3. Post void residual
_____ ml (or volume in bladder _____ ml)
4. Bladder filling (if done)
Capacity: _____ ml
_____ Stable
_____ Involuntary contraction (at _____ ml)
Amount lost: _____ ml
5. Stress maneuvers
Volume in bladder: _____ ml

Supine	Standing	
_____	_____	No leakage
_____	_____	Leak small amount
_____	_____	Leak large amount
_____	_____	Delayed leakage

6. Voided volume
_____ ml
7. Calculated residual
_____ ml
8. Urinalysis
_____ Normal
_____ Hematuria (>2 RBC per high-power field)
_____ Pyuria (>5 WBC per high-power field)
_____ Bacteriuria (>1+)
9. Urine culture
_____ Sterile
_____ Insignificant growth ($<10^5$ colonies/ml)
_____ Significant growth ($>10^5$ colonies/ml)
Organism(s) _____
Sensitive to _____

D. Disposition

_____ Treat reversible factors (describe)
_____ Treat for urge incontinence
_____ Treat for stress incontinence
_____ Treat for mixed incontinence
_____ Manage supportively
_____ Refer for further evaluation
Reason: _____
List specific treatment program
_____
_____

Hospice Northwest Bereavement Assessment

Bereaved	Relationship
Deceased	Date of death
Address	
Phone	
Date of visit/phone call	Length of visit/phone call

GENERAL HEALTH & ABILITY TO FUNCTION: COMMENTS:
Before death of deceased _____
After death of deceased   _____

	Changed	Unchanged
Appetite:	_____	_____
Sleep pattern:	_____	_____
Weight:	_____	_____
Alcohol intake:	_____	_____
Medication:	_____	_____
Living situation:	_____	_____
Finances:	_____	_____
Employment:	_____	_____

SUPPORT SYSTEMS:	Frequent	Infrequent
Family:	_____	_____
Church:	_____	_____
Social:	_____	_____
Accepting of grief:	Yes ____	No ____

PSYCHOLOGICAL/EMOTIONAL:
Verbal expressions of grief:

Crying:	_____	_____
Discussion of loss:	_____	_____
Depressed:	_____	_____
Feelings of guilt:	_____	_____
Feelings of anger:	_____	_____
Suicidal ideation:	Yes ____	No ____

Current affect status:

Appropriate:	_____
Flat:	_____
Labile:	_____

Courtesy Sylvia Harris, Hospice Northwest, Seattle.

EXPECTED COPING LEVEL:

Normal grief and
  recovery: _____

Doubtful, may need help: _____

Requires special help: _____

Professional intervention
  needed: _____

Is bereaved will-
ing to accept
follow-up from
Hospice?

Yes _____

No _____

Plan of Care

Regular:

1. Sympathy card within first week.
2. Grief information packet within 2 weeks.
3. Follow-up phone call/letter within 4 to 5 weeks.
4. Support letters at 6 and 12 months.

High Risk:

1. Includes all of Regular Plan of Care.
2. A list of agencies and community resources which provide individual counseling.
3. Limited individual grief-related counseling provided by the Bereavement Supervisor and/or qualified Bereavement Team Member.
4. More frequent telephone support/contact as agreed upon in consultation with the Bereavement Coordinator.

The survivor will be offered:

_____ Regular Plan of Care

_____ High Risk Plan of Care

Sympathy Card _____

Grief Packet _____

Follow-up phone call/letter _____

6-month letter _____

12-month letter _____

Volunteer _____

Signature: _____

Bereavement Coordinator

Spiritual Assessment

Part I
Meaning or philosophy of life stated by client or family member

Religious affiliation
   Importance   _____ strong   _____ moderate   _____ minimum
   Name and phone of clergy
   Spiritual practices described as important:
      _____ shared prayer
      _____ scriptures
      _____ attendance at worship
      _____ sacraments
      _____ other rituals

Part II
Which of the following themes come up in conversation?

_____ peacefulness, no fear of death	_____ agitation, apprehension
_____ belief in afterlife	_____ no belief in spiritual
_____ felt presence of God, spiritual reality	_____ uncertainty about God
_____ use of prayer, meditation	_____ anger at God, religion
_____ felt meaning in life	_____ lack of meaning, purpose
_____ strong faith	_____ struggling to find meaning
_____ reconciled with family	_____ feeling unloved, estranged
_____ able to forgive self	_____ guilty, self-blaming
_____ able to forgive others	_____ hateful, holding grudges
_____ belief in God's forgiveness	_____ fear of condemnation
	_____ spiritual distress of family

Part III
Spiritual or philosophical needs for which the client asks help

---

Modified from a Hospice of Seattle tool. From Zeruekh J: Home care of the dying. In Martinson I, Widmer J, editors: *Home health nursing care,* Philadelphia, 1989, Saunders.

Barthel Index

The Barthel Index is of value in obtaining baseline functional data and in monitoring improvement in mobility and self-care over time. It measures performance ability in personal care activities of daily living and mobility. The client's ability to perform independently or with help is appraised and scored according to performance in 10 categories of function. The authors of this instrument devised a weighted scoring system that ranges from 0 to 100. A total score of 100 indicates complete independence, independent performance in all 10 domains. To be considered "independent," the client must not require assistance at any time, either before, during, or after the performance of the task.

Modified from Hens MM: Functional evaluation. In Dittmar S, editor: *Rehabilitation nursing*, St Louis, 1989, Mosby.

	With help	Independent
1. Feeding (if food must be in cup, score as "with help")	5	10
2. Moving from wheelchair to bed and return (includes sitting up in bed)	5-10	15
3. Personal toilet (wash face, comb hair, shave, clean teeth)	0	5
4. Getting on and off toilet (handling clothes, wipe, flush)	5	10
5. Bathing self	0	5
6. Walking on level surface	10	15
If unable to walk, propelling wheelchair (score only if unable to walk)	0	5
7. Ascending and descending stairs	5	10
8. Dressing (includes tying shoes, fastening fasteners)	5	10
9. Controlling bowels	5	10
10. Controlling bladder	5	10

From Mahoney FI, Barthel DW: Functional evaluation: the Barthel index, *Md State Med J* 14:2, 1965.

Assessment Data for Persons Experiencing a Loss

Name _____

Date _____

Age _____

1. Nature of the lost object (or person)
2. Meaning the lost object (or person) had for the mourner
3. Mourner's typical coping patterns
4. Mourner's social and cultural milieu
5. Mourner's attitude toward death (if applicable)
6. Special resources (support systems) the mourner possesses for coping with the loss
7. Factors that influence the mourning process:

    Importance of the loss object (or person) as a source of support

    Degree of ambivalence toward the lost object (or person)

    Age of the deceased (if applicable)

    Quantity and quality of other relationships

    Degree of preparation for the loss, which was

        Sudden _____

        Gradual _____

    Mourner's physical health

    Mourner's psychological health

_____

From Detherage KS, Johnson SS: Stress reduction and crisis intervention. In Edelman CL, Mandle CL, editors: *Health promotion throughout the lifespan,* ed 3, St Louis, 1994, Mosby.

◊ Childbearing Assessment
Pregnancy

Postnatal care following pregnancy is a mainstay in the practice of community health nursing. The nurse assists the woman during this critical time by teaching, observing, and supporting her and her family through this usually normal process. A significant contribution of the nurse is early identification of risk. The following tools will help achieve this goal.

Notes

Differential Assessment of Signs and Symptoms of Pregnancy

Symptoms	Possible causes of diagnostic error
Abdominal enlargement	Obesity, abdominal muscle relaxation, tumors, ascites, ventral abdominal hernia
Amenorrhea	Emotional factors: severe emotional shock, tension, fear of or strong desire for pregnancy
	Endocrine factors: adrenal or ovarian neoplasms, thyroid or pituitary disorders, lactation, menopause
	Metabolic factors: anemia, malnutrition, diabetes mellitus, degenerative disorders
	Systemic disease: acute or chronic infection (tuberculosis, brucellosis) or malignancy
	Local causes (cervical obstruction: jogging)
Braxton Hicks' contractions	Contractions of muscles of abdominal wall
Breast sensitivity (mastalgia; mastodynia)	Infectious processes: mastitis, cystic mastitis, premenstrual tension
	Pseudocyesis (false pregnancy)
	Estrogen excess associated with anovulatory periods or ovarian tumors
Cervical and uterine changes in shape, size, consistency	Tumors, adenomyosis, cervical stenosis with hematometra or pyometra, tubo-ovarian cysts
	Normal-size uterus displaced by a pelvic tumor (fibroid or myoma)
Clinical and laboratory findings	Poor thermometer, faulty use of thermometer, inaccurate recording
Elevation of BBT	Corpus luteum cyst
Pregnancy tests	Drug ingestion: progesterone
	False results, incorrect interpretation of results
	Elevation of hCG levels for a few days after spontaneous abortion
	Elevation of hCG: hydatidiform mole, choriocarcinoma
Lassitude and fatigue	Psychological: emotional disorders
	Pathological: anemia, infection, malignant disease
Epulis	Infection, dental calculus, vitamin C deficiency

Hyperpigmentation of skin	Local causes (excessive sunlight, tanning)
	System diseases (Addison's disease)
	Use of oral contraceptives
Leukorrhea	Infections: vaginal, cervical
	Tumors
Nausea or vomiting	Emotional factors: anxiety, pseudocyesis, anorexia nervosa
	Gastrointestinal disorders: hiatal hernia, ulcers, enteritis, appendicitis
	Systemic disease: acute infection—influenza, encephalitis
	Allergies
Nipple discharge (milklike)	Drug ingestion: oral contraceptives, psychotropic drugs
	Tumors
	Syndromes (also associated with amenorrhea): hypothalamic or anterior pituitary disorders
Pseudocyesis	Emotional factors
	Pituitary tumor
Quickening	Peristalsis: "gas"
Souffle	Heard over vascular tumors or aneurysms or in thin women; may be abdominal aortic pulsation

From Bobak IM, Jensen MD, Zalar MK: *Maternity and gynecologic care: the nurse and the family*, ed 4, St Louis, 1989, Mosby.

Assessment of the Family at Risk: Premature Birth

The following questions ask about your experiences after the premature birth of your baby. Please choose the answer that most closely describes your experience and mark an "X" in the box next to the answer.

1. Immediately after the premature birth of your baby, what was the closest contact you had with him or her?

☐ None	☐ Saw my baby	☐ Touched my baby	☐ Held my baby	☐ Took care of my baby

2. After the day of birth, how old was your baby when you next saw him or her?

☐ 1 day	☐ 2 days	☐ 3 days	☐ 4-6 days	☐ 1 week	☐ 2 weeks	☐ 3 or more weeks

3. After the day of birth, how old was your baby when you next touched him or her?

☐ 1 day	☐ 2 days	☐ 3 days	☐ 4-6 days	☐ 1 week	☐ 2 weeks	☐ 3 or more weeks

4. After the day of birth, how old was your baby when you next held him or her?

☐ 1 day	☐ 2-4 days	☐ 5-6 days	☐ 1 week	☐ 2 weeks	☐ 3 weeks	☐ 4 or more weeks

5. How old was your baby when you first got to care for him or her by feeding, diapering, or bathing him or her?

☐ 1 day	☐ 3-6 days	☐ 1 week	☐ 2 weeks	☐ 3 weeks	☐ 4 weeks	☐ 5 or more weeks

6. On the average, how many times a week did you visit your baby while he or she was in the hospital?

☐ Less than once ☐ 1-2 times a week ☐ 3-4 times a week ☐ 5-6 times a week ☐ 7-8 times a week ☐ 9-10 times a week ☐ 11 or more times a week

7. How old was your baby when he or she first came home?

☐ Less than 1 week ☐ 1 week ☐ 2 weeks ☐ 3 weeks ☐ 4 weeks ☐ 5 weeks ☐ 6 or more weeks

8. How old was your baby when you first felt you were really comfortable holding and caring for him or her?

☐ Less than 1 week ☐ 1 week ☐ 2 weeks ☐ 3 weeks ☐ 4 weeks ☐ 5 weeks ☐ 6 or more weeks

9. How old was your baby when you first recognized some traits or behaviors he or she demonstrated that were unique to him or her and not like other babies or traits in your family?

☐ Less than 1 week ☐ 1 week ☐ 2 weeks ☐ 3 weeks ☐ 4 weeks ☐ 5 weeks ☐ 6 or more weeks

10. What was the birth weight of your infant who was born prematurely?

☐ Under 1 lb ☐ 1 lb to 1 lb 15 oz ☐ 2 lb to 2 lb 15 oz ☐ 3 lb to 3 lb 15 oz ☐ 4 lb to 4 lb 15 oz ☐ 5 lb to 5 lb 8 oz ☐ Over 5 lb 8 oz

Continued.

Assessment of the Family at Risk: Premature Birth—cont'd

11. How many weeks early was your baby born?

☐ No weeks early	☐ 1 or 2 weeks	☐ 3 or 4 weeks	☐ 5 or 6 weeks	☐ 7 or 8 weeks	☐ 9 or 10 weeks	☐ More than 10 weeks

12. When you were with your baby in the first 6 weeks after birth, how much did he or she relax or show comfort when you touched or held him or her?

☐ He tensed	☐ No relaxation	☐ Little relaxation	☐ Some relaxation	☐ Moderate relaxation	☐ Full relaxation

13. At the time of the baby's birth, what was your age?

☐ 18 years or less	☐ 18-21 years	☐ 22-25 years	☐ 26-29 years	☐ 30-33 years	☐ 34-37 years	☐ 38 or more years

14. At the time of your baby's birth, what was your marital status?

☐ Single	☐ Married	☐ Divorced	☐ Widowed

15. What is your family's yearly income?

☐ 0 to 6,000 a year	☐ 6,000 to 9,999	☐ 10,000 to 14,999	☐ 15,000 to 19,999	☐ 20,000 to 24,999	☐ 25,000 and above

16. What is your cultural or ethnical background?

☐ White	☐ Black	☐ Hispanic	☐ Asian	☐ Native American	☐ Other

17. At the time of your premature infant's birth, how many other children did you have?

☐ None ☐ 1 ☐ 2 ☐ 3 ☐ 4 ☐ 5 or more

18. Before your infant was born prematurely, had you had any other premature births?

☐ Yes ☐ No

19. Before your infant was born prematurely, had you lost a baby from a previous pregnancy?

☐ Yes ☐ No

20. How many miles was it from your home to the medical center where your baby received special care?

☐ 0-5 miles ☐ 6-10 miles ☐ 11-20 miles ☐ 21-30 miles ☐ 31-50 miles ☐ 51-100 miles ☐ 101 or more miles

21. Was your baby transported to the hospital where he or she received the special care?

☐ Yes ☐ No

Prenatal Assessment Guide

Aspects of Adaptation

Age
Initial response to pregnancy
Planned or unplanned pregnancy
Feelings about pregnancy
Desired family size
Perception of pregnancy affecting present activities and responsibilities
Perception of parenthood affecting future activities and plans
Current developmental task of pregnancy: coping mechanisms, fantasies about pregnancy, changes in mood and effect on others
Sexual functioning during pregnancy: changes, feelings, problems
Nature of verbal interest expressed about self and fetus
Preparations for prenatal classes (type, when completed), place of delivery, other children in mother's absence, and new sibling
Menstrual history: problems, last normal menstrual period, expected date of confinement
Height and prepregnancy weight
Past obstetric history: dates, course, outcomes
Present obstetric status: course, abdominal assessment, quickening, fetal heart sound, blood pressure, urinalysis, weight and pattern of gain, signs of any major complications of pregnancy
Past medical history: illness, date, treatment, outcome, surgery, childhood diseases, current immunization status, allergies, venereal disease, emotional problems
Family medical history: illnesses, emotional problems, genetic defects (both sides of family)
Loss of significant other in past year
Food intolerances (lactose, nausea and vomiting), food cravings, and pica
Iron-vitamin-mineral dietary supplements used
Elimination patterns: changes, problems with remedies used
Pattern of rest, sleep: difficulties, remedies used

Modified from Becker C: *Obstet Gynecol Neonat Nurs,* Nov/Dec 1982. In Hancock LA et al: The prenatal period. In Edelman CL, Mandle CL, editors: *Health promotion throughout the life span,* ed 3, St Louis, 1994, Mosby.

Aspects of Personal Belief System and Life-style

Date first sought prenatal care this pregnancy and in prior pregnancies

Reasons for seeking and receiving prenatal care

Beliefs about pregnancy and childbirth; cultural beliefs about child-bearing (antepartum, intrapartum, postpartum)

Racial, ethnic group

Beliefs about role of father during pregnancy and labor and in child care

Perception of needs of fetus

Perception of needs of infant and proposed methods to meet these needs

Contraceptive history: methods used, failures or problems, knowledge of alternate methods, willingness to use

Patterns of use of tobacco, alcohol, prescription and nonprescription drugs, illegal drugs; perception of effects on health of self and fetus

Patterns of nutrient intake: food dislikes, history and method of dieting

Planned method of infant feeding; why chosen

Occupation: present, former, how long, work requirements, hazards, amenities, plans regarding current occupation

Recreational activities: plans to continue, use of seat belt in car, pets in home

Community activities

Perception of and prior experiences with health care personnel and agencies

Date of last physical examination, including breast examination, Pap smear, chest x-ray films, dental checkup

Breast self-examination done regularly; if not, interested in learning about?

Aspects of Support

Address: how long there, housing accommodations, phone, plans to move (when, where, why?)

Level of education and future plans regarding

Religious preference; normal or active involvement

Marital status: years married

Father of baby: age, occupation, educational level, racial and ethnic group, religious preference

Family composition: household members

Communication patterns with significant others

Communication patterns with health personnel

Perception of support system (mate, family, friends, community agencies): available and willingness to use

Perception of meaning of this pregnancy to significant others; mate's response to news of pregnancy

Type of prenatal service receiving and perception of its adequacy

Available transportation

Social service and community agencies involved with: how long and contact person

Self-concept and perceived ability to cope with life situations

Body-image concept: prepregnant and current; response to physiological changes of pregnancy

Mate's response to body changes in pregnancy

Feelings about parenting woman received as a child; history of separation from mother

Prior experiences with infants; knowledge of infant care

Feelings about previous pregnancies, labor, puerperium, and mothering skills

Knowledge of reproduction, labor and delivery, and puerperium

Notes

Assessment During Pregnancy and Evaluative Criteria

	First and second trimesters (wk 1 through 26)	Third trimester (wk 27 through 38-40 [term])
Schedule of care	After initial contact and preliminary assessments, return visit scheduled for 2 wk, thereafter every 4 wk	Medical and nursing care has been increased to permit detection of any abnormal response, maternal or fetal: woman is examined every 2 wk between 32 and 36 wk and every wk between 36 and 40 wk; if indicated, plan of care is modified
Maternal adaptations		
Physical		
Temperature	Normal range established	Normal range
Pulse	Normal range established	Gradual rise of +8 to +10 by wk 35
Respirations	18-20/min	18-20/min; occasional shortness of breath and sighing breaths may be troublesome at times
Blood pressure	Normal range of less than +30 systolic and +15 diastolic over baseline; may decrease slightly in midpregnancy	Systolic no greater than +30 and diastolic no greater than +15 over baseline, which is normally higher (+6 to +10) as term approaches
Urinalysis	Negative for protein and acetone; no greater than 1+ for glucose; negative for bacteria	Negative for protein and acetone, no greater than 1+ for glucose; lactose is present as hormone prolactin increases

Continued.

From Jenson M, Bobak I: *Maternity and gynecologic nursing,* St Louis, 1985, Mosby.

Assessment During Pregnancy and Evaluative Criteria—cont'd

	First and second trimesters (wk 1 through 26)	Third trimester (wk 27 through 38-40 [term])
Maternal adaptations—cont'd		
Blood tests		
RBC	At sea level for wk 1-13: Hg, 11 g/dl; hematocrit, 37% Wk 12-26: Hg, 10.5 g/dl; hematocrit 35%	At sea level for wk 27 to term: Hg, 10 g/dl; hematocrit, 33% RBC repeated at 32-34 wk
STS* (VDRL)	Negative	Negative
Weight gain	Wk 1-13: about 3-4 lb (1.4-1.8 kg) Wk 12-26: 12-14 lb (5.6-6.3 kg) Approximately 0.5 lb (0.23 kg)/wk	Wk 27 to term: no more than 1 lb (0.45 kg)/wk Approximately 27 ± 4 lb (11 kg) gain over prepregnancy weight (less than 20 lb puts fetus at risk)
Edema	Dependent edema not yet apparent	Dependent edema of lower legs, ankles, and feet
Vagina	Bluish-red hyperemia characteristic of pregnancy, little increase in size No anomalies, including cystocele, rectocele, or relaxed perineum	Highly distensible
Cervix	Long, firm but softening by midpregnancy	Readiness for labor Cervix becomes more softened as term approaches In parous women, external os of cervix may be about 3 cm dilated by wk 35 Discharge persists
	Moderate white mucoid discharge	
Breasts	Early weeks, breasts tender with tingling sensations By wk 8, breasts increase in size, become nodular; veins become visible beneath skin	Striations may appear if increase in size of breasts extensive

	Nipples become larger, more pigmented, and more erectile No secretions from breasts	Areola becomes larger and more deeply pigmented and glands of Montgomery appear Lactogenesis begins with secretion of colostrum; may be expressed by gentle massage Preparation of breasts for breast-feeding begins
Abdomen	Topic of infant feeding introduced Gradual enlargement: see height of fundus	Enlargement continues: see height of fundus Toward end of pregnancy striae gravidarum may occur, in multipara glistening silvery lines of striae from earlier pregnancies may be seen Linea nigra at midline of abdomen
Uterus	Progressive enlargement to accommodate growing products of conception Fundal height at 12-13 wk: felt just above pubic symphysis; 16 wk: 3-4 cm above pubic symphysis; 20 wk: 2-3 cm below umbilicus; 24 wk: at umbilicus	Continued progressive enlargement of uterus Fundal height at 36 wk: almost to xiphoid process; 40 wk: 2 cm below due to "lightening" Readiness for labor: Braxton Hicks' contractions may be felt
Pelvis	Pelvic measurements within normal range (examined at second visit, not repeated); diagonal conjugate 11.5 cm or more Transverse diameter of outlet 8 cm or more Ischial spines not prominent, concavity of sacrum ample, side walls of pelvis do not converge	Pelvic measurements adequate in relation to size of fetus (examined near term)

*Serologic test for syphilis.

Continued.

Assessment During Pregnancy and Evaluative Criteria—cont'd

	First and second trimesters (wk 1 through 26)	Third trimester (wk 27 through 38-40 [term])
Maternal adaptations—cont'd		
Skin	Changes not noticeable	May develop chloasma (mask of pregnancy), vascular spiders, palmar erythema (red palms) Varicose veins may appear in lower legs and vulva
Common problems	Woman or couple verbalizes understanding of physiologic basis and treatment of Nausea and vomiting up to wk 12 Increased skin pigmentation (e.g., linea nigra) Heartburn Constipation Leg cramps Pica	Woman or couple verbalizes understanding of physiologic basis and treatment of Hemorrhoids Varicosities Leg cramps Hypermobility of joints Backache
Abnormal symptoms	Woman or couple verbalizes understanding of physiologic basis, need for immediate treatment, and how to obtain necessary care for Vaginal bleeding Burning or pain on urination Gastroenteritis Exposure to communicable disease (e.g., rubella) Nausea and vomiting beyond wk 12 Abdominal pain	Woman or couple verbalizes understanding of physiologic basis; need for immediate treatment and how to obtain necessary care for Vaginal bleeding; at term rule out brownish spotting occurring 8 hr after vaginal examination or "show" of pinkish mucus Symptoms of preeclampsia-eclampsia: weight gain over 1 lb/wk, generalized edema, persistent headache, dimness or blurring of vision Cessation, noticeable diminution, or acceleration in amount of fetal movement Rupture of membranes

		Burning or pain on urination
		Chills or elevated temperature
		Abdominal pain
		Persistent nausea and vomiting
Psychosocial adaptations	Reactions indicative of positive psychologic response to pregnancy, including birth process and parenthood	Responses typical of normal responses to pregnancy
	During first trimester, woman may be self-centered and concerned with her own adjustment to idea of pregnancy	Interest centered around preparing for parenthood
	During second trimester, woman usually is reasonably free of symptoms; she is more tranquil and at ease; reality of child is now recognized, and most women come to accept their pregnant state; however, feelings of ambivalence come and go	Anxiety may be expressed over pain of labor, behavior during labor, care of other children
	During first and second trimesters family members (spouse, others) adjust in a positive manner to the pregnancy although they may express feelings of being "left out" by mother	Ambivalent feelings persist
	Verbalizes understanding of sexual responses and relates that sexual relationships are mutually accepted and serve as a means of communication	Verbalizes understanding of various modes of sexual expression (which are safe, which to avoid) and of medical acceptance of sexual intercourse with penile penetration until rupture of membrane; feelings of frustration and resentment over abstinence expressed early in third trimester and acceptance expressed toward end of third trimester

Continued.

Assessment During Pregnancy and Evaluative Criteria—cont'd

	First and second trimesters (wk 1 through 26)	Third trimester (wk 27 through 38-40 [term])
Maternal adaptations—cont'd		
	Negative feelings about self-image are recognized as temporary; expresses pride or pleasure about being pregnant	Expresses eagerness to be done with pregnancy; complaints about awkwardness, annoyance about symptoms (shortness of breath and backache) expressed; questions asked about how soon appearance will be back to "normal"
Active participation in care	Verbalizes understanding of plan of care; schedule, need for continuity of care, physical examination to be done, reporting of abnormal symptoms	Verbalizes understanding of preparation for delivery; symptoms of impending labor (i.e., uterine contractions, rupture of membranes, bloody "show"), what to report, and where to go for delivery
		Verbalizes understanding of delivery process; methods to control pain (e.g., analgesia, anesthesia, and breathing-relaxing techniques); responsibilities of spouse, family member, or friend who will be accompanying woman through labor and delivery; and care of newborn (i.e., clothing, feeding, daily hygienic care)
	Complies with care	Complies with care
	Keeps appointments, reports abnormal symptoms promptly, follows diet plan, takes only prescribed medications, refrains from smoking and drinking alcoholic beverages, exercises	Includes behaviors stated earlier
		Demonstrates relaxation, breathing techniques, etc. to be used in labor as taught in prenatal education classes or by prenatal nurse
	Appearance is healthy, grooming adequate, energy level normal	Demonstrates preparation of nipples for breastfeeding

	Discusses techniques of infant feeding	Discusses plans for care of newborn, help at home, preparation of siblings
	Discusses prenatal education classes	
Fetal well-being	FHR heard by Doppler principle (Dopptone) at 8-12 wk, by fetoscope at 17-18 wk	FHR and rhythm are normal (120-160 beats/min) and regular; will be less if fetus is asleep and greater with fetal movement
	Fetal movements felt at 17-19 wk (quickening)	Fetal movements increase with maternal movements, may lessen during fetal sleep; same pattern of movements every 24 hr
	Fetal breathing movements by 18½ wk	Height of fundus, abdominal growth, and estimation of weight within normal limits for the estimated gestational age; presentation, size of infant and maternal pelvic configuration permit vaginal delivery
		Engagement occurs about 2 wk before term in nullipara; may not occur until labor is well established in parous woman

Developmental Tasks of Pregnant Adolescents

Developmental tasks	Actuality of pregnancy
Learn to accept and live comfortably with slowly changing body and associated sexual feelings and desires. Develop positive self-image.	Must deal with gross body changes, particularly huge abdomen and large breasts; skin is marred by chloasma and striae. Sexual feelings and desires may vary in intensity throughout pregnancy. Because of individual's own growth as well as needs of pregnancy, large amounts of food are needed; this is in conflict with the slimness so highly valued in society.
Reorganize thought processes, with thinking becoming less egocentric.	Huge hormonal increases as well as the tasks of pregnancy lead to progressive introspection, dependency, and egocentric thinking and behavior.
Become independent of parents and gradually develop interdependence.	Psychological dependency increases during pregnancy as young woman uses internal resources to cope with tasks of pregnancy. Because most adolescents are unable to support themselves, financial considerations increase dependency on parents; occasionally other extreme occurs—alienation from parents because of pregnancy.

Gain sense of identity through interaction, first with same-sex peers, then with heterosexual friends.

Being pregnant and thus different isolates adolescent from group.

Firm foundation was established incompletely, if at all, with same-sex friends before physical relationship with opposite sex; thus adolescent often is left without peers of either sex.

Take increasing responsibility for own activities.

Critical difference between adolescent and adult is ability to be responsible for oneself and one's activities; financial consequences associated with pregnancy alone can prevent young woman from taking responsibility. Lack of knowledge and maturity also affect ability to parent an infant, although society still tends to hold the teenager more responsible for the pregnancy.

From Hancock LA et al: The prenatal period. In Edelman CL, Mandle CL, editors: *Health promotion throughout the lifespan,* ed 3, St Louis, 1994, Mosby; modified from Bishop B: *The maternity cycle: one nurse's reflections,* Philadelphia, 1980, Davis.

Normal Discomforts Experienced During Pregnancy

Discomforts, probable cause, and nursing suggestions for relief

Discomfort	Known or probable cause	Nursing suggestions for relief
Backache	Changes in posture, such as increased lumbar curve Excessive bending and lifting	Practice good posture Perform pelvic rocking Wear comfortable, low-heeled shoes Squat to lift Avoid prolonged sitting Sleep on firm mattress
Constipation	Pressure of enlarged uterus Slowed peristalsis caused by progesterone Side effect of iron supplement	Increase fluid intake, especially juices Eat high-fiber foods Exercise Drink warm liquids in morning Only if other methods fail, use mild laxative, stool softener, or glycerine suppository
Fatigue	Decreased metabolic rate in early pregnancy	Get full night's sleep Nap or rest during day Share workload when possible "Usually better after first trimester"
Hemorrhoids	Constipation Pressure of enlarged uterus	Relieve constipation with measures just listed Take sitz baths Use ice pack or witch hazel for local relief Reinsert hemorrhoid; do perineal tightening exercises Local preparation for analgesia

Leg cramps	Pressure of large uterus on blood vessels Fatigue or chilling Lack of calcium Sudden stretching or overextension of the foot Excessive phosphorus in diet	Take calcium supplement Practice gentle, steady stretch to relieve cramp Never massage cramping muscle Avoid toe-pointing when exercising
Leukorrhea (increased vaginal discharge)	Increased vascularity of cervix and vagina	Wear cotton crotch panties Wash genital area more frequently If infection develops, have physician treat Do not douche
Nausea and vomiting (may occur any time of day)	Increase in estrogen and progesterone levels Change (especially lowering) of blood glucose level	Eat small, frequent meals Eat dry cracker before getting up in morning Snack at bedtime Usually "stops after first trimester"
Urinary frequency (day and night)	Pressure of uterus on bladder in first and third trimesters Nocturia may result from increased venous return from extremities when lying down	(Explanation of why frequency is occurring) If interfering with sleep, reduce fluids in evening Rest during day
Varicosities	Increased vascularity of pelvic organs Venous return slowed by pressure of uterus Familial tendency Progesterone effect in smooth muscles	Avoid knee socks and tight elastic on underwear Elevate feet for 10 to 15 minutes several times a day Avoid long periods of standing Avoid crossing legs when sitting Wear support stockings

From Edelman CL, Mandle CL: *Health promotion throughout the lifespan*, ed 3, St Louis, 1994, Mosby.

Infancy

An assessment of the infant in the home is an observational and educational function. The mother and family are taught about normal growth and development of the infant as the nurse is carrying out this assessment. The following tools will assist the community health nurse in this activity.

Notes

Guide for Perinatal Assessment of the Newborn

Identification of Risk Factors by Maternal Components
Add the total score and divide by only the number of items checked to get the overall risk index.

(Risk significance: 3 = high risk, 2 = moderate risk, 1 = slight risk)

General information	Risk	General information	Risk	General information	Risk
Age <18 or >40	2	Rh sensitization	3	Ultrasonography: growth retardation >2 wk	3
Marital status		ABO incompatibility	2	Amniocentesis	
Single, separated, divorced, widow	2	**Present pregnancy antepartal course**		L/S ratio <2:1	3
Socioeconomic level		General prenatal information		Bilirubin present	3
Low	2	Prenatal care: little or none	2	Meconium present	3
Low-middle	1	Weight gain ≤15 lb or ≥35 lb	2	Other evidence of immaturity	3
Ethnic-cultural group: minority	2	Medications other than dietary supplement	1	NST: nonreactive	3
Educational level: 10th grade	1	Maternal medical/surgical problems		OCT: positive	3
Hereditary disorder: genetic	3	Diabetes	3	Duration of pregnancy	
Familial health history		Heart disease	2	<37 wk	3
Diabetes	2	Chronic hypertension	1	>42 wk	2
Heart disease	1	Thyroid disease	2	**Present pregnancy intrapartal course**	
Chronic hypertension	1	Other endocrine disorders	2	Onset of labor	
Prepregnancy weight <100 or >200	2	Anemia		Early labor: <37 wk	3
History of infertility		Iron deficiency	1	PROM	3
Para 0, >35 yr	2	Sickle cell	2	Induction	2
Problem conceiving	1				
Pregnancy interval >4 yr	1				
Rx for infertility	2				

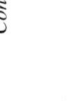

Continued.

From Brodish MS: Perinatal assessment, *JOGN Nurs* 10, January/February, 1981.

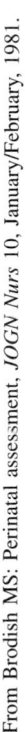

Guide for Perinatal Assessment of the Newborn—cont'd

General information	Risk
Obstetrical history	
Gravida ≥6	2
Parity ≤5	2
Abortions	
≥1 (≤20 wk)	3
Gravida <1 + para	3
Stillbirths ≥1 (≥37 wk)	3
Prematurity <37 wk	3
SGA	
<37 wk	3
37 to 41 wk	2
≥42 wk	2
LGA	
<37 wk	3
37 to 41 wk	2
≥42 wk	2
Neonatal death ≤4 wk	3
History of congenital anomalies	2
History of neonatal asphyxia	2
Previous prenatal history	
Preeclampsia	2
Eclampsia	3
PROM	2
Ectopic pregnancy	2

General information	Risk
Present pregnancy antepartal course—cont'd	
Other	3
Pulmonary disease	2
Chronic renal disease	2
Neurologic disease	2
PID	2
Pelvic surgery	2
Habits/Present pregnancy	
Heavy smoker: ≥20 cigarettes/day	2
Alcohol	
Moderate use	1
Heavy use	2
Abuse	2
Drug abuse	3
Complications	
Preeclampsia	2
Eclampsia	3
Hyperemesis gravidarum	3
Early bleeding ≤20 wk	2
Late bleeding ≥20 wk	3
Bleeding with pain	2
Hydramnios	2

General information	Risk
Present pregnancy intrapartal course—cont'd	
Cesarean section	2
Duration of labor	
1st stage >16 hr	2
2nd stage >2 hr	3
2nd stage <10 min	3
Total >20 hr	2
<3 hr	2
Identified intrapartal problems CPD	2
Preeclampsia	2
Eclampsia	3
Rx $MgSO_4$ >25 g	3
Meconium staining	3
Placenta previa	3
Placenta abruptio	3
Cord compression	2
Prolapsed cord	3
Uterine inertia	3
Uterine tetany	3
Multiple birth	3
Maternal fever ≥100°F	3
Fetal heart monitoring	3
Baseline FHR <100 or >160	3

Item	Score
Placenta previa	2
Placenta abruptio	2
CPD	3
Uterine dystocia	3
Cesarean section	2
Induction	1
Demerol >25 mg IM within 1 hr of delivery	3
Course of delivery	
Presentation	
Breech	3
Transverse lie	3
Position: vertex other than OA	2
Forceps	
Outlet	1

Delivery room assessment

Item	Score
Apgar score: 1 min	
1-4	3
7-8	1
5-7	2
Apgar score: 5 min	
1-4	3
5-7	3
7-8	2

Item	Score
Oligohydramnios	2
Rubella infection (8 to 12 wk)	2
Venereal disease	3
Other infections	3
Maternal FUO	2
Rh sensitization	1
Antepartal diagnostic tests	
Estriol level: no rise >36 wk	3
Low	2
Mid or >	3
Vacuum extraction	3
Identified problems	3
Shoulder dystocia	2
Nuchal cord × 1	
≥ × 2	1
Short cord	
Cesarean section	
Repeat	

Admission nursery assessment

Item	Score
Variation of Dubowitz from dates >2 wk	2
Size/gestational age	
SGA	3
LGA	2

Item	Score
Tachycardia >30 min	3
Tachycardia ≥30 min	3
Poor beat-to-beat variability	3
Increasing number of variables	3
Late decelerations	3
Analgesia	
Total Demerol >200 mg	3
Demerol >25 mg IV within ½ hr of delivery	3
Emergency	3
Episiotomy: none, with laceration	1
Anesthesia	
General	3
Spinal 15 min before delivery	2
Maternal bonding	
No bonding	2
Inappropriate affect	2

Admission nursery assessment

Item	Score
2 Vessels	3
Meconium stained	3

Newborn physical examination

Item	Score
Skin	
Ecchymoses	2

Continued.

Guide for Perinatal Assessment of the Newborn—cont'd

General information	Risk	General information	Risk	General information	Risk
Delivery room assessment—cont'd		**Admission nursery assessment—cont'd**		**Newborn physical examination—cont'd**	
Temperature regulation: <97°F	2	Measurements		Petechiae	2
Resuscitation measures		Weight <5 lb (2000 g)	3	Plethoric	2
Intubation	3	>9 lb (3500 g)	2	Pustules	3
Sustained O$_2$	3	Length <18 in (45 cm)	3	Edematous	2
Bagging	3	Head circumference		Head	
Drug administration	3	<12½ in (32 cm)	3	Circumference <32 cm	3
Respiratory effort		>14 in (36 cm)	3	or >36 cm	
See-saw respiration	3	Chest circumference <12 in	3	Enlarged fontanels	2
Retractions	3	(30 cm)		Bulging fontanels	3
Chin-tug	3	Head circumference < or >1 in	3	Sunken fontanels	2
Expiratory grunt	3	(2 cm) of chest		Facial asymmetry	1
Flaring nares	2	Dextrostix ≤30 mg/100 ml	2	Excessive molding	1
Tachypnea >60	2	Color		Cephalhematoma	2
Noisy respiration (rales)	1	Pale	2	Eyes	
No initial spontaneous	3	Cyanotic	1	Dull	3
respiration		Jaundiced	3	Nonreactive	3
Maternal bonding		Axillary temperature		Fixed	3
No bonding	2	97° to 96°F	2	Nose patency: obstruction	2
Inappropriate affect	2	<96°F	2	Mouth	
		Heart rate: <100 or >160	3	Cleft lip/cleft palate	2

Admission nursery assessment

Item	Score
Gestational age by dates	
<37 wk	3
>42 wk	2
Gestational age by Dubowitz	
<37 wk	3
>42 wk	2

Newborn physical examination

Item	Score
Poor muscle tone	2
Distention	3
Enlarged liver	3
Enlarged kidney	3
Enlarged spleen	3
Inguinal hernia	2
Umbilical hernia	1
Omphalocele	3
Urogenital	
Undescended testes	1
Hydrocele	1
Hypospadius	2
Enlarged clitoris	1
Ectopic bladder	3
No voiding	3
Spine	
Curvature	2
Sacral dimple	1

Item	Score
Respiratory rate: <40 or >60	3
Respiratory effort	
Flaring nares	3
Rales	2
See-saw respiration	
Retractions	3
Chin-tug	2
Expiratory grunt	
Cry	
Weak	2
Shrill	3
Umbilical cord	3

Newborn physical examination

Item	Score
Gross malformation	2
Fractured clavicle	1
Reflexes	3
Absence of any of the normal reflexes (Moro, sucking, rooting, swallowing, tonic neck, gag, grasp, walking, Babinskin)	1

Nursery activity patterns (first 24 hours)

Item	Score
Sleeping pattern	2
>20 to 22 hr	1

Item	Score
Frenulum linguae	1
Chest	
Circumference <12 in (30 cm)	3
Heart rate <100 or >160	3
Heart murmur	3
Respiratory rate <40 or >60	2
Breath sounds (rales)	2
Retractions	3
Abdomen	

Nursing activity patterns (first 24 hours)

Item	Score
Warming unit necessary to maintain body temperature	2
Color	
Pale	2
Cyanotic	1
Jaundiced	3
Heart rate	
<100 or >160	3
Murmur present	3
Respirations	
Rate <40 or >60	3
Breath sounds (rales)	2
Retractions	3
Flaring nares	2
See-saw respiration	3

Continued.

Guide for Perinatal Assessment of the Newborn—cont'd

General information	Risk	General information	Risk	General information	Risk
Newborn physical examination—cont'd		**Nursery activity patterns (first 24 hours)—cont'd**		**Nursing activity patterns (first 24 hours)—cont'd**	
Spina bifida	3	No quiet alert states	3	Chin-tug	3
Extremities		Constantly fussy	3	Expiratory grunt	3
Paralysis	2	Flaccid	3	Parental bonding	
Deviation in position and ROM	2	Feeding pattern		Calling baby "it"	2
Extra gluteal creases	2	Inability to suck, swallow, or	3	Refusal to touch	3
Hip click	2	retain		No desire to see	3
Club feet	1	Poor intake		No interest in caring for	3
Polydactyly		Voiding pattern: no voiding	2	No eye-to-eye contact	3
		Bowel elimination: no stooling	3	Disappointment in sex of	2
		Weight loss 1st day: >4 oz	2	Anxiety about breast-feeding	1
		Temperature regulation			
		Axillary temperature <97°F	2		

Neonatal Perception Inventory

The Neonatal Perception Inventory is easily and quickly administered by telling the mother: "We are interested in learning more about the experiences of mothers and their babies during the first few weeks after delivery. The more we can learn about mothers and their babies, the better we will be able to help other mothers with their babies. We would appreciate it if you would help us to help other mothers by answering a few questions."

The procedures are identical for administering the Average Baby form of the NPI on the first or second postpartum day and the NPI at 1 month of age. The mother is handed the Average Baby form while the individual administering the inventory says: "Although this is your first baby, you probably have some ideas of what most little babies are like. Will you please check the blank you *think* best describes what *most* little babies are like."

The tester waits until the mother has completed the Average Baby form and takes it from the mother and then hands the mother the Your Baby form.*

The procedure for administering the Your Baby forms of the NPI is the same at Time I and Time II. However, the instructions given to the mother vary slightly to take into account the time factor. At Time I the tester tells the mother: "While it is not possible to know for certain what your baby will be like, you probably have some ideas of what your baby will be like. Please check the blank you *think* best describes what *your* baby will be like."

At Time II, she says:

"You have had a chance to live with your baby for a month now. Please check the blank you think best describes your baby."

Method of Scoring

The Average Baby Perception form elicits the mother's concept of the average baby's behavior. The Your Baby Perception form elicits her rating of her own baby. Each of these instruments consists of six single-item scales. Values of 1 to 5 are assigned to each of these scales for each of the inventories. The blank signified none is valued as 1 and a great deal has a value of 5. The lower values on the scale represent the most desirable behavior.

The six scales are totaled with no attempt at weighing the scales for each of the inventories separately. Thus a total score is obtained for the Average Baby and a total score is obtained for the Your Baby.

---

*The tester remains with the mother during the entire administration procedure.

The total score of Your Baby Perception form is then subtracted from the Average Baby Perception form. The discrepancy constitutes the Neonatal Perception Inventory score.

The inventories have shown both construct and criterion validity.

Neonatal Perception Inventory 1
Average baby

Although this is your first baby, you probably have some ideas of what most little babies are like. Please check the blank you think best describes the average baby.

How much crying do you think the average baby does?

| a great deal | a good bit | moderate amount | very little | none |

How much trouble do you think the average baby has in feeding?

| a great deal | a good bit | moderate amount | very little | none |

How much spitting up or vomiting do you think the average baby does?

| a great deal | a good bit | moderate amount | very little | none |

How much difficulty do you think the average baby has in sleeping?

| a great deal | a good bit | moderate amount | very little | none |

How much difficulty does the average baby have with bowel movements?

| a great deal | a good bit | moderate amount | very little | none |

How much trouble do you think the average baby has in settling down to a predictable pattern of eating and sleeping?

| a great deal | a good bit | moderate amount | very little | none |

Your baby

While it is not possible to know for certain what your baby will be like, you probably have some ideas of what your baby will be like. Please check the blank that you think best describes what your baby will be like.

From Stanhope M, Lancaster J: *Community health nursing: promoting health of aggregates, families, and individuals,* ed 4, St Louis, 1996, Mosby.

How much crying do you think your baby will do?

——————— ——————— ——————————— ——————— ———
a great deal   a good bit   moderate amount   very little   none

How much trouble do you think your baby will have feeding?

——————— ——————— ——————————— ——————— ———
a great deal   a good bit   moderate amount   very little   none

How much spitting up or vomiting do you think your baby will do?

——————— ——————— ——————————— ——————— ———
a great deal   a good bit   moderate amount   very little   none

How much difficulty do you think your baby will have sleeping?

——————— ——————— ——————————— ——————— ———
a great deal   a good bit   moderate amount   very little   none

How much difficulty do you expect your baby to have with bowel movements?

——————— ——————— ——————————— ——————— ———
a great deal   a good bit   moderate amount   very little   none

How much trouble do you think your baby will have settling down to a predictable pattern of eating and sleeping?

——————— ——————— ——————————— ——————— ———
a great deal   a good bit   moderate amount   very little   none

Neonatal Perception Inventory II

Note: Same inventory for average baby is given again.

Your baby

You have had a chance to live with your baby for a month now. Please check the blank you think best describes your baby.

How much crying has your baby done?

——————— ——————— ——————————— ——————— ———
a great deal   a good bit   moderate amount   very little   none

How much trouble has your baby had feeding?

——————— ——————— ——————————— ——————— ———
a great deal   a good bit   moderate amount   very little   none

How much spitting up or vomiting has your baby done?

——————— ——————— ——————————— ——————— ———
a great deal   a good bit   moderate amount   very little   none

How much difficulty has your baby had sleeping?

——————— ——————— ——————————— ——————— ———
a great deal   a good bit   moderate amount   very little   none

How much difficulty has your baby had with bowel movements?

a great deal	a good bit	moderate amount	very little	none

How much trouble has your baby had in settling down to a predictable pattern of eating and sleeping?

a great deal	a good bit	moderate amount	very little	none

Degree of bother inventory

Listed below are some of the things that have sometimes bothered mothers in caring for their babies. We would like to know if you were bothered about any of these. Please place a check in the blank that best describes how much you were bothered by your baby's behavior in regard to these.

Crying

a great deal	somewhat	very little	none

Spitting up or vomiting

a great deal	somewhat	very little	none

Sleeping

a great deal	somewhat	very little	none

Feeding

a great deal	somewhat	very little	none

Elimination

a great deal	somewhat	very little	none

Lack of a predictable schedule

a great deal	somewhat	very little	none

Other (specify):

a great deal	somewhat	very little	none

a great deal	somewhat	very little	none

a great deal	somewhat	very little	none

Information regarding the NPI can be obtained from Broussard ER, Hartner S: Further considerations regarding maternal perception of the first born. In Hellmuth J, editor: *Exceptional infant: studies in abnormalities,* vol 2, New York, 1971, Brunner/Mazel.

Assessment of Infant Reflexes

Reflex	Expected behavioral response	Deviation
Localized		
Eyes		
Blinking or corneal reflex	Infant blinks at sudden appearance of a bright light or at approach of an object toward the cornea; should persist throughout life	Absent or asymmetric blink suggests damage to cranial nerves II, IV, and V
Pupillary	Pupil constricts when a bright light shines toward it, should persist throughout life	Unequal constriction Fixed dilated pupil
Doll's eye	As the head is moved slowly to the right or left, eyes normally do not move; should disappear as fixation develops	Asymmetric in abducens paralysis
Nose		
Sneeze	Spontaneous response of nasal passages to irritation or obstruction; should persist throughout life	Absent or continuous sneezing
Glabellar	Tapping briskly on glabella (bridge of nose) causes eyes to close tightly	Absence

From Wong DL, Whaley LF: *Clinical manual of pediatric nursing*, ed 3, St Louis, 1990, Mosby.

Continued.

Assessment of Infant Reflexes—cont'd

Reflex	Expected behavioral response	Deviation
Mouth and throat		
Sucking	Infant should begin strong sucking movements of circumoral area in response to stimulation; should persist throughout infancy, even without stimulation, such as during sleep	Weak or absent suck
Gag	Stimulation of posterior pharynx by food, suction, or passage of a tube should cause infant to gag; should persist throughout life	Absence of gag suggests damage to glossopharyngeal nerve
Rooting	Touching or stroking the cheek along the side of the mouth will cause infant to turn the head toward that side and begin to suck; should disappear at about age 3 to 4 months, but may persist for up to 12 months	Absence, especially when infant is not satiated
Extrusion	When tongue is touched or depressed, infant responds by forcing it outward; should disappear by age 4 months	Constant protrusion of tongue may suggest Down syndrome
Yawn	Spontaneous response to decreased oxygen by increasing amount of inspired air; should persist throughout life	Absence
Cough	Irritation of mucous membranes of larynx or tracheobronchial tree causes coughing; should persist throughout life; usually present after first day of birth	Absence

Extremities		
Grasp	Touching palms of hands or soles of feet near base of digits causes flexion of hands and toes; palmar grasp should lessen after age 3 months, to be replaced by voluntary movement; plantar grasp lessens by 8 months of age	Asymmetric flexion may indicate paralysis
Babinski	Stroking outer sole of foot upward from heel and across ball of foot causes toes to hyperextend and hallux to dorsiflex; should disappear after age 1 year	Persistence indicates a pyramidal tract lesion
Ankle clonus	Briskly dorsiflexing foot while supporting knee in partially flexed position results in one to two oscillating movements ("beats"); eventually no beats should be felt	Several beats
Mass		
Moro	Sudden jarring or change in equilibrium causes sudden extension and abduction of extremities and fanning of fingers, with index finger and thumb forming a C shape, followed by flexion and abduction of extremities; legs may weakly flex; infant may cry; should disappear after age 3 to 4 months, usually strongest during first 2 months	Persistence of Moro reflex past age 6 months may indicate brain damage Asymmetric Moro reflex may suggest injury to brachial plexus, clavicle, or humerus

Continued.

Assessment of Infant Reflexes—cont'd

Reflex	Expected behavioral response	Deviation
Mass—cont'd		
Startle	A sudden loud noise causes abduction of the arms with flexion of the elbows; the hands remain clenched; should disappear by age 4 months	Absence indicates hearing loss
Perez	While infant is prone on a firm surface, thumb is pressed along spine from sacrum to neck; infant responds by crying, flexing the extremities, and elevating the pelvis and head; lordosis of the spine, as well as defecation and urination, may occur; should disappear by age 4 to 6 months	Significance is similar to that of Moro reflex
Asymmetric tonic neck	When infant's head is quickly turned to one side, arm and leg extends on that side, and opposite arm and leg flex; should disappear by age 3 to 4 months, to be replaced by symmetric positioning of both sides of body	Absence or persistence may indicate central nervous system damage
Neck-righting	While infant is supine, head is turned to one side; shoulder and trunk turns toward that side, followed by pelvis; disappears at age 10 months	Absence; significance is similar to that of asymmetric tonic neck reflex
Otolith-righting	When body of an erect infant is tilted, head is returned to upright, erect position	Absence; significance is similar to that of asymmetric tonic neck reflex

Trunk incurvation (Galant)	Stroking infant's back alongside spine causes hips to move toward stimulated side; should disappear by age 4 weeks	Absence may indicate spinal cord lesion
Dance or step	If infant is held so that sole of foot touches a hard surface, there is a reciprocal flexion and extension of the leg, simulating walking; should disappear after age 3 to 4 weeks, to be replaced by deliberate movement	Asymmetry of stepping
Crawling	Infant, when placed on abdomen, makes crawling movements with the arms and legs; should disappear at about age 6 weeks	Asymmetry of movement
Placing	When infant is held upright under arms and dorsal side of foot is briskly placed against hard object, such as table, leg lifts as if foot is stepping on table; age of disappearance varies	Absence

Nursing Interventions to Assist in Stressful Situations During Infancy

Attempt to meet the infant's needs promptly.

Allow favorite toy or item of security to be present during stressful experiences.

Allow familiar caregiver to be present to calm infant.

Attempt to keep the number of strangers interacting with infant to a minimum.

Attempt to provide a warm and accepting environment for the infant.

Allow freedom of expression (crying) to reduce tension in the infant.

Identify the infant's established daily routine and try to follow through.

Reinforce the infant's need for expression.

Establish a trust relationship with the infant.

Provide opportunity for play so that the infant can "vent" fears.

Provide emotional support for the parents so they may in turn give support to their infant.

From Edelman CL, Mandle CL: *Health promotion throughout the lifespan,* ed 3, St Louis, 1994, Mosby.

Nursing Interventions to Prevent Aspiration of Foreign Objects by Infants

Keep all small objects out of an infant's reach.

Avoid propping bottles and making large holes in nipples to prevent aspiration of formula into the infant's lungs.

Discourage the use of powder for infants to reduce risk of aspiration pneumonia from inhalation of zinc stearate.

Burp the infant well before placing into the crib; place on abdomen or prop on right side.

Older children should not give food to the infant, who may choke on it. An adult should be close by to supervise children around infants.

Adults should not set a bad example by putting pins or other objects in their mouths; older infants mimic them and may do likewise.

Inspect all toys for loose, removable parts that potentially could reach the infant's mouth.

From Edelman CL, Mandle CL: *Health promotion throughout the lifespan,* ed 3, St Louis, 1994, Mosby.

Clinical Manifestations of Dehydration

	Isotonic (loss of water and salt)	Hypotonic (loss of salt in excess of water)	Hypertonic (loss of water in excess of salt)
Skin			
Color	Gray	Gray	Gray
Temperature	Cold	Cold	Cold or hot
Turgor	Poor	Very poor	Fair
Feel	Dry	Clammy	Thickened, doughy
Mucous membranes	Dry	Slightly moist	Parched
Tearing and salivation	Absent	Absent	Absent
Eyeball	Sunken	Sunken	Sunken
Fontanel	Sunken	Sunken	Sunken
Body temperature	Subnormal or elevated	Subnormal or elevated	Subnormal or elevated
Pulse	Rapid	Very rapid	Moderately rapid
Respirations	Rapid	Rapid	Rapid
Behavior	Irritable to lethargic	Lethargic to comatose; convulsions	Marked lethargy with extreme hyperirritability on stimulation

From Wong D: *Whaley and Wong's nursing care of infants and children,* ed 5, St Louis, 1995, Mosby.

Postnatal Care

Ideally a woman should be followed prenatally through home visits, but frequently the community health nurse first meets a woman postnatally, especially if the pregnancy is uneventful. The following tools will assist the nurse in making appropriate observations during the postnatal period.

MIST: Mother/Infant Screening Tool

The Mother Infant Screening Tool assesses mother-infant bonding. It includes four areas for evaluation: tactile, visual, auditory, and feeding. Circle the answer under A, B, C, D that best describes the *mother's* behavior. Circle the answer under A, B, C, D that best describes the *infant's* behavior. Add the numbers under each A, B, C, D for mothers and infants separately. The more A's mother and baby have, the more attachment that has occurred. The more D's mother and baby have, the less attachment. Use as a guide for planning care.

Notes

	A	B	C	D
T	**Mother** Holds infant close to her body	Holds infant on forearm	Holds infant away from body	Doesn't hold infant
A	**Infant** Curls up close to mother	Keeps some distance	Moves away when touched	Stiffens-up when held
C **T**	**Mother** Comfortable touching infant, strokes head or face	Looks comfortable, pats infant's back	Tentative when touching infant	Avoids touching infant
I **L** **E**	**Infant** At ease; turns toward mother's touch	Looks at ease	Looks tense	Cries when touched
V	**Mother** Establishes eye contact	Looks at infant's face	Does not look at infant's face	Does not look at infant
I **S**	**Infant** Establishes eye contact	Looks at mother's face	Does not look at mother's face	Does not look at mother
U **A**	**Mother** Smiles and makes faces in play	Smiles	No special facial expressions	Looks unhappy
L	**Infant** Laughs or big smile	Smiles	No special facial expressions	Looks unhappy

From Reiser SL: A tool to facilitate mother-infant attachment, *JOGN Nursing* 10:297, 1981.

Continued.

The letters in the left margin read vertically: **A U D I T O R Y** and **F E E D I N G**.

	A	B	C	D
A **Mother**	Talks to infant in soothing or playful way	Talks to infant in calm way	Talks but just gives directions	Doesn't talk to infant
U **Infant**	Infant makes happy sounds, coos and goos	Makes ah-ah sounds	Cries	Doesn't talk
D **Mother**	Understands meaning of infant's cries	Differentiates most of infant's cries	Seldom differentiates infant's cries	Never differentiates infant's cries
I **Infant**	Exhibits different cries	Usually exhibits different cries	Seldom exhibits different cries	Never exhibits different cries
T O **Mother**	Shows signs of pleasure during feeding—smiles, rocks, sings	Looks content during feeding	Acts unsure during feeding—stops and starts	Agitated or irritable
R Y E D **Infant**	Shows pleasure in being fed—smiles, coos	Looks content during feeding	Restless during feeding	Agitated—cries during feeding
I N **Mother**	Looks pleased after feeding	Looks satisfied after feeding	Looks uneasy after feeding	Looks agitated after feeding
G **Infant**	Looks happy after feeding	Looks satisfied after feeding	Looks restless after feeding	Looks agitated after feeding

Total score Mother _____

Total score Infant _____

Date _____

Observations to be Made at Postpartum Checkups and Pediatric Checkups

1. Does the mother have fun with the baby?
2. Does the mother establish eye contact (direct in face position) with the baby?
3. How does the mother talk to her baby? Is everything she expresses a demand?
4. Are most of her verbalizations about the child negative?
5. Does she remain disappointed over the child's sex?
6. What is the child's name? Where did it come from? When did they name the child?
7. Are the mother's expectations for the child's development far beyond the child's capabilities?
8. Is the mother very bothered by the baby's crying? How does she feel about the crying?
9. Does the mother see the baby as too demanding during feedings? Is she repulsed by the messiness? Does she ignore the baby's demands to be fed?
10. What is the mother's reaction to the task of changing diapers?
11. When the baby cries, does she or can she comfort him or her?
12. What was/is the husband's and/or family's reaction to the baby?
13. What kind of support is the mother receiving?
14. Are there sibling rivalry problems?
15. Is the husband jealous of the baby's drain on the mother's time and affection?
16. When the mother brings the child for checkups does she get involved and take control over the baby's needs and what's going to happen (during the examination and while in the waiting room), or does she relinquish control to the physician or nurse (undressing the child, holding the child, allowing the child to express his or her fears, etc.)?
17. Can attention be focused on the child in the mother's presence? Can the mother see something positive for herself in that?
18. Does the mother make nonexistent complaints about the baby? Does she describe to you a child that you don't see there at all? Does she call with strange stories that the child has, for example, stopped breathing, turned color, or is doing something "on purpose" to aggravate the parent?
19. Does the mother make emergency calls for very small things, not major things?

From Stanhope M, Lancaster J: *Community health nursing: promoting health of aggregates, families, and individuals,* ed 4, St Louis, 1996, Mosby; modified from Kempe CH: Approaches to preventing child abuse, *Am J Dis Child* 130, 1976, copyright 1976, American Medical Association.

Postpartum Period Evaluation Criteria

Area assessed	First 2 wks	By wk 4 to 6
Temperature	Temperature is elevated to 38°C (100.4°F) in first 24 hr after delivery. This is not unusual, and if unaccompanied by other symptoms, e.g., pain in the calf or leg or a foul odor of lochia, it is considered to be caused by dehydration. If temperature elevation begins after 24 hr or persists for 48 hr, it is considered abnormal.	Returns to prepregnant level.
Pulse	Pulse rate falls a short time after delivery (range of 50 to 70 beats/min), and bradycardia may persist for 6 to 8 days even in absence of stress.	Returns to prepregnant level.
Respirations	Rate remains within normal limits.	
Blood pressure	Blood pressure remains in accord with previous normal readings.	
Breasts	For 2 to 3 days after delivery breasts secrete colostrum in increasing amounts. By second day in multiparas and by third day in primiparas, breasts become engorged, firm, tense, and tender. This is caused by venous or lymphatic stasis, and in 36 to 48 hr pain disappears as swelling spontaneously subsides. Fever does not accompany this process. Soon after onset of this engorgement, true milk is formed and let-down reflex in response to suckling of infant or manual manipulation causes expression of milk.	Breasts do not reveal soreness, tenderness, or masses. If woman is not breast-feeding, no milk or only a small amount of milk may be expressed. If woman is breast-feeding, lactation is well established; nipples are intact.

Uterus	Involution of uterus progresses normally.	Uterus is only slightly larger than in prepregnant state and anteverted. If retroverted, it has developed free mobility.
	Size of uterus diminishes. Immediately after delivery, uterus weighs about 1 kg; its size approximates that of pregnancy of 16 wk gestation; its position is below level of umbilicus, in midline or slightly to right of midline; it descends into pelvic cavity 1 cm/day.	
	Uterine tone is maintained by contraction and retraction of uterine muscles.	
	Uterus feels firm and contracts readily after massage; there is expulsion of clots. During first 12 hr after delivery contractions are strong, regular, and coordinated. Thereafter intensity, frequency, and regularity decrease. After-pains occur for 2 or 3 days and are more noticeable in multipara than in primipara and during suckling of infant.	
Lochia	Color and consistency of lochia change.	Uterine bleeding (lochia) decreases until about third or fourth week and then ceases; vaginal discharge is minimum; small period (menstruation) may have occurred during fourth or fifth week after delivery.
	Lochia rubra contains blood, placental and decidual debris, and clots and is dark red. It persists from delivery through third day.	
	Lochia serosa is thin, serous, and brownish and lasts from fourth to tenth day.	
	Lochia alba, a yellowish-white discharge, contains an increased number of leukocytes and lasts from tenth day to as long as sixth week.	
	Odor remains characteristically "fleshy" rather than foul.	
	Amount of discharge is moderate for first 2 to 3 days and then is scant. Some women may have none after 2 wk; in others discharge persists until sixth wk.	

From Jensen MD, Bobak IM: *Maternity and gynecologic care: the nurse and the family,* ed 3, St Louis, 1985, Mosby.

Continued.

Postpartum Period Evaluation Criteria—cont'd

Area assessed	First 2 wks	By wk 4 to 6
Cervix	Cervix regains its shape in few days, and external os is contracted by 2 wk (introduction of 1-cm probe is difficult) and cervical mucosa is restored.	Cervix is healed; external os has assumed typical transverse slit of parous woman. Occasionally glandular epithelium lining cervical canal visualized as bright red area surrounding external os. Papanicolaou smear reveals normal estrogen pattern.
Vagina	Vagina remains distensible; introitus gapes when intraabdominal pressure is increased by bearing-down effort or by coughing.	Pelvic floor has essentially regained its tone, permitting only a mild degree of uterine prolapse, cystocele, or rectocele. Vulva and perineal area show no evidence of infection. Episiotomy or laceration usually healed without undue contraction; introitus adequate to permit coitus without discomfort.

Abdomen	Abdominal wall is lax and weak in midline, where abdominal muscles may be widely separated. Muscles feel like masses on either side of abdomen and are not to be confused with fundus of uterus.	Muscles of abdomen reveal some degree of laxity, but tone is returning to prepregnant level.
Weight	There is an immediate weight loss; then as excess tissue is eliminated, there is further loss in first 3 to 4 days. Further decrease occurs as uterus involutes and plasma volume contracts.	Woman will retain about 60% of weight gained in excess of 11 kg (24 lb).
Urinary system	Most women void spontaneously by 8 hr following delivery and thereafter void copious amounts frequently for 48 hr as retained tissue fluids are released.	There are no symptoms of urinary tract infection (e.g., frequency, urgency, dysuria, urinary incontinence). Urinalysis reveals normal findings; proteinuria has disappeared. Lactose may be present if woman is breast-feeding, but no pus cells are present. Culture reveals no organisms.
Gastrointestinal system	Most women are hungry and have good appetites.	Appetite is good. Diet is adjusted for weight maintenance or weight loss (averages 2000-2500 cal/day). If woman is breast-feeding, caloric intake is increased by 500 cal and fluid increased by 500 ml.

Continued.

Postpartum Period Evaluation Criteria—cont'd

Area assessed	First 2 wks	By wk 4 to 6
Gastrointestinal system—cont'd	Some women defecate spontaneously by third day. Others reestablish regular habits only with aid of laxatives or enemas in addition to added roughage in diet and fluids.	Regular bowel habits are reestablished without fecal incontinence or fistula formation.
Vascular system	Although a normal concentration of blood occurs as retained tissue fluids are released and tendency to clot increases as number of platelets increases, thrombi rarely develop. Hematocrit reading by third postdelivery day is within normal range (42% ± 5%). There is no evidence of thromboembolism.	Hemorrhoids are reduced. Varicosities have disappeared. Woman wears support hose, if necessary. Hemoglobin level is 12 g/dl or greater, and hematocrit level is 37% ± 5%.
Pain or discomfort	Many women feel stress and strain of labor and delivery for 1 or 2 days, and discomfort associated with an episiotomy, hemorrhoids, engorgement of breasts, or other conditions may act to impede recovery for 3 to 5 days.	Discomfort from episiotomy is gone.
Emotional response	New mothers exhibit typical dependent behaviors for 24 to 48 hr. These usually are superseded by mixture of dependent-independent behaviors, which in turn give way to interdependent behaviors. Depressive reactions may begin by end of second postdelivery day and persist for 1 to 3 days. Mother-child relationships may be positive immediately or show a "maternal lag," which may not interfere unduly with child care activities. Parents talk freely about their birthing experience.	Emotional response has stabilized. Family roles are in the process of change through negotiation. Client is able to discuss client-centered problems.

Child care	Skill in child care activities increases with physical recovery and practice.	Becoming skilled in child care activities, less apprehensive, able to ask questions.
Health maintenance	Couple is aware of contraception techniques available. Postdelivery immunization is completed (i.e., rubella vaccination and prevention of Rh isoimmunization), if appropriate. Woman is aware of need for rest, exercise, and nutrition. Couple is aware of danger signals, safety measures, and whom to contact: Hemorrhage Infection Thromboembolism Hypertension or hypotension Depressive states Couple is aware of need for medical examination 4 to 6 wk.	Couple has begun practicing their chosen method of family planning. Woman has established schedule for adequate rest and exercise. Woman is aware of need for a medical reexamination in 6 mo. Parents have chosen health care supervision for infant and have arranged for first examination.
Records	Records are complete. Discharge summary is available for 4 to 6 wk examination.	Record keeping is completed to date.

Brief Screening Inventory for Postpartum Adaptation

Below is an example of a proposed brief screening inventory. Items will be rated on a scale from 0 to 10 to indicate low versus high degree of disturbance.

1. My sleep is disrupted to the degree that it is interfering with my ability to manage care of the household, family, baby, and myself.
2. I am not able to eat one to two complete, adequate meals each day.
3. My mood swings last more than 2 or 3 days at a given time.
4. My mood swings do not occur in response to something specific happening to me or in my environment.
5. Fatigue interferes with my ability to perform everyday activities.
6. I have frequent thoughts about childbirth events, and that preoccupation is interfering with my ability to function well on a daily basis.
7. I am ambivalent or experience uncomfortable feelings about my childbirth experiences.
8. I experience uncomfortable feelings while with my baby.
9. I frequently feel "something bad" will happen to my baby.
10. I become increasingly uncomfortable as I do the tasks necessary in caring for the baby.
11. I have doubts that this mothering role is good for me.
12. My relationship with the baby's father has deteriorated and is posing a problem for me at this time.
13. I do not have time to socialize with other adults.
14. I feel I am not receiving adequate emotional support from others.
15. I make more critical judgments about myself now than before the baby's arrival.
16. I feel I am not attractive anymore.
17. My predominant mood is not positive.
18. My outlook for the future is not favorable.
19. I experience depressive feelings most of the time.
20. Thoughts of suicide have crossed my mind more than once or twice.

Given that mothers postpartum are experiencing early hospital discharge and community health nurses will not be able to conduct home visits for them all, initial screening to identify those at risk is imperative. The list above is designed as a brief self-report instrument that can be given to women upon hospital discharge or mailed to them between the second and fourth postpartum weeks, with instructions for its completion and return in preaddressed envelopes. The inventory can help identify women who need further assessments and also facilitate their reentry into the health care system by eliminating the waiting period for the routine 6-week examination that

From Affonso D: Assessment of maternal postpartum adaptation, *Public Health Nurs* 4(1), 1987. Reprinted with permission of Blackwell Scientific Publications, Inc.

focuses only on physiologic indexes of well-being. For those who require more evaluation, a follow-up home visit can be planned to target the following sample questions:

1. Daily activities

    How are you managing your own daily activities with respect to eating properly, getting adequate sleep, replenishing your energy, and stabilizing your moods?

    How are you managing such concerns for your baby?

    How would you rate your effectiveness now in managing all that you must do?

2. Impact of childbirth events

    What thoughts and feelings do you have when you look back at your childbirth experience?

    Describe how you think you handled your childbirth experience?

    What aspects of your childbirth experience stand out for you and why?

3. Mother-infant interactions

    How do you feel about yourself as a mother?

    What do you think is your baby's attitude toward you as his or her mother?

    What thoughts and feelings do you have while you are with your baby?

    What concerns do you have regarding your baby's health and safety?

    How do you handle these concerns?

4. Social activities and supports

    How are you doing in return to or resumption of your social activities and responsibilities with other adults?

    How is your relationship with the baby's father?

    Describe the social activities you have engaged in that were pleasurable or not pleasurable to you since the baby's birth?

5. Self-worth

    How would you rate yourself at this time with respect to goodness?

    In your opinion, how are you adjusting at this time?

    What thoughts and feelings do you have regarding your physical attractiveness since the baby's birth?

    What is your predominant mood these days?

    How do you view your future?

Answers indicate how each woman views herself and her many relationships, such as with the baby, family and household, and others. Study results indicated that negative answers to these questions were related to women's self-reports of depressive symptomatology.

Protocol for Postpartum Home Visit

Previsit Interventions

1. Contact family to arrange details for home visit.
   a. Identify self, credentials, and agency role.
   b. Review purpose of home visit follow-up.
   c. Schedule convenient time for visit.
   d. Confirm address and route to family home.
2. Review and clarify appropriate data.
   a. All available assessment data for mother and infant (i.e., referral forms, hospital discharge summaries, family-identified learning needs).
   b. Review records of any previous nursing contacts.
   c. Contact other professional caregivers, as necessary to clarify data (i.e., obstetrician, nurse midwife, pediatrician, referring nurse).
3. Identify community resources and teaching materials appropriate to meet needs already identified.
4. Plan the visit, and prepare bag with equipment, supplies, and materials necessary for assessments of mother and infant, actual care anticipated for mother and infant, and client teaching.

In-home Interventions: Establishing a Relationship

1. Reintroduce self and establish purpose of postpartum follow-up visit for mother, infant, and family; offer family opportunity to clarify their expectations of contact.
2. Spend brief time socially interacting with family to become acquainted and establish trusting relationship.

In-home Interventions: Working with Family

1. Conduct systematic assessment of mother and newborn to determine physiological adjustment and any existing complications.
2. Throughout visit, collect data to assess the emotional adjustment of individual family members to newborn and life-style changes. Note evidence of family-newborn bonding and sibling rivalry; note relationships among mother, father, children, and grandparents.

From Bobak IM: *Maternity and gynecologic care,* ed 5, St Louis, 1993, Mosby.

3. Determine adequacy of support system.
   a. To what extent does someone help with cooking, cleaning, and other home-management tasks?
   b. To what extent is help being provided in caring for the newborn and any other children?
   c. Are support persons encouraging the new mother to care for herself and get adequate rest?
   d. Who is providing helpful information? Emotional support?
4. Throughout the visit, observe home environment for adequacy of the following resources:
   a. Space: privacy, safe play of children, sleeping
   b. Overall cleanliness and state of repair
   c. Number of steps new mother must climb
   d. Adequacy of cooking arrangements
   e. Adequacy of refrigeration and other food storage areas
   f. Adequacy of bathing, toileting, and laundry facilities
   g. Arrangements in home for newborn: sleeping, bathing, formula preparation (if needed), layette items, and diapers
5. Throughout the visit, observe home environment for overall state of repair and existence of the following safety hazards:
   a. Storage of medications, household cleaners, and other substances hazardous to children
   b. Presence of peeling paint on furniture, walls, or pipes
   c. Factors that contribute to falls, such as dim lighting, broken steps, scatter rugs
   d. Presence of vermin
   e. Use of crib or playpen that fails to meet safety guidelines
   f. Existence of emergency plan in case of fire; fire alarm or extinguisher
6. Provide care to mother or newborn as prescribed by their respective primary caregiver or in accord with agency protocol.
7. Provide client teaching on basis of previously identified needs.
8. Refer family to appropriate community agencies or resources, such as warm lines and support groups.
9. Ascertain that client knows potential problems to watch for and whom to call if they occur.
10. Ensure that used disposable items have been handled appropriately and that reusable items are cleaned and repacked appropriately in the nurse's bag.

In-home Interventions: Ending the Visit*

1. Summarize the activities and main points of the visit.
2. Clarify future expectations, including schedule of next visit.
3. Review teaching plan, and provide major points in writing.
4. Provide information about reaching the nurse or agency if needed before the next scheduled visit.

Postvisit Interventions

1. Document the visit thoroughly, using the necessary agency forms to serve as a legal record of the visit and to allow third-party reimbursement, as possible.
2. Initiate the plan of care on which the next encounter with the client/family will be based.
3. Communicate appropriately (by telephone, letter, progress notes, or referral form) with primary caregiver, other health professionals, or referral agencies in behalf of client/family.

---

*If this is the nurse's final planned encounter with the client/family, it is important to recognize that both the client and nurse may have feelings evoked by ending a meaningful relationship and by saying goodbye. Such feelings as anger, denial, and sadness are normal in this situation. Freely expressing these feelings at the end of the relationship is encouraged. Often clients are encouraged to do so if the nurse shares such feelings first.

PART THREE
SCREENING TOOLS

Screening tools are valuable instruments for identifying and planning appropriate interventions for clients of all ages. The instruments in this section primarily address mechanisms for the nurse to diagnose client problems that are seen in the community as a basis for assessing client needs and planning care. They may be used or adapted to the practice of the nurse in ways that are most useful to a specific setting or agency.

Clinical Decision-Making Guides

The nurse in the home often finds it necessary to plan care based on physiological changes that occur suddenly or insidiously. Appropriate clinical decision making is essential in order to initiate proper referrals or to plan interventions. The following selected tools will assist the nurse in the home.

Signs and Symptoms of Congestive Heart Failure

- **Right ventricular failure**
    Peripheral edema (pitting)
    Liver enlargement with right upper quadrant pain
    Ascites
    Distended neck veins

From Phipps WJ et al: *Medical-surgical nursing: concepts and clinical practice,* ed 5, St Louis, 1995, Mosby.

- **Left ventricular failure**
  Dyspnea
  Orthopnea
  Paroxysmal nocturnal dyspnea (PND)
  Cheyne-Stokes respirations
  Fatigue
  Auscultatory crackles

Assessment
Subjective data

Data to be collected to assess the client with congestive heart failure concern the person's perception of breathing ability, fluid retention, response to activity, and knowledge of and response to the cardiac failure, including the following:

Shortness of breath and presence of cough
Presence of orthopnea (number of pillows needed for sleep)
Recent weight gain
Edema, especially pedal
Dizziness or confusion
Fatigue
Exercise or heat intolerance
Discomfort: anginal or abdominal pain
Appetite
Usual bowel patterns
Concerns, anxieties
Knowledge of condition
Usual coping skills

Objective data

Objective data focus primarily on signs of fluid retention and include the following:

Respiratory distress, increased effort, and respiratory rate
Neck vein distention: presence, degree
Adventitious breath sounds
Heart sounds: presence of S_3 or gallop rhythm
Edema: site and degree of pitting
Coolness of extremities
Pulse changes
Abdominal distention
Daily weights
Level of consciousness
Character of stools

Signs and Symptoms of TIA

The major importance of TIAs is that they warn the client and health care professional of the existence of an underlying pathologic condition. At least one third of clients who have TIAs will have a CVA in 2 to 5 years. A person with a TIA needs to be aggressively assessed to determine if preventive measures can be taken.

Assessment
Subjective data

1. Client's understanding of disease or symptoms
2. Characteristics of onset of symptoms
3. Presence of headache—nature and location
4. Any sensory deficits
5. Visual ability—presence of diplopia, blurred vision
6. Ability to think clearly
7. Any other concomitant symptom

Objective data

1. Motor strength—paresis or plegia is common
2. Change in level of consciousness, including unconsciousness
3. Signs of increased intracranial pressure
4. Respiratory status
5. Ability to verbalize—presence of aphasia

The exact clinical picture varies depending on the area of the brain affected. The most common focal signs and symptoms are caused by disruption of flow through the midcerebral artery. These symptoms include the following:

1. Contralateral paralysis or paresis
2. Contralateral sensory loss
3. Sensory and motor loss most noticeable in face, neck, and upper extremities
4. Dysphasia or aphasia; occurs if dominant hemisphere is affected (left hemisphere in right-handed persons and most left-handed persons)
5. Spatial-perceptual problems, changes in judgment and behavior, neglect of paralyzed side, and inability to recognize paralyzed extremity as own (*anosognosia*) if nondominant hemisphere is affected
6. Contralateral *homonymous hemianopsia*

From Phipps WJ et al: *Medical-surgical nursing: concepts and clinical practice,* ed 5, St Louis, 1995, Mosby.

Aphasia is a disorder of language caused by damage to the speech-controlling areas of the brain. It includes all areas of language, including speech, reading, writing, and understanding. These abnormalities can occur in a variety of ways as follows:

1. **Sensory aphasia**—inability to comprehend spoken word (also called receptive aphasia)
2. **Motor aphasia**—inability to use the symbols of speech (also called expressive aphasia)
3. **Global aphasia**—inability to understand the spoken word, as well as to speak

Warning Signs of Stroke

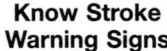

**Know Stroke
Warning Signs**

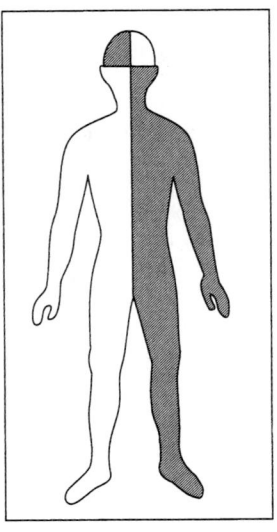

W ooziness or temporary unsteadiness.

A sudden temporary dimness or loss of vision, particularly in one eye.

R ecent, severe headaches or change in pattern of headaches.

N umbness or weakness in face, arm, or leg.

I ncidence of double vision.

N otable, recent change in personality or mental ability.

G arbled speech or trouble understanding speech.

A stroke in one hemisphere of the brain affects the functioning of the opposite side of the body.

Classification of Cerebral Aneurysms

Symptoms of an intracranial hemorrhage include sudden explosive headache, photophobia, neck rigidity (if subarachnoid), nausea and vomiting, loss of consciousness (usually), convulsions, signs and symptoms of increased intracranial pressure, respiratory distress, and shock.

The following system of grading has been developed to classify the clinical state of the client with intracranial bleeding by level of consciousness and neurological deficit.

Grade I—minimal bleeding, alert, no neurological deficit
Grade II—mild bleeding, alert, minimal neurological deficit such as third nerve palsy and stiff neck
Grade III—moderate bleeding, drowsy or confused, stiff neck with or without neurological deficit
Grade IV—moderate or severe bleeding; semicoma with or without neurological deficit
Grade V—severe bleeding, coma, decerebrate movement

Additional grades are added for clients older than 50 years of age and those with major heart, lung, kidney, and liver conditions that increase risk for procedures.

From Phipps WJ et al: *Medical-surgical nursing: concepts and clinical practice,* ed 5, St Louis, 1995, Mosby.

Comparison of Expressive
and Receptive Aphasia

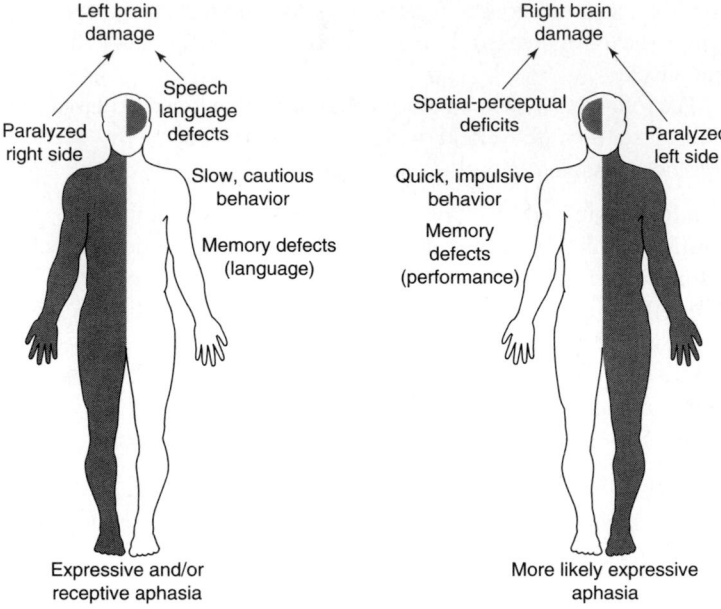

Receptive and expressive aphasia arising from right and left brain damage.

From Ebersole P, Hess P: *Toward healthy aging: human needs and nursing response,* ed 4, St Louis, 1994, Mosby. (Illustration by Joseph Pierre. Modified from Fowler R, Fordyce W: *Stroke: why do they behave that way?* Dallas, 1974, American Heart Association.)

Types of Aphasia

Type	Definition	Site of lesion	Clinical manifestations	Client awareness
Wernicke's	Type of fluent aphasia	Wernicke's area of left hemisphere	Fluent speech with normal and rapid rate; grammar and rhythm are in tact, but with little content to speech Paraphasias, neologisms, and verbal non-words occur	Not aware of mistake
Anomic	Type of fluent aphasia	Area of angular gyrus	Speech is fluent but client cannot name objects or places; may define or describe what he or she is trying to name	Is aware
Conduction	Type of fluent aphasia	Arcuate fasciculus	Speech characterized by literal paraphasia but comprehension is intact	Is aware
Fluent	Impairment of ability to comprehend spoken language or written language			
Nonfluent	Loss of ability to express one's thoughts in speech or writing (motor, Broca's, expressive)	Motor cortex at Broca's area	Problems in selecting, organizing, and initiating motor speech patterns Speech halting, with effort to produce each word Limited vocabulary Telegraphic speech—omission of small grammatic words	Knows what he or she wishes to say and comprehends disability Often frustrated
Global	Occurs with extensive left damage and involves several speech areas Few intact language skills	Several sites	Nonfluent speech, poor comprehension, limited ability to name objects or repeat words	Cannot comprehend world around him or her

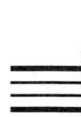

From Phipps WJ et al: *Medical-surgical nursing: concepts and clinical practice*, ed 5, St Louis, 1995, Mosby.

Communicating with Aphasic Clients

- Explain situations, treatments, and anything else that is pertinent to client as he or she may understand; the sounds of normal speech tend to be rehabilitative even if the words are not understood. Talk as if the person understands.
- Avoid patronizing and childish phrases.
- The aphasic client may be especially sensitive to feelings of annoyance; remain calm and patient.
- Speak slowly, ask one question at a time, and wait for a response.
- Ask questions in a way that can be answered with a nod or the blink of an eye; if the client cannot verbally respond instruct him or her in nonverbal responses.
- Speak of things familiar and of interest to client.
- Use visual cues, objects, pictures, and gestures as well as words.
- Organize environment to be as predictable as possible.
- Encourage articulation even if words convey no meaning.
- Show interest in the client as an individual.

From Ebersole P, Hess P: *Toward healthy aging: human needs and nursing response,* ed 4, St Louis, 1994, Mosby.

Precipitating Causes of Hyperosmolar Coma

Clinical Condition	Pharmacologic Agents (Especially in the Elderly)
Myocardial infarction	
Infection	Diuretic
Pancreatitis	Glucocorticoid
Renal failure/dialysis	Beta-blockers
Surgery	Dilantin
Burns	Diazoxide
Hyperalimentation	Immunosuppressants
Thyrotoxicosis	Mannitol

From Bergenstal R: Acute and chronic complications of diabetes, *Caring* 3(11), 1988.

Comparison of Delirium, Depression, and Dementia

	Delirium	Depression	Dementia
Onset	Rapid (hours to days)	Rapid (weeks to months)	Gradual (years)
Course	Wide fluctuations; may continue for weeks if cause not found	May be self-limited or may become chronic without treatment	Chronic; slow but continuous decline
Level of consciousness	Fluctuates from hyperalert to difficult to arouse	Normal	Normal
Orientation	Client is disoriented, confused	Client may seem disoriented	Client is disoriented, confused
Affect	Fluctuating	Sad, depressed, worried, guilty	Labile; apathy in later stages
Attention	Always impaired	Difficulty concentrating; client may check and recheck all actions	May be intact; client may focus on one thing for long periods
Sleep	Always disturbed	Disturbed; excess sleeping or insomnia, especially early-morning waking	Usually normal
Behavior	Agitated, restless	Client may be fatigued, apathetic; may occasionally be agitated	Client may be agitated or apathetic; may wander
Speech	Sparse or rapid; client may be incoherent	Flat, sparse, may have outbursts; understandable	Sparse or rapid; repetitive; client may be incoherent
Memory	Impaired, especially for recent events	Varies day to day; slow recall; often short-term deficit	Impaired, especially for recent events

From Holt J: *Am J Nurs* 93:32, 1993.

Continued.

Comparison of Delirium, Depression, and Dementia—cont'd

	Delirium	Depression	Dementia
Cognition	Disordered reasoning	May seem impaired	Disordered reasoning and calculation
Thought content	Incoherent, confused, delusions, stereotyped	Negative, hypochondriac, thoughts of death, paranoid	Disorganized, rich content, delusional, paranoid
Perception	Misinterpretations, illusions, hallucinations	Distorted; client may have auditory hallucinations; negative interpretation of people and events	No change
Judgment	Poor	Poor	Poor; socially inappropriate behavior
Insight	May be present in lucid moments	May be impaired	Absent
Performance on mental status exams	Poor but variable; improves during lucid moments and with recovery	Memory impaired; calculation, drawing, following directions usually not impaired; frequent "I don't know" answers	Consistently poor; progressively worsens; client attempts to answer all questions

The Four Phases of Alzheimer's Disease

Phase	Observable changes
I	Onset is insidious.
	Spontaneity, energy, and initiative are decreased; slowness is increased.
	Word-finding is difficult.
	Learning times and reacting are slower.
	Anger is easier.
	Familiarity is sought and preferred.
II	Supervision with detailed activities such as banking is needed.
	Speech and understanding are much slower.
	Train of thought is lost.
III	Personality change is marked (can be depressed).
	Directions must be specific and repeated for safety.
	Recent memory is poor.
	Disorientation is easy.
	People are incorrectly identified.
	Behavior is lethargic.
IV	Apathy is noticeable.
	Memory is poor or absent.
	Person can't be alone.
	Urinary incontinence is present.
	Individuals aren't recognized.

From Edelman CL, Mandle CL: *Health promotion throughout the lifespan,* ed 3, St Louis, 1994, Mosby.

Criteria for Clinical Diagnosis of Alzheimer's Disease

I.   The criteria for the clinical diagnosis of *probable* Alzheimer's disease include the following:

Dementia established by clinical examination and documented by the Mini-Mental Test, Blessed Dementia Scale, or some similar examination, and confirmed by neuropsychological tests

Deficits in two or more areas of cognition

Progressive worsening of memory and other cognitive functions

No disturbance of consciousness

Onset between ages 40 and 90, most often after age 65

Absence of systemic disorders or other brain diseases that in and of themselves could account for the progressive deficits in memory and cognition

II.   The diagnosis of *probable* Alzheimer's disease is supported by the following:

Progressive deterioration of specific cognitive functions such as language (aphasia), motor skills (apraxia), and perception (agnosia)

Impaired activities of daily living and altered patterns of behavior

Family history of similar disorders, particularly if confirmed neuropathologically

Laboratory results of normal lumbar puncture as evaluated by standard techniques; normal pattern or nonspecific changes in EEG, such as increased slow-wave activity; and evidence of cerebral atrophy on CT with progression documented by serial observation

III. Other clinical features consistent with the diagnosis of *probable* Alzheimer's disease, after exclusion of causes of dementia other than Alzheimer's disease, include the following:

Plateaus in the course of progression of the illness

Associated symptoms of depression, insomnia, incontinence, delusions, illusions, hallucinations, catastrophic verbal, emo-

From McKhann G et al: Clinical diagnosis of Alzheimer's disease: a report of the NINCDS-ADRDA work group under the auspices of the Department of Health and Human Services Task Force on Alzheimer's disease, *Neurology* 34:940, 1984.

tional, or physical outbursts, sexual disorders, and weight loss

Other neurological abnormalities in some clients, especially with more advanced disease and including motor signs such as increased muscle tone, myoclonus, or gait disorder

Seizures in advanced disease

CT normal for age

IV.   Features that make the diagnosis of *probable* Alzheimer's disease uncertain or unlikely include the following:

Sudden, apoplectic onset

Focal neurological findings such as hemiparesis, sensory loss, visual field deficits, and incoordination early in the course of the illness

Seizures or gait disturbances at the onset or very early in the course of the illness

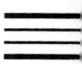

V.   Clinical diagnosis of *possible* Alzheimer's disease:

May be made on the basis of the dementia syndrome, in the absence of other neurological, psychiatric, or systemic disorders sufficient to cause dementia, and in the presence of variations in the onset, in the presentation, or in the clinical course

May be made in the presence of a second systemic or brain disorder sufficient to produce dementia, which is not considered to be *the* cause of the dementia

Should be used in research studies when a single, gradually progressive severe cognitive deficit is identified in the absence of other identifiable cause

VI.   Criteria for diagnosis of *definite* Alzheimer's disease are as follows:

The clinical criteria for probable Alzheimer's disease

Histopathologic evidence obtained from a biopsy or autopsy

VII.   Classification of Alzheimer's disease for research purposes should specify features that may differentiate subtypes of the disorder, such as the following:

Familial occurrence

Onset before age of 65

Presence of trisomy-21

Coexistence of other relevant conditions, such as Parkinson's disease

Characteristics of Seizures

Etiology	Characteristics	Clinical signs	Aura	Postictal period
Grand mal				
Most common type	Generalized, characterized by loss of consciousness for several minutes	Aura Cry Loss of consciousness Fall Tonic-clonic movements Incontinence	Present Flashing lights Smells Spots before eyes Dizziness	Present Need for sleep for 1 to 2 hr Headache common
Petit mal				
Usually occurs during childhood and adolescence Frequency decreases as child gets older	Sudden impairment in or loss of consciousness with little or no tonic-clonic movement Occurs without warning Has tendency to appear a few hours after arising or when person is quiet	Sudden vacant facial expression with eyes focused straight ahead All motor activity ceases except perhaps for slight symmetric twitching about eyelids Possible loss of muscle tone Consciousness returns	None	None

Psychomotor				
Occurs at any age	Sudden change in awareness associated with complex distortion of feeling and thinking and partially coordinated motor activity Longer than petit mal	Behaves as if partially conscious Often appears intoxicated May perform antisocial acts such as exposing self or carrying out violent acts Autonomic complaints may occur: Chest pain Respiratory distress Tachycardia Gastrointestinal distress Urinary incontinence	Present Complex hallucinations or illusions	Present Confusion Amnesia Need for sleep
Jacksonian, or focal				
Occurs almost entirely in clients with structural brain disease	Depends on site of focus May or may not be progressive	Typically begins in hand, foot, or face May end in grand mal seizure	Present Numbness Tingling Crawling feeling	Present

Continued.

From Phipps WJ et al: *Medical-surgical nursing: concepts and clinical practice*, ed 5, St Louis, 1995, Mosby.

Characteristics of Seizures—cont'd

Etiology	Characteristics	Clinical signs	Aura	Postictal period
Myoclonic May antedate grand mal by months or years	May be very mild or may cause rapid, forceful movements	Sudden involuntary contraction of muscle group, usually in extremities or trunk No loss of consciousness	None	None
Akinetic Uncommon	Peculiar generalized tonelessness	Person falls in flaccid state Unconscious for 1 or 2 min	Rarely present	None

Common Causes of
Transient Urinary Incontinence

Potential causes	Comment
Delirium (confusional state)	In the delirious client, incontinence is usually an associated symptom that will abate with proper diagnosis and treatment of the underlying cause of confusion.
Infection (symptomatic urinary tract infection)	Dysuria and urgency from symptomatic infection may defeat the older person's ability to reach the toilet in time. Asymptomatic infection, although more common than symptomatic infection, is rarely a cause of incontinence.
Atrophic urethritis or vaginitis	Atrophic urethritis may present as dysuria, dyspareunia, burning on urination, urgency, agitation (in demented clients), and occasionally as incontinence. Both disorders are readily treated by conjugated estrogen administered either orally (0.3 to 1.25 mg/day) or locally (2 g or fraction/day).
Pharmaceuticals	
Sedative hypnotics	Benzodiazepines, especially long-acting agents such as flurazepam and diazepam, may accumulate in elderly clients and cause confusion and secondary incontinence. Alcohol, frequently used as a sedative, can cloud the sensorium, impair mobility, and induce a diuresis, resulting in incontinence.
Diuretics	A brisk diuresis induced by loop diuretics can overwhelm bladder capacity and lead to polyuria, frequency, and urgency, thereby precipitating incontinence in a frail older person. The loop diuretics include furosemide, ethacrynic acid, and bumetanide.

From DHHS, PNS, AHCPR: *Urinary incontinence in adults: the quick reference guide for clinicians,* Publication #AHCRR 92-0041, Rockville, Md, 1992.

Continued.

Common Causes of
Transient Urinary Incontinence—cont'd

Potential causes	Comment
Anticholinergic agents Antihistamines Antidepressants Antipsychotics Disopnamide Opiates Antispasmodics (dicyclomine and Donnatal) Anti-parkinsonian agents (trihexyphenidyl and benztropine mesylate)	Nonprescription (over-the-counter) agents with anticholinergic properties are taken commonly by older clients for insomnia, coryza, pruritus, and vertigo, and many prescription medications also have anticholinergic properties. Anticholinergic side effects include urinary retention with associated urinary frequency and overflow incontinence. Besides anticholinergic actions, antipsychotics such as thioridazine and haloperidol may cause sedation, rigidity, and immobility.
Alpha-adrenergic agents Sympathomimetics (decongestants) Sympatholytics (e.g., prazosin, terazosin, and doxazosin)	Sphincter tone in the proximal urethra can be decreased by alpha antagonists and increased by alpha agonists. An older woman, whose urethra is shortened and weakened with age, may develop stress incontinence when taking an alpha antagonist for hypertension. An older man with prostate enlargement may develop acute urinary retention and overflow incontinence when taking multicomponent "cold" capsules, which contain alpha agonists and anticholinergic agents, especially if a nasal decongestant and a nonprescription hypnotic antihistamine are added.
Calcium-channel blockers	Calcium-channel blockers can reduce smooth muscle contractility in the bladder and occasionally can cause urinary retention and overflow incontinence.
Psychological	Severe depression may occasionally be associated with incontinence, but is probably less frequently a cause in older clients.

Potential causes	Comment
Excessive urine production	Excess intake, endocrine conditions that cloud the sensorium and induce a diuresis (e.g., hypercalcemia, hyperglycemia, and diabetes insipidus); expanded volume states such as congestive heart failure, lower extremity venous insufficiency, drug-induced ankle edema (e.g., nifedipine, indomethacin); and low albumen states cause polyuria and can lead to incontinence.
Restricted mobility	Limited mobility is an aggravating or precipitating cause of incontinence that can frequently be corrected or improved by treating the underlying condition (e.g., arthritis, poor eyesight, Parkinson's disease, or orthostatic hypotension). A urinal or bedside commode and scheduled toileting often help resolve the incontinence that results from hospitalization and its environmental barriers (e.g., bed rails, restraints, and poor lighting).
Stool impaction	Clients with stool impaction have either urge or overflow incontinence and may have fecal incontinence as well. Disimpaction restores continence.

Types of Urinary Incontinence

Description	Causes	Symptoms
Total		
Total uncontrolled and continuous loss of urine	Neuropathy of sensory nerves; trauma or disease of spinal nerves or urethral sphincter; fistula between bladder and vagina	Constant flow of urine at unpredictable times, nocturia, unawareness of bladder filling or incontinence
Functional		
Involuntary, unpredictable passage of urine in client with intact urinary and nervous systems	Change in environment; sensory, cognitive, or mobility deficits	Strong urge to void that causes loss of urine before reaching appropriate receptacle
Stress		
Increased intraabdominal pressure that causes leakage of small amount of urine	Coughing, laughing, vomiting, or lifting with full bladder; obesity; full uterus in third trimester; incompetent bladder outlet; weak pelvic musculature	Dribbling of urine with increased intraabdominal pressure, urinary urgency and frequency
Urge		
Involuntary passage of urine after strong sense of urgency to void	Decreased bladder capacity; irritation of bladder stretch receptors; alcohol or caffeine ingestion; increased fluid intake	Urinary urgency, abdominal frequency (more often than every 2 hr), bladder contracture or spasm, nocturia, voiding in small (less than 100 ml) or large (more than 550 ml) amounts
Reflex or overflow		
Involuntary loss of urine occurring at somewhat predictable intervals when specific bladder volume is reached	Upper spinal cord injury or disease involving area above reflex arc, blocking cerebral awareness Lower spinal cord injury blocking impulses to reflex arc	Unawareness of bladder filling, lack of urge to void, uninhibited bladder contraction or spasm at regular intervals

Elements of an Incontinence Assessment

History	Details of present problem
	Medical history
	Surgical history
	Urological procedures/problems
	Dietary and bowel patterns
	Fluid intake
Environmental review	Location of toilet facility
	Assistive devices needed
	Factors that impede (rugs, stairs, layout of living area)
Medications	
Physical examination with limited neurological examination	Gross motor functions
	Fine motor movement
	Mental status
	Rectal tone
	Presence/absence fecal impaction
Females	Inspection outer perineal area
	Look for pelvic descent
	Internal examination
Males	Check prostate
Functional examination	Determine mobility; ability to handle devices
	Observe clothing, how client manages now—*important to see how individual functions*
Urinalysis	Detect associated conditions such as hematuria, glycosuria, proteinuria, bacteria or white cells

From *Clinical practice guidelines: urinary incontinence in adults,* USDHHS, AHCPR, Rockville, Md, 1992.

Elements of a Supplemental
Urinary Incontinence Assessment

Use of a voiding record
Evaluation of environmental and social factors
Observing voiding
Blood tests
Urine cytology
Urodynamic tests
Endoscopic tests
Imaging tests of upper tract and/or lower tract with and without voiding

From *Clinical practice guidelines: urinary incontinence in adults,* USDHHS, AHCPR, Rockville, Md, 1992.

Assessment of Bowel Function

Premorbid elimination pattern and practices
Elimination pattern for past 2 weeks (usual time, frequency, consistency)
Usual diet
Fluid intake
Activity level and mobility
Current medications
Medical conditions affecting elimination
Neurological impairment
Cognitive perceptual deficits
Communication deficits
Physical assessment bowel sounds, palpation, rectal exam, testing of perianal sensation and reflexes
Client preference

From Hennig L, May L: Rehabilitation in the home. In Martinson I, Widmer J, editors: *Home health care nursing,* Philadelphia, 1989, Saunders.

Causes of Fecal Incontinence

Abnormal delivery of feces to rectum

Drug-induced (that is, cathartics, antibiotics, and so forth)
Metabolic (that is, diabetic diarrhea)
Blind loop syndrome
Inflammatory bowel disease
Infectious disease
Celiac sprue

Sphincter dysfunction

Trauma (disruption of nerves or musculature, surgical or obstetric trauma, or injury)
Radiation proctitis
Diabetes mellitus
Inflammatory bowel disease

Reduced rectal compliance

Rectal ischemia and fibrosis
Fecal impaction
Proctitis (inflammatory, infectious, or radiation-induced)
Infiltrating diseases or malignancy
Hirschsprung's disease

From Hanauer SB, Sable KS: Pathology of fecal incontinence. In Doughty DB, editor: *Urinary and fecal incontinence: nursing management,* St Louis, 1991, Mosby.

Anatomic derangement

Obstetric or surgical trauma
Injury
Congenital malformations of anorectum
Inflammatory bowel disease (that is, fistula, abscess, or perianal disease)
Rectal prolapse
Third-degree hemorrhoids
Tumor

Neurological impairment

Central nervous system
   Stroke
   Trauma
   Tumor
   Degenerative disease (that is, dementia)
   Encephalopathy
   Mental retardation
   Psychiatric disorders (that is, depressive disorders)
   Drug reaction or intoxication
Spinal
   Multiple sclerosis
   Tumor
   Trauma
   Meningomyelocele (spina bifida)
   Degenerative disease (that is, severe vitamin B_{12} deficiency)
Peripheral nervous system
   Diabetes (polyneuropathy)
   Shy-Drager syndrome
   Tabes dorsalis
   Cauda equina lesions
   Guillain-Barré syndrome
   Toxic neuropathy
   Idiopathic fecal incontinence
   Perineal descent syndrome

Muscular and neuromuscular disorders

Congenital or hereditary myopathy
Myasthenia gravis
Idiopathic fecal incontinence
Perineal descent syndrome

Behavioral and developmental dysfunctions

Childhood encopresis
Mental retardation
Psychiatric disorders (rarely)

Fecal Incontinence Assessment

History

Characteristics of incontinence
Relevant medical history
Medication review
Diet history
Activity patterns
Client/caregiver perception
Environmental characteristics

Physical examination

Abdomen
Neurological
Rectal

Functional assessment of mobility status

Bowel record (1 week)

Laboratory and other tests as needed

From Ebersole P, Hess P: *Toward healthy aging: human needs and nursing response,* ed 4, St Louis, 1994, Mosby.

Notes

Types of Skin Lesions

Observed skin changes	Differentiation	Term	Example
Change in color or texture			
Spot	Circumscribed; flat; color change	Macule	Freckle
Discoloration (reddish purple)	Bleeding beneath the surface; injury to tissue	Contusion	Bruise
Soft whitening	Caused by repeated wetting of skin	Maceration	Between toes after soaking
Flake	Dry cells of surface	Scale	Dandruff; psoriasis
Roughness from dried fluid	Dry exudate over lesions	Crust	Eczema, impetigo
Roughness from cells	Leathery thickening of outer skin layer	Lichenification	Callus on foot
Change in shape			
Fluid-filled lesions	Less than 1 cm; clear fluid	Vesicle	Blister; chickenpox
	Greater than 1 cm; clear fluid	Bulla	Large blister; pemphigus
	Small, thick yellowish fluid (pus)	Pustule	Acne
Solid mass, *cellular* growth	Less than 5 mm	Papule	Small mole; raised rash
	5 mm to 2 cm	Nodule	Enlarged lymph node
	Greater than 2 cm	Tumor	Benign or malignant tumor
	Excess connective tissue over scar	Keloid	Overgrown scar
Swelling of tissue	Generalized swelling; fluid between cells	Edema	Inflammation; swelling of feet
	Circumscribed surface edema; transient; some itching	Wheal ("hive")	Allergic reaction

From Long BC: Assessment of the skin. In Phipps WJ et al, editors: *Medical-surgical nursing: concepts and clinical practice,* ed 5, St Louis, 1995, Mosby.

Continued.

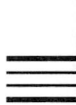

Types of Skin Lesions—cont'd

Observed skin changes	Differentiation	Term	Example
Breaks in skin surfaces			
Oozing, scraped surface	Loss of superficial structure of skin	Abrasion	"Floor burn"; scrape
Scooped-out depression	Loss of deeper layers of skin	Ulcer	Decubitus or stasis ulcer
Superficial linear skin breaks	Scratch marks, frequently by fingernails	Excoriations	Scratching
Linear cracks or cleft	Slit or splitting of skin layers	Fissure	Athlete's foot
Jagged cut	Tearing of skin surface	Laceration	Accidental cut by blunt object
Linear cut, edges approximated	Cutting by sharp instrument	Incision	Knife cut
Vascular lesions			
Small, flat, round, purplish, red spot	Intradermal or submucous hemorrhage	Petechia	Bleeding tendency; vitamin C deficiency
Spiderlike, red, small	Dilation of capillaries, arterioles, or venules	Telangiectasis	Liver disease, vitamin B deficiency
Discoloration, reddish purple	Escape of blood into tissue	Ecchymosis	Trauma to blood vessels

Characteristics of Pressure Sores

Anatomical Terms

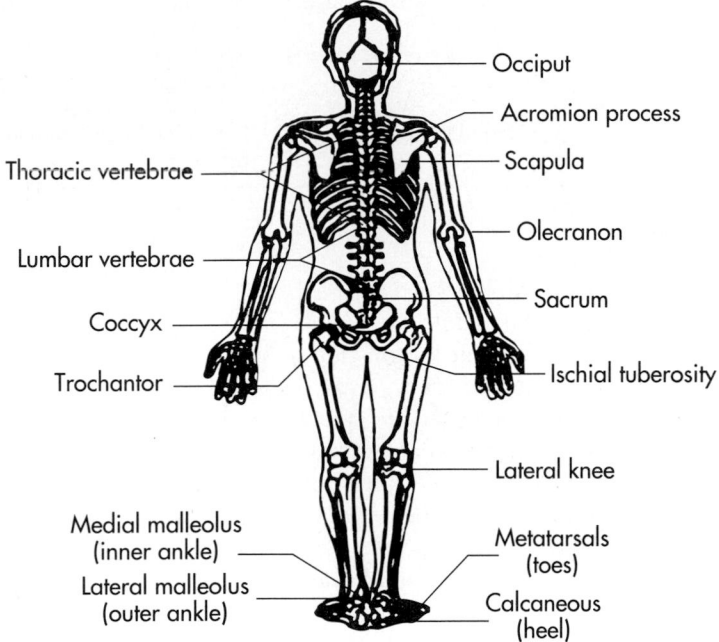

Occiput
Acromion process
Scapula
Thoracic vertebrae
Olecranon
Lumbar vertebrae
Sacrum
Coccyx
Trochantor
Ischial tuberosity
Lateral knee
Medial malleolus (inner ankle)
Metatarsals (toes)
Lateral malleolus (outer ankle)
Calcaneous (heel)

Pressure Sore Assessment

- Location
- Dimensions
- Stage
- Exudate: color, consistency, amount
- Condition: base, surrounding skin, sinus tracts
- Signs or symptoms: local versus systemic odor

Interventions

- Pressure relief devices turn schedule
- Nutritional support
- Cleansing
- Treatment
- Teaching

From *Medicare home health agency manual,* Health Care Financing Administration, Transmittal No 203, December 1987.

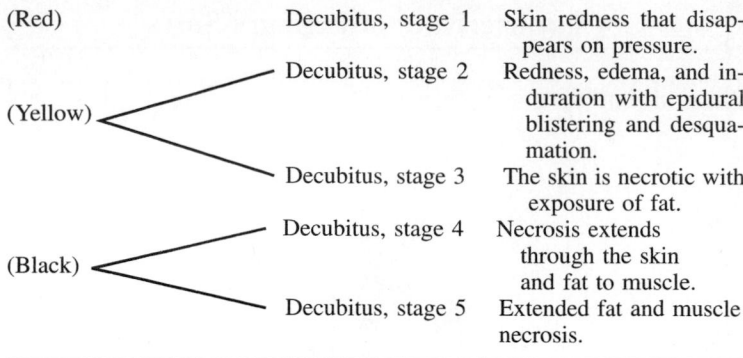

(Red)	Decubitus, stage 1	Skin redness that disappears on pressure.
(Yellow)	Decubitus, stage 2	Redness, edema, and induration with epidural blistering and desquamation.
	Decubitus, stage 3	The skin is necrotic with exposure of fat.
(Black)	Decubitus, stage 4	Necrosis extends through the skin and fat to muscle.
	Decubitus, stage 5	Extended fat and muscle necrosis.

Prevention

- Inspect the skin daily in good light.
- Keep the skin clean and dry.
- Consult a nutritionist for information on proper nutrition.
- Help the client exercise joints, arms, and legs, if possible.
- Turn the client often (every ½ hour to every 2 or more hours, depending on the person's condition), or arrange a trapeze over the bed to enable the person to shift positions.
- Use a footboard and keep the bed at less than a 30-degree angle to prevent "shearing" (damage from the skin being stretched and torn from sliding down the bed or wheelchair).
- Use pull and draw sheets for turning or lifting.
- Make sure bed linen is smooth and soft, without crumbs, wrinkles, or folds to irritate the skin.
- Contact a medical supply dealer for information on pressure- and friction-relieving products, such as sheepskin, elbow and heel protectors, cushions, and pads that provide equal weight and pressure distribution for wheelchair users.

Pressure Sore Risk Assessment

Norton Scale

A Physical condition	B Mental state	C Activity	D Mobility	E Incontinence	Total score
4 Good	4 Alert	4 Ambulant	4 Full	4 Not	
3 Fair	3 Apathetic	3 Walks with help	3 Slightly limited	3 Occasional	
2 Poor	2 Confused	2 Chairbound	2 Very limited	2 Usually urine	
1 Bad	1 Stupor	1 Bedrest	1 Immobile	1 Double incontinence	

Norton Plus Scale

(For determining high risk for pressure sores)

Check ONLY if YES   <u>YES</u>

Diagnosis of diabetes   _____

Diagnosis of hypertension   _____

Hematocrit (M) <41%   _____

      (F) <36%

Hemoglobin (M) <14 g/dl   _____

      (F) <12 g/dl

Albumin level <3.3 g/dl   _____

Febrile >99.6°F   _____

5 or more medications   _____

Changes in mental status to confused, lethargic within 24 hours   _____

TOTAL Number of Checkmarks

Norton Scale Score   _____

Minus total from above   _____

Norton Plus Score   _____

From Norton D, McLaren R, Exton-Smith AN: *An investigation of geriatric nursing problems in hospital*, Edinburgh, 1975, Churchill Livingstone. Maximum score = 20 (good physical condition); minimum score = 5; high risk for pressure ulcers = 12 or below.

Diagnostic tests

There are no specific laboratory tests to assist with diagnosis of pressure sores. Related laboratory examinations pertinent to risk factors have been included in the previous discussion of risk factors.

Medication

There are no particular medications for pressure ulcers. Antibiotics are used if an infection is present.

Treatment

More than 100 products exist as purported treatment measures for pressure sores.

Diet

Clients with wounds require additional protein and calorie intake to assist with tissue regeneration on a cellular level. A well-balanced diet is sufficient to maintain healthy skin; however, most clients with any identified risk factors are not eating a well-balanced diet. Protein supplementation in balanced amounts is helpful. Only a registered dietitian can determine accurately a balance of demand and replacement that will be therapeutic for the client. Research also suggests that supplemental vitamin C and zinc, as well as a multiple vitamin with iron, are all helpful agents to stimulate wound healing on a cellular level.

Activity

The more independently active the client is, the lower the risk of pressure sore formation and the greater the chances of wound healing. If the client is unable to assume an active role in mobility, it *must* be assumed by the nurse for the client. The key factor related to wound healing is the removal of the causative agent(s). Regardless of the treatment prescribed for wound care, if the pressure is not relieved by the client or passively by the nurse, wound healing will not occur.

From Phipps WJ et al: *Medical-surgical nursing: concepts and clinical practice,* ed 5, St Louis, 1995, Mosby.

Referral/Consultation

In some settings the nurse assumes responsibility for making referrals to other services. Many disciplines have become involved with wound healing modalities. Physical therapists receive some education about wound healing. Nurses and physicians receive minimal education about products and principles of wound healing. A nursing specialty has evolved over the past 25 years called *enterostomal therapy (ET) nursing*. ET nurses are nationally recognized as leaders in the wound care arena and are an active part of the NPUAP. If your institution does not have an ET nurse on staff, the Wound, Ostomy and Continence Nurses Society in California can refer you to the closest person by calling 714-476-0268.

Pressure Sore Products Identified by Categories, Examples, and Manufacturers

Category	Example	Manufacturer
Exudate absorption		
Dextronomer beads	Debrisan	Johnson & Johnson Medical, Inc.
Copolymer starch dressings	Absorption dressing Duoderm granules	Bard ConvaTec
Calcium alginates (absorb exudate, as well as release calcium on a cellular level—stimulates angiogenesis)	Kaltostat Sorbsan Algosteril	Calgon Vestal Laboratories Dow B. Hickman, Inc. Johnson & Johnson Medical, Inc.
Debridement		
Enzymatic	Elase ointment Travase Santyl Panafil Biozyme C	Parke-Davis Flint Knoll Pharmaceuticals Rystan Pharmaceuticals Armour Pharmaceuticals
Wet-to-dry dressings*	Gauze in many forms (4 × 4, kerlex)	Multiple manufacturers

From Phipps WJ et al: *Medical-surgical nursing: concepts and clinical practice,* ed 5, St Louis, 1995, Mosby.

NOTE: Research suggests that wounds heal most effectively if there is a moist, natural environment, with a clean, debris- and necrotic-free wound area. Dressings and interventions are all designed with these principles in mind. Several have other added benefits that are discussed separately within each category.

*Solutions used vary according to preference of physician; most common solution is normal saline.

Continued.

Pressure Sore Products Identified by
Categories, Examples, and Manufacturers—cont'd

Category	Example	Manufacturer
Wound protection, insulation and mild absorption		
Hydrocolloids (waxy pectin adhesive dressings that provide an optimal wound environment)	Duoderm Restore Tegasorb Ultec	ConvaTec Hollister, Inc. 3M Health Care Sherwood Medical
Transparent dressings (thin, adhesive dressings that support the microenvironment for cellular regeneration)	Tegaderm Bioclusive OpSite Acu-Derm Polyskin	3M Health Care Johnson & Johnson Medical, Inc. Smith & Nephew United, Inc. Acme United Corp. Kendall Healthcare
Polyurethane foam dressings (nonadhesive; some assist with odor control)	Allevyn Lyofoam EpiLock	Smith & Nephew United, Inc. Acme United Corp. Calgon Vestal Laboratories
Hydrogel dressings (nonadherent; have a topical soothing effect; varied in thickness)	Elasto-Gel Vigilon Second Skin	Southwest Technologies Bard Patient Care Spenco

Screening for Common Orthopedic Problems in Infancy and Childhood

Deformity	Screening
Congenital hip dislocation (CHD)	
Complete or partial displacement of femoral head out of the acetabulum.	Barlow's maneuver (for dislocation of femoral head): flex hip to 90 degrees; grasp symphysis in front and sacrum in back with one hand; with other hand, apply lateral pressure to medial thigh with thumb and longitudinal pressure to knee with palm; abduct flexed hip. A positive sign is sensation of abnormal movement. Reverse hands for examining other hip. See Fig. 2.

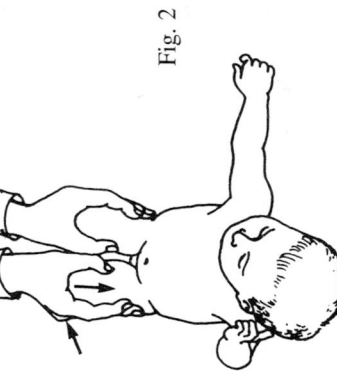

Fig. 2

From Stanhope M, Lancaster J: *Community health nursing: promoting health of aggregates, families, and individuals*, ed 4, St Louis, 1996, Mosby.

Continued.

Screening for Common Orthopedic Problems in Infancy and Childhood—cont'd

Deformity	Screening
Congenital hip dislocation (CHD)—cont'd Complete or partial displacement of femoral head out of the acetabulum—cont'd.	Ortolani's maneuver (for reduction of femur): abduct hip to 80 degrees, lifting proximal femur anteriorly with fingers placed on lateral thigh. A positive sign is sensation of a jerk or snap with reduction into socket. See Fig. 3. Limited full abduction of hips: with child flat on back, abduct hips one at a time, then together. See Fig. 4 for degrees of hip abduction. Apparent shortening of femur: 1. Allis' sign: with child lying on back, pelvis flat, knees flexed and feet planted firmly, observe knees. If the knee projects further anteriorly, femur is longer; if one knee is higher, the tibia is longer. 2. With child on back, both legs are extended out with pressure on knees. Heels are matched and observed for equal or unequal length. 3. Trendelenburg sign: with child standing on one leg, observe pelvis. When child stands on abnormal leg, the pelvis drops on normal side. See Fig. 5.
Metatarsus adductus (varus) Adduction or turning in of forefoot with high longitudinal arch and wide space between first and seond toes. Commonly associated with tibial torsion.	Test foot for flexibility and elicit tonic foot reflexes. Rigidity is indicated by eversion or inversion when foot does not move beyond neutral position or does not respond to toe grasping or by dorsiflexing. Signs of metatarsus adductus are illustrated in Fig. 6.

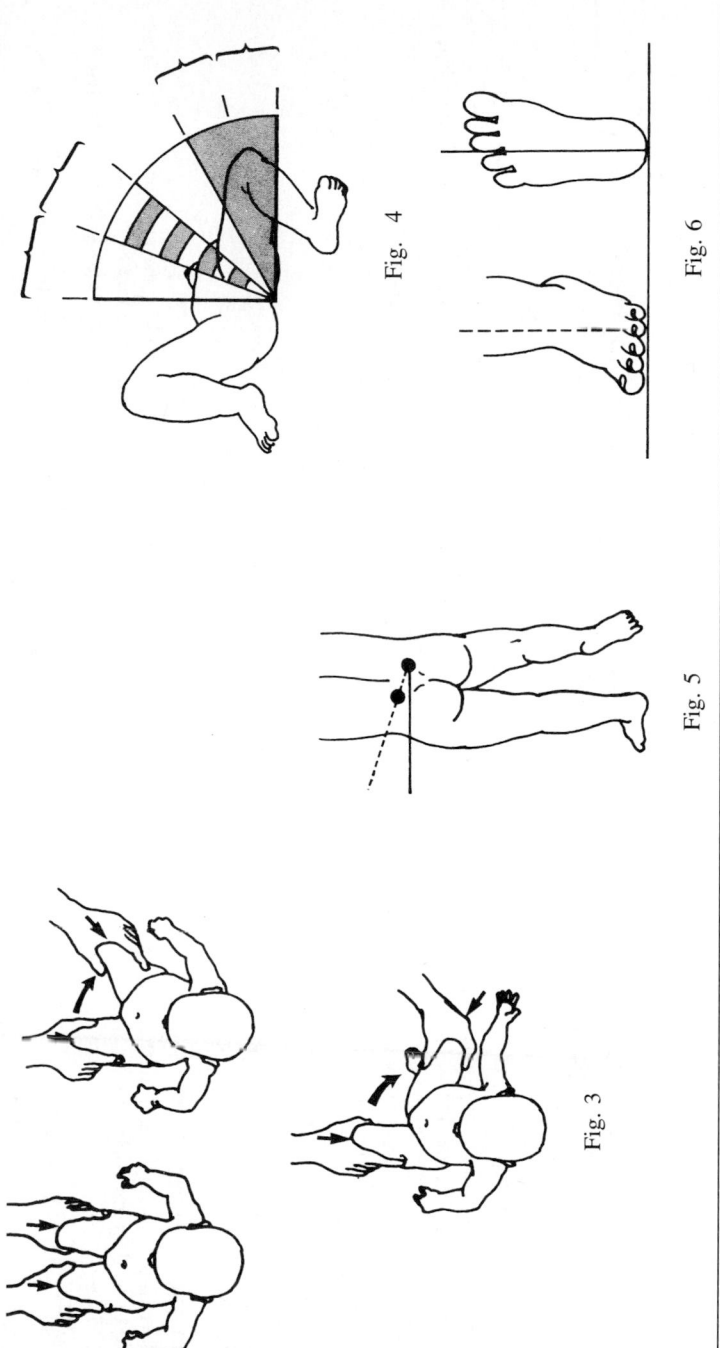

Fig. 3

Fig. 4

Fig. 5

Fig. 6

Continued.

Screening for Common Orthopedic Problems in Infancy and Childhood—cont'd

Deformity	Screening
Pes planus (flat feet)	
When child is weight bearing, longitudinal arch of foot appears flat on floor.	1. Observe feet in weighted and unweighted position.
1. Pseudo flat feet: very common until ages 2 to 3; created by plantar fat pad. Feet are flexible, exhibit hypermobility of joint, and have a low arch.	2. Stand child on toes. Arch disappears with weight bearing in flexible flat foot and reappears when on toes. See Fig. 7.
	3. Elicit dorsal and plantar flexion to rule out tight heel cord.
	4. Elicit eversion and inversion flexion to rule out tarsal coalition.
2. Rigid flat feet: uncommon; created by tightness of heel cord or tarsal coalition (a cartilaginous fibrous or bony connection between bones).	Same as for preceding No. 1 (pseudo flat feet).
Genu valgum (knock-knees)	
A deviant axis of thighs and calves of more than 10 to 15 degrees; (normal from ages 2 to 6).	1. Observe axis of thighs and calves with child standing. Normally axis are parallel with 10 to 15 degrees deviance. See Fig. 8.
	2. Observe space between the knees from front to back. Normal spacing is 1½ inches.
	3. Observe space between ankles from front and back. Normal spacing between medial malleoli at heel is 2 inches.

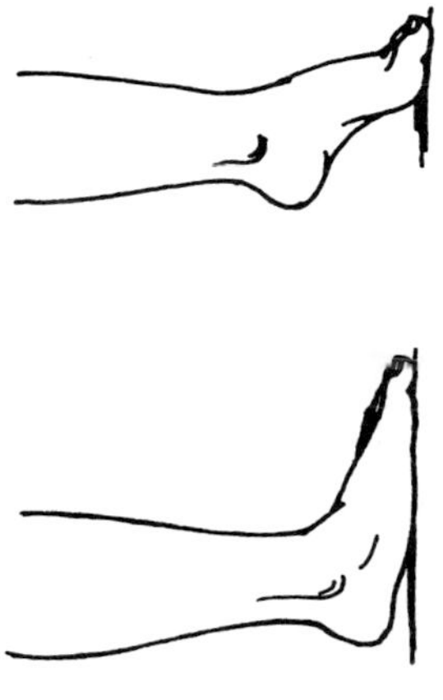

Fig. 7

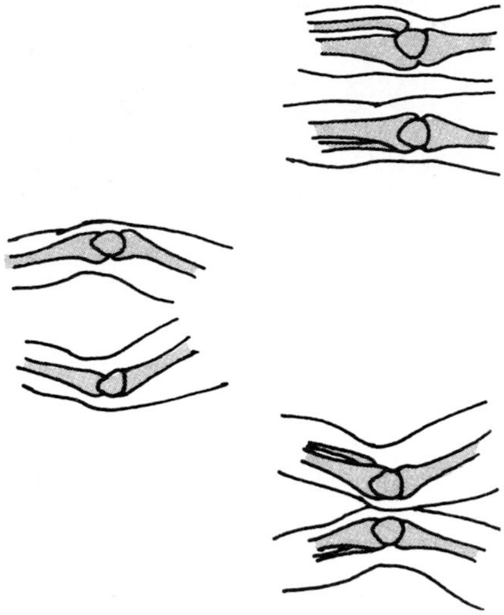

Fig. 8

Continued.

Screening for Common Orthopedic Problems in Infancy and Childhood—cont'd

Deformity	Screening
Genu varum (bowlegs)	Same for genu valgum.
Deviant axis of thighs and calves.	
1. Physiological: normal until ages 2 to 3; occurs with internal tibial torsion and genu valgum.	
2. Pathological.	
Internal tibial torsion	1. Examine legs for range of motion, flexibility of ankle and elicit tonic foot reflexes.
Twisting or torsion of tibia usually accompanied by metatarsus adductus.	2. Holding knee firmly with foot in neutral position, observe medial and lateral malleoli. The normal angle between them is approximately 15 to 20 degrees. See Fig. 9.
	3. Have child sit on examining table and draw a circle over patellar and external malleoli. With patella facing forward only anterior edge of malleolar circle should be seen. See Fig. 10.
Scoliosis	Screening is implemented as follows:
S-shaped lateral curvature of spine with rotation of vertical bodies.	1. Ask the child to bend forward in a 50% flexing position with shoulders drooping forward, arms and head dangling. Observe the spine from above the head and inspect for any lateral curvature or prominent projection of the rib cage on one side. See Fig. 11.

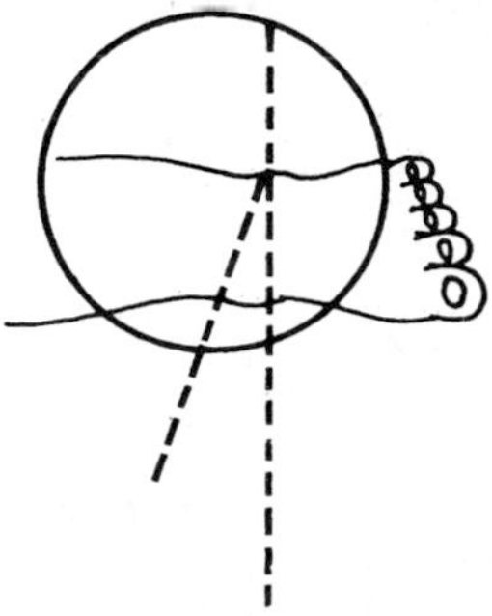

Fig. 11

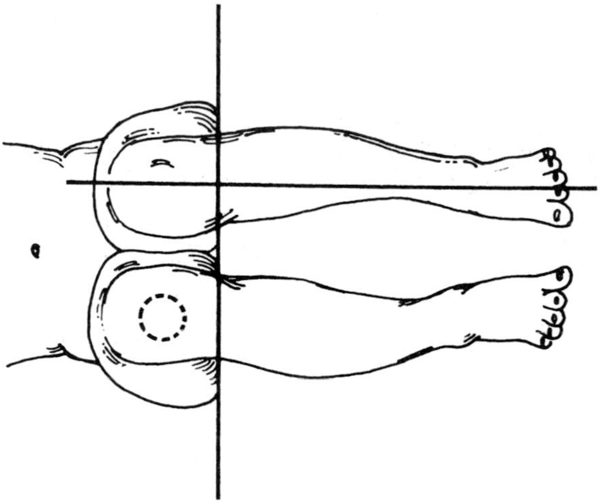

Fig. 10

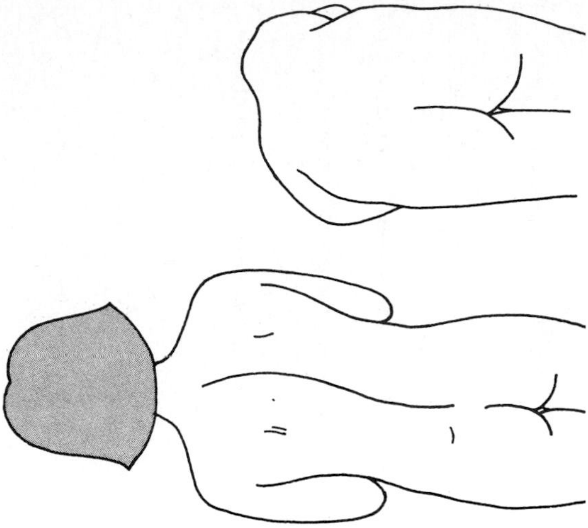

Fig. 9

Continued.

Screening for Common Orthopedic Problems in Infancy and Childhood—cont'd

Deformity	Screening

Scoliosis—cont'd
S-shaped lateral curvature of spine with rotation of vertical bodies—cont'd.
	2. While the child is standing erect with weight equal on both feet, observe for:
	    difference in levels of shoulders, scapula, and hips.
	    differences in the size of the spaces between the arms and the trunk.
	    prominence of either scapula or hip.
	    a curve in the vertebral spinous process alignment.
	3. Ask the child to walk and make observations discussed in No. 2 and observe for the presence of a waddle, limp, or tilt.

Example of a Grading System for Muscle Strength in Immobile Elderly Clients

Grade		Observed strength
Normal	5	
Good	4	Muscle produces movements against gravity and can overcome some resistance
Fair	3	Muscle produces movements against gravity but cannot overcome any resistance
Poor	2	Muscle produces movements but not against gravity
Trace	1	Muscle tightens but cannot produce movement, even after gravity is eliminated
None	0	Muscle does not contract at all

From Kane R et al: *Essentials of clinical geriatrics,* ed 3, New York, 1994, McGraw-Hill.

Signs and Symptoms of Depression

Depression is a normal response to illness, once the illness has been accepted. The person may describe feelings of sadness or unhappiness. Some common signs of depressed behavior include the following:

1. Decreased interaction with others
2. Lack of interest in activities or environment
3. Voiced concern about illness and amount of care required
4. Expressed wish for or concerns about dying
5. Dependent behavior
6. Decreased activity
7. Complaints of fatigue or inability to sleep
8. Crying spells
9. Change in appetite

Any expressions about suicide should be taken seriously and the person referred for counseling.

Approaches useful when working with a person exhibiting depressed behavior include the following:

1. Approach the client in a serious mood.
2. Convey by action and communication an understanding of what the person must be feeling.
3. Help the person express feelings.
4. Convey acceptance of the right to feel sad.
5. Listen to the person so that the anger can be turned outward.

From Phipps W et al: *Medical surgical nursing: concepts and clinical practices,* ed 5, St Louis, 1995, Mosby.

Effects of Alcohol on Organ Systems

Body system	Effects	Late effects
Central nervous system	Depression leading to loss of memory and ability to concentrate Lessening of inhibitory functions Self-control and judgment lessened	Unprovoked seizures Wernicke-Korsakoff's syndrome Brain atrophy Sleep disturbances Neuronal damage Neuropathies
Cardiovascular system	Increased pulse rate Vasomotor depression and vasodilation of cutaneous vessels with hypotension Hypertension	Cardiomyopathy (irreversible) Hyperlipidemia Hyperuricemia Coronary artery disease
Skeletal muscles	Lessening awareness of fatigue Reduced muscular capacity for work	Skeletal myopathy
Immunological system	Increased susceptibility to infection	Infections and communicable diseases
Gastrointestinal system	Stimulation of gastric secretions and gastric acid production Irritation of GI mucosa Constipation or diarrhea Vomiting	Pancreatitis Gastritis Nutritional and vitamin deficiencies Cancer of mouth and esophagus Skin syndrome Wernicke-Korsakoff's syndrome

Hepatic system	Few liver changes in acute ingestion	Cirrhosis of the liver Cellular damage Cell necrosis Vitamin depletion (especially B complex vitamins) Cell fibrosis Liver failure Interferes with clotting factors
Renal system	Diuretic effect from inhibition of antidiuretic hormone	
Pancreas	Epigastric pain: vomiting and rigidity of abdominal muscles	Pancreatitis
Hematologic system		Anemia Thrombocytopenia Bone marrow depression Prolonged clotting time

From Phipps WJ et al: *Medical-surgical nursing: concepts and clinical practice,* ed 5, St Louis, 1995, Mosby.

Levels of Intensity of Hallucinations

Level	Characteristics	Observable client behaviors
Stage 1: Comforting **Moderate level of anxiety** Hallucination is generally of a pleasant nature.	The hallucinator experiences intense emotions, such as anxiety, loneliness, guilt, and fear, and tries to focus on comforting thoughts to relieve anxiety. The individual recognizes that thoughts and sensory experiences are within conscious control if the anxiety is managed. **Nonpsychotic**	Grinning or laughter that seems inappropriate Moving lips without making any sounds Rapid eye movements Slowed verbal responses as if preoccupied Silent and preoccupied
Stage II: Condemning **Severe level of anxiety** Hallucination generally becomes repulsive.	Sensory experience of any of the identified senses is repulsive and frightening. The hallucinator begins to feel a loss of control and may attempt to distance self from the perceived source. Individual may feel embarrassed by the sensory experience and withdraw from others. **Nonpsychotic**	Increased autonomic nervous system signs of anxiety such as increased heart rate, respiration, and blood pressure Attention span begins to narrow Preoccupied with sensory experience and may lose ability to differentiate hallucination from reality

Stage III: Controlling
Severe level of anxiety
Sensory experiences become omnipotent.

Hallucinator gives up trying to combat the experience and gives in to it. Content of hallucination may become appealing. Individual may experience loneliness if sensory experience ends. **Psychotic**

- Directions given by the hallucination will be followed, rather than objected to
- Difficulty relating to others
- Attention span of only a few seconds or minutes
- Physical symptoms of severe anxiety such as perspiring, tremors, inability to follow directions

Stage IV: Conquering
Panic level of anxiety
Generally becomes elaborate and interwoven with delusions.

Sensory experiences may become threatening if individual doesn't follow commands. Hallucinations may last for hours or days if there is no therapeutic intervention. **Psychotic**

- Terror-stricken behaviors such as panic
- Strong potential for suicide or homicide
- Physical activity that reflects content of hallucination such as violence, agitation, withdrawal, or catatonia
- Unable to respond to complex directions
- Unable to respond to more than one person

From Stuart GW, Sundeen SJ: *Principles and practice of psychiatric nursing*, ed 5, St Louis, 1995, Mosby.

Language Disorders

The following responses from clients indicate an organic or mental health problem that necessitates follow-up by an appropriate health provider. Should a client develop one of the following, the nurse should contact the client's physician immediately.

Notes

From Rawlins RP, Williams SR, Beck CK: *Mental health–psychiatric nursing: a wholistic life-cycle approach,* ed 3, St Louis, 1993, Mosby.

Language Disorders

Language change	Definition	Example
Asyndetic expression	A language disorder manifested by a juxtaposition of elements or meanings without adequate linkage	A client, when asked the name of the president, responds, "White House."
Metonymic speech	The use of imprecise terms or words with approximate meaning	"I have eaten three meals" becomes "I have had three menus."
Echolalia	The purposeless repetition of a word or phrase just stated by another individual	The nurse says, "Turn on the lights," and the client responds, "The lights, the lights, the lights, the lights."
Neologisms	A private word or phrase coined by the speaker that has special meaning to the speaker and cannot be understood by others	A client responds to a question by saying, "Ethuel tanigram."
Clang associations	The repetition of words or phrases that have a similar sound but no other relationship	The nurse says, "What would you like to eat?" The client's response is "Eat, feet, meet, beat."
Word salad	The linking of ordinary words and phrases in a meaningless, illogical, disconnected manner	A client, pacing the hallway, says, "Vanilla reason lopsided can go left and right he is."

Diagnostic Criteria for Attention-Deficit Hyperactive Disorder (ADHD)

Note: Consider a criterion met only if the behavior is considerably more frequent than that of most people of the same mental age.

A. A disturbance of at least 6 months during which at least eight of the following are present:
  1. Often fidgets with hands or feet or squirms in seat (in adolescents, may be limited to subjective feelings of restlessness)
  2. Has difficulty remaining seated when required to do so
  3. Is easily distracted by extraneous stimuli
  4. Has difficulty awaiting turn in games or group situations
  5. Often blurts out answers to questions before they have been completed
  6. Has difficulty following through on instructions from others (not caused by oppositional behavior or failure of comprehension), for example, fails to finish chores
  7. Has difficulty sustaining attention in tasks or play activities
  8. Often shifts from one uncompleted activity to another
  9. Has difficulty playing quietly
  10. Often talks excessively
  11. Often interrupts or intrudes on others, for example, butts into other children's games
  12. Often does not seem to listen to what is being said to him or her
  13. Often loses things necessary for tasks or activities at school or at home (e.g., toys, pencils, books, assignments)
  14. Often engages in physically dangerous activities without considering possible consequences (not for the purpose of thrill-seeking), for example, runs into street without looking
B. Onset before the age of 7
C. Does not meet the criteria for a pervasive developmental disorder

From Edelman CL, Mandle CL: *Health promotion throughout the lifespan,* ed 3, St Louis, 1994, Mosby; modified from American Psychiatric Association: *Diagnostic and statistical manual of mental disorders,* ed 3, revised (DSM-III-R), Washington, DC, 1987, The Association.

Major Developmental Characteristics of Hearing

Age (months)	Development
Birth	Responds to loud noise by startle reflex
	Responds to sound of human voice more readily than to any other sound
	Low-pitched sounds, such as lullaby, metronome, or heartbeat, have quieting effect
2-3	Turns head to side when sound is made at level of ear
3-4	Locates sound by turning head to side and looking in same direction
4-6	Can localize sounds made below ear, which is followed by localization of sound made above ear; will turn head to the side and then look up or down
	Begins to imitate sounds
6-8	Locates sounds by turning head in a curving arc
	Responds to own name
8-10	Localizes sounds by turning head diagonally and directly toward sound
10-12	Knows several words and their meaning, such as "no," and names of members of the family
	Learns to control and adjust own response to sound, such as listening for sound to occur again
18	Begins to discriminate between harshly dissimilar sounds, such as sound of doorbell and train
24	Refines gross discriminative skills
36	Begins to distinguish more subtle differences in speech sounds, such as between "e" and "er"
48	Begins to distinguish such similar sounds as "f" and "th" or between "f" and "s"
	Listening becomes considerably refined
	Able to be tested with an audiometer

From Wong DL, Whaley LF: *Clinical manual of pediatric nursing,* ed 3, St Louis, 1990, Mosby; modified from Illingworth RS: *The development of the infant and young child,* New York, 1975, Churchill Livingstone; Weiss CE, Lillywhite HS: *Communicative disorders: prevention and early intervention,* ed 2, St Louis, 1981, Mosby.

Assessment of Child
for Hearing Impairment

Family History
Genetic disorders associated with hearing impairment
Family members, especially siblings, with hearing disorders

Prenatal History
Miscarriages
Illnesses during pregnancy (rubella, syphilis, diabetes)
Drugs taken
Exposure to childhood diseases
Eclampsia

Delivery
Duration of labor, type of delivery
Fetal distress
Presentation (especially breech)
Drugs used
Blood incompatibility

Birth History
Birth weight <1500 g
Hyperbilirubinemia at level exceeding indications for exchange
  transfusion
Severe asphyxia
Congenital perinatal infection (cytomegalovirus, rubella, herpes,
  syphilis, toxoplasmosis)
Congenital anomalies involving head and neck

Past Health History
Immunizations
Serious illness (e.g., bacterial meningitis)
Convulsions
High unexplained fevers
Ototoxic drugs
No history (adopted child)
Colds, ear infections, allergies

From Wong DL, Whaley LF: *Clinical manual of pediatric nursing,* ed 3, St Louis,
1990, Mosby.

Treatment of ear problems
Visual difficulties
Exposure to excessive noise

Hearing

Parental concerns regarding hearing loss (what cues, at what age)
Response to name calling, loud noises, sounds of different frequencies
  (crinkling paper, whisper, bell, rattle)
Results of previous audiometric testing

Speech Development

Age of babbling, first meaningful words, phrases
Intelligibility of speech
Present vocabulary

Motor Development

Age of sitting, standing, walking
Level of independence in self-care, feeding, toileting, grooming

Adaptive Behavior

Play activities
Socialization with other children
Behaviors: temper tantrums, stubbornness, self-vexation, vibratory
  stimulus
Educational achievement
Recent behavioral or personality changes

Hearing Screening

Tuning Fork Tests

Tests and Steps	Rationale
Weber's test (lateralization of sound) Hold fork at its base and tap it lightly against heel of palm. Place base of vibrating fork on top of client's head or middle of forehead (see Fig. at right). Ask client where sound is heard (one or both sides).	Client with normal hearing hears sound equally in both ears or in midline of head. In conduction deafness, sound is heard in impaired ear. In unilateral sensorineural hearing loss, sound is identified only in normal ear.

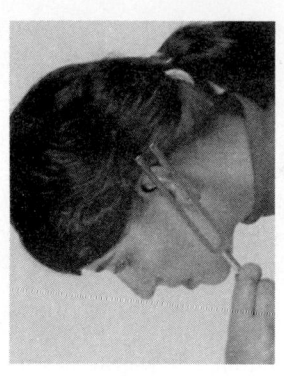 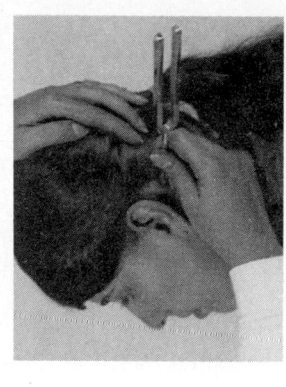

Rinne test (comparison of air and bone conduction)

Strike tuning fork against heel of palm.

First hold vibrating fork with tines parallel to auricle and their tips 2 cm from the external meatus* (see Fig. at right, top).

Place stem of vibrating fork on bone of mastoid process (see Fig. at right, bottom).

Ask client to inform you if sound is louder by air conduction or bone conduction.

If client is believed to have conduction deficit, referral for audiometry is appropriate.

Client first confirms that sound can be heard. Normally, sound can be heard louder through bone than through air (positive test). In conduction deafness, sounds through bone conduction can be heard longer than through air conduction (negative test). In sensorineural deafness, sound is reduced and heard longer through air.

From Potter PA, Perry AG: *Fundamentals of nursing: concepts, process, and practice,* ed 3, St Louis, 1993, Mosby. Illustrations from Seidel HM et al: *Mosby's guide to physical examination,* ed 2, St Louis, 1991, Mosby.
*Data from Swan IRC: *Hosp Pract* Sept 30, 1989, p 99.

Clues for Detecting Hearing Impairment

Orientation Response

Lack of startle or blink reflex to a loud sound
Persistence of Moro reflex beyond 4 months of age (associated with mental retardation)
Failure to be awakened by loud environmental noises during early infancy
Failure to localize a source of sound by 6 months of age
General indifference to sound
Lack of response to the spoken word; failure to follow verbal directions
Response to loud noises as opposed to the voice

Vocalizations and Sound Production

Monotone quality, unintelligible speech, lessened laughter
Normal quality in central auditory loss
Lessened experimental sound play and squealing
Normal use of jargon during early infancy in central auditory loss, with persistent use later on
Absence of babble or inflections in voice by age 7 months
Failure to develop intelligible speech by age 24 months
Vocal play, head banging, or foot stamping for vibratory sensation
Yelling or screeching to express pleasure, annoyance, or need

Visual Attention

Augmented visual alertness and attentiveness
Responding more to facial expression than verbal explanation
Being alert to gestures and movement
Use of gestures rather than verbalization to express desires, especially after age 15 months
Marked imitativeness in play

Social Rapport and Adaptations

Less interest and involvement in vocal nursery games
Intense preoccupation with things rather than persons
Avoidance of social interactions; often puzzled and unhappy in such situations

---

From Wong DL, Whaley LF: *Clinical manual of pediatric nursing,* ed 3, St Louis, 1990, Mosby.

Inquiring, sometimes confused facial expression
Suspicious alertness, sometimes interpreted as paranoia, alternating
   with cooperation
Marked reactivity to praise, attention, and physical affection
Shows less interest than peers in casual conversation
Is often inattentive unless the environment is quiet and the speaker is
   close to the child
Is more responsive to movement than to sound
Intently observes the speaker's face, responding more to facial
   expression than verbalization
Often asks to have statements repeated
May not follow directions exactly

Emotional Behavior

Use of tantrums to call attention to self or needs
Frequently stubborn because of lack of comprehension
Irritable at not making self understood
Shy, timid, and withdrawn
Often appears "dreamy," "in a world of his or her own," or markedly
   inattentive

Major Developmental Characteristics of Language and Speech

Age (years)	Normal language development	Normal speech development	Intelligibility
1	Says two to three words with meaning Imitates sounds of animals	Omits most final and some initial consonants Substitutes consonants "m," "w," "p," "b," "k," "g," "n," "t," "d," and "h" for more difficult sounds Height of unintelligible jargon at age 18 months	Usually no more than 25% intelligible to unfamiliar listener
2	Uses two- to three-word phrases Has vocabulary of about 300 words Uses "I," "me," "you"	Uses above consonants with vowels but inconsistently and with much substitution Omission of final consonants Articulation lags behind vocabulary	At age 2 years, 65% intelligible in context
3	Says four- to five-word sentences Has vocabulary of about 900 words Uses "who," "what," and "where" in asking questions Uses plurals, pronouns, and prepositions	Masters "b," "t," "d," "k," and "g"; sounds "r" and "l" may still be unclear, omits or substitutes "w" Repetitions and hesitations common	At age 3 years, 70% to 80% intelligible

4 to 5	Has vocabulary of 1500 to 2100 words Able to use most grammatic forms correctly such as past tense of verb with "yesterday" Uses complete sentences with nouns, verbs, prepositions, adjectives, adverbs, and conjunctions	Masters "f" and "v"; may still distort "r," "l," "s," "z," "sh," "ch," "y," and "th" Little or no omission of initial or last consonant
5 to 6	Has vocabulary of 3000 words, comprehends "if," "because," and "why"	Masters "r," "l," and "th"; may still distort "s," "z," "sh," "ch," and "j" (usually mastered by age 7½ to 8 years)	Speech is totally intelligible, although some sounds are still imperfect

From Wong DL, Whaley LF: *Clinical manual of pediatric nursing*, ed 3, St Louis, 1990, Mosby.

Vital Signs Along the Age Continuum

Age	Temperature	Sex	Pulse	Respiratory rate	Blood pressure (upper limits)
Newborn	99.1	Male	120	35	110/75
	99.1	Female	120	35	110/75
1 year	99.1	Male	120	30	110/75
	98.8	Female	120	30	110/75
2 years	99.0	Male	110	25	110/75
	98.8	Female	110	25	110/75
4 years	98.6	Male	100	23	110/75
	98.5	Female	100	23	110/75
6 years	98.4	Male	100	21	120/80
	98.5	Female	100	21	120/80
8 years	98.3	Male	90	20	120/80
	98.3	Female	90	20	120/80
10 years	98.0	Male	90	19	125/85
	98.1	Female	90	19	125/85

		Temperature	Pulse	Respiration	Blood Pressure
12 years	Male	97.8	85	19	125/85
	Female	97.9	90	19	125/85
14 years	Male	97.6	80	18	135/90
	Female	97.9	85	18	135/90
16 years	Male	97.3	75	17	135/90
	Female	97.8	80	17	135/90
18 years	Male	97.2	70	16-18	135/90
	Female	97.9	75	16-18	135/90
Adults		97.3	60-90	12-20	
Older Adults		More sensitive to temperature	Slows with age	No variation	

Modified from Yaladian I, Porter D: *Physical growth and development*, Boston, 1977, Little, Brown; Thompson JM et al: *Clinical nursing*, St Louis, 1986, Mosby; US Department of Health and Human Services: *The 1984 report of the Joint National Committee on detection, evaluation, and treatment of high blood pressure*, NIH Pub No 84-1088, Bethesda, MD, 1984.

Tools and Measurements

Lesion Size Measurement

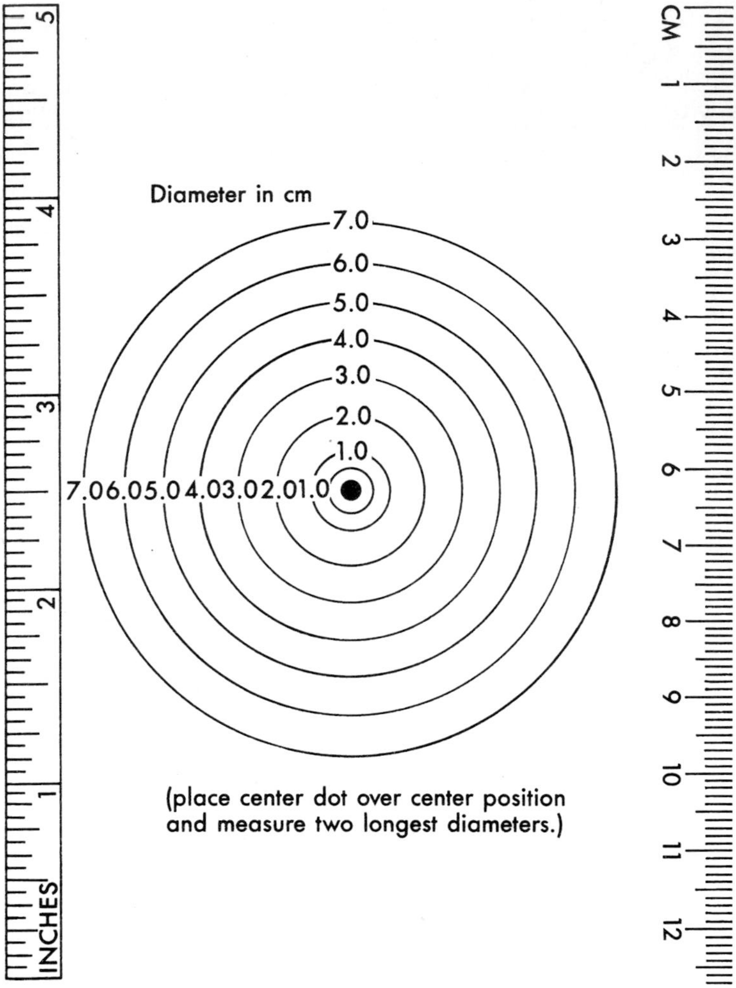

Diameter in cm

7.0
6.0
5.0
4.0
3.0
2.0
1.0

7.06.05.04.03.02.01.0 ●

(place center dot over center position
and measure two longest diameters.)

CM
1
2
3
4
5
6
7
8
9
10
11
12

5
4
3
2
1
INCHES

Redrawn from ConvaTec, a Bristol-Meyers Squibb Company, Princeton, N.J.

PULSES Profile

The PULSES Profile (see below and on p. 280) is a global functional assessment instrument that yields a broad view of a client's well-being. Each letter in the acronym PULSES represents a domain of measurement. The "P" represents general physical condition; "U," use of the upper extremities; "L," use of the lower extremities; first "S," sensory status in the realms of vision, hearing, and speech; "E," excretory status; and second "S," mental and emotional status. Each domain of measurement has four descriptor items that are weighted and scored. A number "1" descriptor item assigned to a domain represents no abnormality or restriction of function, and "2," "3," and "4" descriptor items, respectively, indicate increasing levels of dysfunction from minor to severe. The cumulative domain scores provide the PULSES Profile of the individual and give a broad picture of function.

The original PULSES Profile, as well as a later adapted version by Granger and Greer, has been used to assess, study, and monitor the functional status of clients involved in rehabilitation. The original authors have shown that the PULSES Profile is useful in classifying clients according to level of function over time and in predicting level of function in relation to medical diagnosis.

PULSES Profile*

P. Physical condition, including diseases of the viscera (cardiovascular, pulmonary, gastrointestinal, urological, and endocrine) and cerebral disorders that are not enumerated in the lettered categories below
1. No gross abnormalities considering age of individual
2. Minor abnormalities not requiring frequent medical or nursing supervision
3. Moderately severe abnormalities requiring frequent medical or nursing supervision yet still permitting ambulation
4. Severe abnormalities requiring constant medical or nursing supervision or confining individual to bed or wheelchair

---

Modified from Hens MM: Functional evaluation. In Dittmar S, editor: *Rehabilitation nursing,* St Louis, 1989, Mosby.
*From Moskowitz E, McCann CB: *J Chronic Dis* 5:343, 1957.

U. Upper extremities, including shoulder girdle, cervical, and upper dorsal spine
   1. No gross abnormalities considering age of individual
   2. Minor abnormalities with fairly good range of motion and function
   3. Moderately severe abnormalities but permitting performance of daily needs to a limited extent
   4. Severe abnormalities requiring constant nursing care
L. Lower extremities, including pelvis, lower dorsal, and lumbosacral spine
   1. No gross abnormalities considering age of individual
   2. Minor abnormalities with fairly good range of motion and function
   3. Moderately severe abnormalities permitting limited ambulation
   4. Severe abnormalities confining individual to bed or wheelchair

S. Sensory components relating to speech, vision, and hearing
   1. No gross abnormalities considering age of individual
   2. Minor deviations insufficient to cause any appreciable functional impairment
   3. Moderate deviations sufficient to cause appreciable functional impairment
   4. Severe deviations causing complete loss of hearing, vision, or speech
E. Excretory function, that is, bowel and bladder control
   1. Complete control
   2. Occasional stress incontinence or nocturia
   3. Periodic bowel and bladder incontinence or retention alternating with control
   4. Total incontinence, either bowel or bladder
S. Mental and emotional status
   1. No deviations considering age of individual
   2. Minor deviations in mood, temperament, and personality not impairing environmental adjustment
   3. Moderately severe variations requiring some supervision
   4. Severe variations requiring complete supervision

Profile

P	U	L	S	E	S

Quadriplegia Index of Function

The Quadriplegia Index of Function was developed by an interdisciplinary team for the sole purpose of measuring the functional status of persons with quadriplegia. The index measures degree of performance ability in transfers, grooming, bathing, feeding, dressing, wheelchair mobility, and bed activities. It also measures degree of performance ability in management of bladder and bowel programs. Scoring criteria are meticulously outlined, thereby reducing observer bias.

Domains of measurement and descriptor items. Client who voids voluntarily on toilet.

Domain of measurement for bladder program (28 points)
Score inapplicable routine as 9.

	4	3	2	1	0	9
A. 1. Voluntary voiding: toilet		3				
2. Voluntary voiding: commode						9
B. Intermittent catheterization program						9
C. Automatic bladder program						9
D. Indwelling catheter						9
E. Ileal diversion						9
F. Credé maneuver						9

From Gresham GE et al: *Arch Phys Med Rehabil* 61:355-358, 1980.

Continued.

Modified from Hens MM: Functional evaluation. In Dittmar S, editor: *Rehabilitation nursing,* St Louis, 1989, Mosby.

Descriptor items for bladder program: scoring criteria

A. Voluntary voiding
  1. Toilet
     4 = Client is completely independent, that is, needs no help in transfers, managing clothes, and cleaning self afterward.
     3 = Client is independent in transfers but may require assistance in *only* one of the following: managing clothes or cleaning self afterward.
     2 = Client is independent in transfers but requires assistance in managing clothes and in cleaning self afterward.
     1 = Client needs help in transfers *and* in one of the following: managing clothes or cleaning self afterward.
     0 = Client cannot do *any* of the above. Completely dependent.
  2. Commode
     3 = Client is independent, that is, can get commode, requires no assistance in managing clothes or cleaning self afterward.
     2 = Client can prepare commode but requires assistance in either managing clothes or cleaning afterward but not both.
     1 = Client can prepare commode but requires assistance in managing clothes *and* in cleaning afterward.
     0 = Client cannot do any of the above.

B. Intermittent catheterization program
     3 = Client needs *no* assistance in preparing, positioning, and disposing of equipment, manages clothes, and cleans self afterward.
     2 = Client can manage clothes but needs assistance in *only* one of the following: preparing, positioning, and disposing of equipment and in cleaning self afterward.
     1 = Client needs help in all of the above but is able to instruct others in the necessary procedure.
     0 = There is no bladder program, or client does not possess sufficient knowledge to instruct others in the necessary procedure.

C. Automatic bladder program
     3 = Client is completely independent, that is, manages clothes, prepares, applies, and removes external device, *and* cleans self afterward without help.
     2 = Client manages clothes but needs help in one of the following: preparing, applying, and removing external device and cleaning self afterward.
     1 = Client cannot do any of the above but can instruct someone in the necessary procedure.
     0 = Client cannot do any of the above.

D. Indwelling catheter
     3 = Client needs no help in managing clothes, changing bags and catheters, positioning, and cleaning self afterward.
     2 = Client needs help in no more than two of the following: managing clothes, preparing catheters, changing bags, positioning, and cleaning self.
     1 = Client needs help in three or more of the above areas *but* can instruct someone in the necessary procedure.
     0 = Client is completely dependent and cannot instruct someone in the necessary procedure.

E. Ileal diversion
  3 = Client needs no help in managing clothes, changing bags, and cleaning self afterward.
  2 = Client needs help in one of the above.
  1 = Client needs help in two or more of the above *but* can also instruct someone in the necessary procedure.
  0 = Client cannot instruct someone in the necessary procedure.
F. Credé maneuver
  3 = Client needs no help in managing clothes, preparing supplies, doing Credé maneuver, and cleaning afterward.
  2 = Client needs help in only *one* of the above.
  1 = Client needs help in two or more of the above but can also instruct someone in necessary procedure.
  0 = Client cannot instruct someone in the necessary procedure.

Pain Measurement

The following scales show various ways to help quantify the amount of pain a client feels. Different approaches to quantification will be appropriate with different clients. Factors such as age and intellectual ability should be considered when choosing a scale.

Initial Pain Assessment Tool

Date _____

Client's Name _____ Age _____ Room _____
Diagnosis _____ Physician _____
Nurse _____

I.   LOCATION: Client or nurse mark drawing.

II.   INTENSITY: Client rates the pain. Scale used _____
       Present: _____
       Worst pain gets: _____
       Best pain gets: _____
       Acceptable level of pain: _____
III.   QUALITY: (Use client's own words, e.g., prick, ache, burn, throb, pull, sharp.) _____
       _____
IV.   ONSET, DURATION, VARIATIONS, RHYTHMS: _____

V.   MANNER OF EXPRESSING PAIN: _____
       _____

VI.   WHAT RELIEVES THE PAIN? _____
       _____

VII.   WHAT CAUSES OR INCREASES THE PAIN? _____
       _____

VIII. EFFECTS OF PAIN: (Note decreased function, decreased quality of life.)
       Accompanying symptoms (e.g., nausea) _____
       Sleep _____
       Appetite _____
       Physical activity _____
       Relationship with others (e.g., irritability) _____
       Emotions (e.g., anger, suicidal, crying) _____
       Concentration _____
       Other _____
IX.   OTHER COMMENTS: _____
       _____

X.   PLAN: _____
       _____

From McCaffrey M, Beebe A: *Pain: clinical manual for nursing practice,* St Louis, 1989, Mosby.

What Does Your Pain Feel Like?

Some of the words below describe your *present* pain. Circle *ONLY* those words that best describe it. Leave out any category that is not suitable. Use only a single word in each appropriate category—the one that applies best.

Sensory domain

Temporal
Flickering
Quivering
Pulsing
Throbbing
Beating
Pounding

Spatial
Jumping
Flashing
Shooting

Punctated pressure
Pricking
Boring
Drilling
Stabbing
Lancinating

Incisive pressure
Sharp
Cutting
Lacerating

Constrictive pressure
Pinching
Pressing
Gnawing
Cramping
Crushing

Traction pressure
Tugging
Pulling
Wrenching

Thermal
Hot
Burning
Scalding
Searing

Brightness
Tingling
Itchy
Smarting
Stinging

Dullness
Dull
Sore
Hurting
Aching
Heavy

Miscellaneous
Tender
Taut
Rasping
Splitting

Affective domain

Tension
Tiring
Exhausting

Autonomic
Sickening
Suffocating

Fear
Fearful
Frightful
Terrifying

Punishment
Punishing
Grueling
Cruel
Vicious
Killing

Evaluative/cognitive domain
Annoying
Miserable
Unbearable
Troublesome
Intense

Miscellaneous
Spreading
Radiating
Penetrating
Piercing
Tight
Numb
Drawing
Squeezing
Tearing
Cool
Cold
Freezing
Nagging
Nauseating
Agonizing
Dreadful
Torturing

From Barker E: *Neuroscience nursing,* St Louis, 1994, Mosby.

How Intense Is Your Pain?

People agree that the following five words represent pain of increasing intensity. They are:

CATEGORY SCALE Representing pain intensity:

1	2	3	4	5
Mild	Discomforting	Distressing	Horrible	Excruciating

PATTERN OF PAIN As it changes with time:

1	2	3
Continuous	Rhythmic	Brief
Steady	Periodic	Momentary
Constant	Intermittent	Transient

Modified from Barker E: *Neuroscience nursing,* St Louis, 1994, Mosby.

To answer each question below, write the number of the most appropriate word in the space beside the question.

1. Which word describes your pain right now? _____
2. Which word describes it at its worst? _____
3. Which word describes it when it is the least? _____
4. Which word describes the worst toothache you ever had? _____
5. Which word describes the worst headache you ever had? _____
6. Which word describes the worst stomachache you ever had? _____

Modified from Jacox A: *Pain: a source book for nurses and other health professionals,* Boston, 1977, Little, Brown.

Visual Analog Scales

A mark is placed on the line to represent the status of pain and pain relief at the time:

Pain Scale

No
Pain

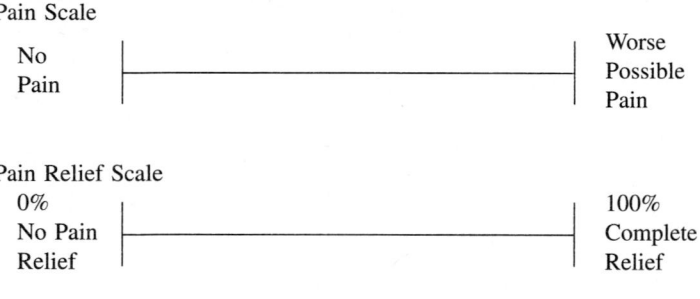

Worse
Possible
Pain

Pain Relief Scale
0%
No Pain
Relief

100%
Complete
Relief

From Barker E: *Neuroscience nursing,* St Louis, 1994, Mosby.

Faces Scale

Explain to child that each face is for a person who feels happy because there is no pain (hurt) or sad because there is some or a lot of pain. Face 0 is very happy because there is no hurt. Face 1 hurts just a little bit. Face 2 hurts a little more. Face 3 hurts even more. Face 4 hurts a whole lot, but Face 5 hurts as much as you can imagine, although you don't have to be crying to feel this bad. Ask child to choose face that best describes own pain. May be used with children as young as 3 years.

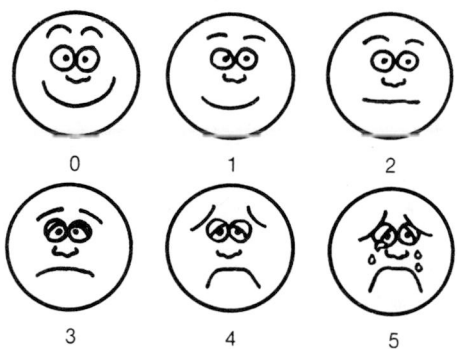

From Whaley LF, Wong DL: *Whaley and Wong's nursing care of infants and children,* ed 5, St Louis, 1995, Mosby.

Guidelines for Referral Regarding Communication Impairment

Age	Assessment findings
2 years	Failure to speak any meaningful words spontaneously Consistent use of gestures rather than vocalizations Difficulty in following verbal directions Failure to respond consistently to sound
3 years	Speech is largely unintelligible Failure to use sentences of three or more words Frequent omission of initial consonants Use of vowels rather than consonants
5 years	Stutters, stammers, or has any other type of dysfluency Sentence structure noticeably impaired Substitutes easily produced sounds for more difficult ones Omits word endings (plurals, tenses of verbs, and so on)
School age	Poor voice quality (monontonous, loud, or barely audible) Vocal pitch inappropriate for age Any distortions, omissions, or substitutions of sounds after age 7 years Connected speech characterized by use of unusual confusions or reversals
General	Any child with signs that suggest a hearing impairment Any child who is embarrassed or disturbed by own speech Parents who are excessively concerned or who pressure the child to speak at a level above that appropriate for the child's age

From Wong DL, Whaley LF: *Clinical manual of pediatric nursing,* ed 3, St Louis, 1990, Mosby.

Glasgow Coma Scale

The most widely recognized level-of-consciousness assessment tool is the Glasgow Coma Scale (GCS). This scored scale is based on evaluation of three categories: eye opening, verbal response, and best motor response.

The best possible score on the GCS is 15, and the lowest score is 3. Generally a GCS of 8 or less indicates coma. Originally the scoring system was developed to assist with general communication of the severity of neurological injury. Adapted and modified, this scale has become the basis of many neurological assessment flow sheets.

When using the GCS for serial assessment, one should remember several points. The GCS is a level-of-consciousness assessment tool only and should *never* be considered a complete neurological examination. It is not a sensitive tool for evaluation of altered sensorium. The GCS does not account for possible aphasia.

Notes

From Barker E: *Neuroscience nursing,* St Louis, 1994, Mosby.

Glasgow coma scale

Category	Response	Score
Eye opening	Spontaneous—eyes open spontaneously without verbal or noxious stimulation	4
	To speech—eyes open with verbal stimuli but not necessarily to command	3
	To pain—eyes open with various forms of noxious stimuli	2
	None—no eye opening with any type of stimulation	1
Verbal response	Oriented—aware of person, place, time, reason for hospitalization, and personal data	5
	Confused—answers not appropriate to question but correct use of language	4
	Inappropriate words—disorganized, random speech, no sustained conversation	3
	Incomprehensible sounds—moans, groans, and mumbles incomprehensibly	2
	None—no verbalization, even to noxious stimulation	1
Best motor response	Obeys commands—performs simple tasks on command and able to repeat task on command	6
	Localizes to pain—organized attempt to localize and remove painful stimuli	5
	Withdraws from pain—withdraws extremity from source of painful stimuli	4
	Abnormal flexion—decorticate posturing that occurs spontaneously or in response to noxious stimuli	3
	Extension—decerebrate posturing that occurs spontaneously or in response to noxious stimuli	2
	None—no response to noxious stimuli; flaccid	1

Modified from Teasdale G, Jennett B: *Lancet* 2:81, 1974.

Rancho Los Amigos Scale of Cognitive Levels and Expected Behaviors

The Ranchos Los Amigos scale of cognitive functioning was developed as a behavioral rating scale to aid in assessment and treatment of the head-injured person. It represents the progression of recovery of cognitive abilities as demonstrated through behavioral change. The tool is used to assess the client and to give some structure to interventions.

For purposes of client management, eight levels of cognitive functioning are grouped in the following four basic recovery phases and intervention strategies:

Level	Recovery phase	Approach
II, III	Decreased response	Stimulation
IV	Agitated response	Structure
V, VI	Confused response	Structure
VII, VIII	Automatic response	Community

Levels of cognitive functioning*
(Rancho Los Angeles Amigos scale)

I. NO RESPONSE
Client is completely unresponsive to any stimuli.
   II. GENERALIZED RESPONSE
Client reacts inconsistently and nonpurposefully to stimuli in nonspecific manner.
   III. LOCALIZED RESPONSE
Client reacts specifically but inconsistently to stimuli.
   IV. CONFUSED—AGITATED
Client is in heightened state of activity with severely decreased ability to process information.
   V. CONFUSED—INAPPROPRIATE
Client appears alert and is able to respond to simple commands fairly consistently.
   VI. CONFUSED—APPROPRIATE
Client shows goal-directed behavior but depends on external input for direction.
   VII. AUTOMATIC—APPROPRIATE
Client appears appropriate and oriented within hospital and home setting, goes through daily routine automatically, with minimal to absent confusion and has shallow recall of actions.
VIII. PURPOSEFUL—APPROPRIATE
Client is alert and oriented, is able to recall and integrate past and recent events, and is aware of and responsive to culture.

From Phipps WJ, Sands J, Lehman MK, Cassmeyer V: *Medical-surgical nursing: concepts and clinical practice,* ed 5, St Louis, 1995, Mosby.
*From Malkmus D et al: *Rehabilitation of the head-injured adult—comprehensive cognitive management,* Downey, Calif, 1980, Professional Staff Association of Rancho Los Amigos Hospital, Inc.

Normal Values of Cellular Blood Components

Type	Normal values
Red blood cells	Male: 4.6-6.1 million/mm^3 Female: 4.0-5.4 million/mm^3
Hematocrit (Hct)	Male: 45%-52% Female: 37%-48%
Hemoglobin (Hgb)	Male: 13-18 g/100 ml Female: 12-16 g/100 ml
Mean corpuscular volume (MCV)	80-90 μm^3
Mean corpuscular Hgb concentration (MCHC)	32%-36%
White blood cells	5000-10,000/mm^3
Neutrophils	55%-70% ⎫
Eosinophils	1%-4% ⎪
Basophils	0%-1% ⎬ Differential blood cell
Monocytes	2%-6% ⎪ count—totals 100%
Lymphocytes	25%-40% ⎭
Platelets	150,000/mm^3

From Phipps WJ et al: *Medical-surgical nursing: concepts and clinical practice,* ed 5, St Louis, 1995, Mosby.

Diagnostic Tests for Phenylketonuria

Test	Method	Use
Urine tests		
Diaper test	10% ferric chloride dropped on freshly wet diaper; green spot (positive); probable PKU	Inexpensive; useful in screening large groups of infants but not of value until infant is at least 4 to 6 wk of age
Phenistix test	Prepared test stick pressed against wet diaper or dipped in urine; green color reaction: probable PKU	Simple; more accurate than diaper test; useful in screening large groups of infants but not of value until after infant is 6 wk of age
Serum phenylalanine tests		
Guthrie inhibition assay methods	Drops of blood placed on filter paper; laboratory uses bacterial growth inhibition test; phenylalanine level above 8 mg/dl blood: diagnostic of PKU	Effective in newborn period; used also to monitor PKU diet; blood easily obtained by heel or finger puncture; inexpensive; used for wide-scale screening
LaDu-Michael method	5 ml of blood; serum separated and tested for phenylalanine; level above 8 mg/dl blood: PKU; in persons with PKU, phenylalanine level above 8 to 12 mg/dl blood: loss of dietary control	Useful diagnostic tool and to monitor PKU diet; requires blood drawn from person; laboratory method difficult (test not available in many laboratories)
McCarnan and Robins fluorometric method	5 ml of blood; serum separated and tested for phenylalanine; level above 8 mg: PKU or loss of dietary control	Diagnostic and diet monitoring tool; laboratory procedure more simple than LaDu-Michael method; test not available in many laboratories

Modified from Williams SR: *Nutrition and diet therapy,* ed 4, St Louis, 1989, Mosby; *Diagnostic and laboratory test reference,* St Louis, 1992, Mosby.

PART FOUR
NUTRITION GUIDES

Good nutrition is integral to a healthy life for everyone. Nutrition balance is the goal for all ages, and the nurse should assist clients in a practical and informed way. The following instruments will aid the nurse in gathering appropriate data from across the lifespan.

Guides for Children

Diet History for Children

What are the family's usual mealtimes?
Do family members eat together or at separate times?
Who does the family grocery shopping and meal preparation?
How much money is spent to buy food each week?
How are most foods prepared—baked, broiled, fried, other?
How often does the family or your child eat out?
   What kinds of restaurants do you go to?
   What kinds of food does your child typically eat at restaurants?
Does your child eat breakfast regularly?
Where does your child eat lunch?
What are your child's favorite foods, beverages, and snacks?
   What are the average amounts eaten per day?
   What foods are artificially sweetened?
   What are your child's snacking habits?
   When are sweet foods usually eaten?
   What are your child's toothbrushing habits?

From Wong D, Whaley L: *Clinical manual of pediatric nursing,* ed 3, St Louis, 1990, Mosby.

What special cultural practices are followed?
  What ethnic foods are eaten?
What foods and beverages does your child dislike?
How would you describe your child's usual appetite (hearty eater, picky eater)?
What are your child's feeding habits (breast, bottle, cup, spoon, eats by self, needs assistance, any special devices)?
Does your child take vitamins or other supplements; do they contain iron or fluoride?
Are there any known or suspected food allergies; is your child on a special diet?
Has your child lost or gained weight recently?
Are there any feeding problems (excessive fussiness, spitting up, colic, difficulty sucking or swallowing); any dental problems or appliances, such as braces, that affect eating?
What types of exercise does your child do regularly?
Is there a family history of cancer, diabetes, heart disease, high blood pressure, or obesity?

Additional Questions for Parents of Infants

What was the infant's birth weight; when did it double, triple?
Was the infant premature?
Are you breast-feeding or have you breast-fed your infant? For how long?
If you use a formula, what is the brand?
  How long has the infant been taking it?
  How many ounces does the infant drink a day?
Are you giving the infant cow's milk (whole, low fat, skimmed)? When did you start?
  How many ounces does the infant drink a day?
Do you give your infant extra fluids (water, juice)?
If your infant takes a bottle to bed at nap or nighttime, what is in the bottle?
At what age did you start cereal, vegetables, meat or other protein sources, fruit/juice, finger food, table food?
Do you make your own baby food or use commercial foods, such as infant cereal?
Does the infant take a vitamin/mineral supplement? If so, what type?
Has the infant shown an allergic reaction to any foods? If so, list the foods and describe the reaction.
Does the infant spit up frequently, have unusually loose stools, or have hard, dry stools? If so, how often?
How often do you feed your infant?
How would you describe your infant's appetite?

Clinical Assessment of Nutritional Status in Children

Evidence of adequate nutrition	Evidence of deficient or excess nutrition	Deficiency/excess*
General growth		
Within 5th and 95th percentiles for height, weight, and head circumference	Below 5th or above 95th percentiles for growth	Protein, calories, fats, and other essential nutrients, especially vitamin A, pyridoxine, niacin, calcium, iodine, manganese, zinc
Steady gain with expected growth spurts during infancy and adolescence	Absence of or delayed growth spurts; poor weight gain	
Sexual development appropriate for age	Delayed sexual development	Excess vitamin A, D
Skin		
Smooth, slightly dry to touch	Hardening and scaling	Vitamin A
Elastic and firm	Seborrheic dermatitis	Excess niacin
Absence of lesions	Dry, rough, petechiae	Riboflavin
Color appropriate to genetic background	Delayed wound healing	Vitamin C
	Scaly dermatitis on exposed surfaces	Riboflavin, vitamin C, zinc
	Wrinkled, flabby	Niacin
	Crusted lesions around orifices, especially nares	Protein and calories
		Zinc
	Pruritus	Excess vitamin A, riboflavin, niacin
	Poor turgor	Water, sodium
	Edema	Protein, thiamin
		Excess sodium

From Wong D, Whaley L: *Clinical manual of pediatric nursing*, ed 3, St Louis, 1990, Mosby.
*Nutrients listed are deficient unless specified as excess.

Continued.

Clinical Assessment of Nutritional Status in Children—cont'd

Evidence of adequate nutrition	Evidence of deficient or excess nutrition	Deficiency/excess*
Skin—cont'd		
	Yellow tinge (jaundice)	Vitamin B$_{12}$
		Excess vitamin A, niacin
	Depigmentation	Protein, calories
	Pallor (anemia)	Pyridoxine, folic acid, vitamin B$_{12}$, C, E (in premature infants), iron
		Excess vitamin C, zinc
	Paresthesia	Excess riboflavin
Hair		
Lustrous, silky, strong, elastic	Stringy, friable, dull, dry, thin	Protein, calories
	Alopecia	Protein, calories, zinc
	Depigmentation	Protein, calories, copper
	Raised areas around hair follicles	Vitamin C
Head		
Even molding, occipital prominence, symmetric facial features	Softening of cranial bones, prominence of frontal bones, skull flat and depressed toward middle	Vitamin D
Fused sutures after 18 months	Delayed fusion of sutures	Vitamin D
	Hard tender lumps in occiput	Excess vitamin A
	Headache	Excess thiamin

Neck		
Thyroid not visible, palpable in midline	Thyroid enlarged; may be grossly visible	Iodine
Eyes		
Clear, bright	Hardening and scaling of cornea and conjunctiva	Vitamin A
Conjunctiva—pink, glossy	Burning, itching, photophobia, cataracts, corneal vascularization	Riboflavin
Good night vision	Night blindness	
Ears		
Tympanic membrane—pliable	Calcified (hearing loss)	Excess vitamin D
Nose		
Smooth, intact nasal angle	Irritation and cracks at nasal angle	Riboflavin
		Excess vitamin A
Mouth		
Lips—smooth, moist, darker color than skin	Fissures and inflammation at corners	Riboflavin
		Excess vitamin A
Gums—firm, coral pink color, stippled	Spongy, friable, swollen, bluish-red or black color, bleed easily	Vitamin C
Mucous membranes—bright pink, smooth, moist	Stomatitis	Niacin
Tongue—rough texture, no lesions, taste sensation	Glossitis	Niacin, riboflavin, folic acid
	Diminished taste sensation	Zinc

Continued.

Clinical Assessment of Nutritional Status in Children—cont'd

Evidence of adequate nutrition	Evidence of deficient or excess nutrition	Deficiency/excess*
Mouth—cont'd		
Teeth—uniform white color, smooth, intact	Brown mottling, pits, fissures	Excess fluoride
	Defective enamel	Vitamin A, C, D, calcium, phosphorus
	Caries	Excess carbohydrates
Chest		
In infants, shape is almost circular	Depressed lower portion of rib cage	Vitamin D
In children, lateral diameter increases in proportion to anteroposterior diameter	Sharp protrusion of sternum	
Smooth costochondral junctions	Enlarged costochondral junctions	Vitamin C, D
Breast development—normal for age	Delayed development	See General growth on p. 297, especially zinc
Cardiovascular system		
Pulse and blood pressure (BP) within normal limits	Palpitations	Thiamin
	Rapid pulse	Potassium
		Excess thiamin
	Arrhythmias	Magnesium, potassium
		Excess niacin, potassium
	Increased BP	Excess sodium
	Decreased BP	Thiamin
		Excess niacin

Abdomen

In young children, cylindric and prominent	Distended, flabby, poor musculature	Protein, calories
Older children, flat	Prominent, large	Excess calories
Normal bowel habits	Potbelly, constipation	Vitamin D
	Diarrhea	Niacin
		Excess vitamin C
	Constipation	Excess calcium, potassium

Musculoskeletal system

Muscles—firm, well-developed, equal strength bilaterally	Flabby, weak, generalized wasting	Protein, calories
	Weakness, pain, cramps	Thiamin, sodium, chloride, potassium, phosphorus, magnesium
		Excess thiamin
	Muscle twitching, tremors	Magnesium
	Muscular paralysis	Excess potassium
	Kyphosis, lordosis, scoliosis	Vitamin D
Spine—cervical and lumbar curves (double S curve)		
Extremities—symmetric; legs straight with minimum bowing	Bowing of extremities, knock-knees	Vitamin D, calcium, phosphorus
	Epiphyseal enlargement	Vitamin A, D
	Bleeding into joints and muscles, joint swelling, pain	Vitamin C

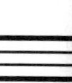

Continued.

Clinical Assessment of Nutritional Status in Children—cont'd

Evidence of adequate nutrition	Evidence of deficient or excess nutrition	Deficiency/excess*
Musculoskeletal system—cont'd		
Joints—flexible, full range of motion, no pain or stiffness	Thickening of cortex of long bones with pain and fragility, hard tender lumps in extremities	Excess vitamin A
	Osteoporosis of long bones	Calcium
		Excess vitamin D
Neurological system		
Behavior—alert, responsive, emotionally stable	Listless, irritable, lethargic, apathetic (sometimes apprehensive, anxious, drowsy, mentally slow, confused)	Thiamin, niacin, pyridoxine, vitamin C, potassium, magnesium, iron, protein, calories
		Excess vitamin A, D, thiamin, folic acid, calcium
	Masklike facial expression, blurred speech, involuntary laughing	Excess manganese
Absence of tetany, convulsions	Convulsions	Thiamin, pyridoxine, vitamin D, calcium, magnesium
		Excess phosphorus (in relation to calcium)
Intact peripheral nervous system	Peripheral nervous system toxicity (unsteady gait, numb feet and hands, fine motor clumsiness)	Excess pyridoxine
Intact reflexes	Diminished or absent tendon reflexes	Thiamin, vitamin E

A Diet History Questionnaire
for Infants through Teenagers

Questionnaire I—Infants (Birth to 1 Year)*

Date _____   Age _____

Name _____   Birth date _____

Please answer the following questions by checking the appropriate box or filling in the blank. Answer only those questions that apply to you or your child. All information is confidential.

1. Is the baby breast-fed?   Yes _____ No _____
   If yes, does he or she also receive milk or formula?
   Yes _____ No _____
   If yes, what kind? _____

2. Does the baby receive formula?   Yes _____ No _____
   If yes: Ready-to-feed   _____
   Concentrated liquid _____
   Powdered   _____
   Evaporated milk   _____
   Other _____
   How is formula prepared? _____
   Is the formula iron fortified? _____
   Yes _____ No _____
   Don't know _____

3. Does the baby drink milk?   Yes _____ No _____
   If yes: Whole milk   _____
   2% milk   _____
   Skim milk   _____
   Other _____

4. Does the baby drink any fluids other than milk or formula?
   Yes _____ No _____
   If yes, what? _____

5. How many times does the baby eat each day, including milk or formula feedings? _____

6. Does the baby usually take a bottle to bed?
   Yes _____ No _____
   If yes, what is usually in the bottle? _____

7. If the baby drinks milk or formula, what is the usual amount in a day?
   Less than 16 oz (2 cups)   _____
   16 to 32 oz   _____
   More than 32 oz (1 quart)   _____

From Stanhope M, Lancaster J: *Community health nursing: process and practice for promoting health,* ed 4, St Louis, 1996, Mosby.
*From Bureau of Maternal and Child Health/Nutrition: *Diet history questionnaire for infants,* Washington, DC, 1978.

8. Does the baby take vitamin or iron drops?
   Yes _____ No _____
   If yes, how often? _____   What kind? _____
9. Is the baby on a special diet now?   Yes _____ No _____
   If yes: Allergy   _____
           Weight reduction   _____
           Other _____
   Who recommended the diet? _____
10. Does the baby eat clay, paint chips, dirt, paper, or anything else that is
    not considered food?
    Yes _____ No _____
    If yes, what? _____   How often? _____
11. Do you think the baby has a feeding problem?
    Yes _____ No _____
    If yes, describe _____
12. Who usually feeds the baby? _____
    Does the person have the use of:
       Working stove   _____
       Refrigerator   _____
       Piped water   _____
13. Does the family participate in:
       Food stamp program   Yes _____ No _____
       WIC program   Yes _____ No _____
       Day care food program Yes _____ No _____
14. Please check which, if any, of the following foods the baby eats and how
    often.

	Less than once a week	Not daily but at least once a week	Every day or nearly every day
Cheese, yogurt, ice cream, pudding	_____	_____	_____
Milk or formula	_____	_____	_____
Eggs	_____	_____	_____
Dried beans, peas, peanut butter, nuts	_____	_____	_____
Meat, fish, poultry, wild game	_____	_____	_____
Bread, rice, grits, cereal, tortillas, noodles, spaghetti	_____	_____	_____
Fruits or fruit juices	_____	_____	_____
Vegetables (including potatoes)	_____	_____	_____
Candy, desserts, sweets	_____	_____	_____

15. If the baby eats fruits or drinks fruit juices every day or nearly every day, which ones does he or she eat or drink most often (not more than three)?

_____   _____   _____

16. If the baby eats vegetables every day or nearly every day, which ones does he or she eat most often (not more than three)?

_____   _____   _____

17. Does the baby eat:

    Sticky or sweet foods   Yes _____ No _____

    Salty foods   Yes _____ No _____

    If yes, what are the foods? _____

_____

    Is salt added to the baby's food? Yes _____ No _____

18. Below list the foods and beverages the baby has had during the last 24 hours.

Time	Food eaten	Amount	How is this food prepared?

Questionnaire II—Preschool and Young School-Age Child (Guardian Responds)

Date _____   Age _____

Name _____   Birth date _____

    Please answer the following questions by checking the appropriate box or filling in the blank. Answer only those questions that apply to you or your child. All information is confidential.

  1. Does the child drink milk?   Yes _____ No _____

    If yes: Whole milk   _____

           2% milk   _____

           Skim milk   _____

           Other _____

    If yes: Less than 8 oz (1 cup) _____

           8 to 32 oz   _____

           More than 32 oz (1 quart) _____

2. Does the child drink anything from a bottle?
   Yes _____ No _____
   If yes: Milk _____
           Other _____
   Does the child take a bottle to bed?   Yes _____ No _____
   If yes, what is usually in the bottle?

   _____

3. How many times a day does the child usually eat, including snacks?

   _____
   Does the child eat anything after he or she has gone to bed?
   Yes _____ No _____
   If yes, what? _____

4. Does the child take vitamins or iron?
   Yes _____ No _____
   If yes, how often? _____
   What kind? _____

5. Is the child on a special diet now?   Yes _____ No _____
   If yes: Allergy   _____
           Weight reduction   _____
           Other _____
   Who recommended the diet? _____

6. Does the child eat clay, paint chips, dirt, paper, or anything else not
   usually considered food?
   Yes _____ No _____
   If yes, what? _____ How often? _____

7. How would you describe the child's appetite?
         Good   _____
         Fair   _____
         Poor   _____
         Other (specify) _____

8. Who usually feeds the child? _____
   Does this person have use of:
         Working stove _____
         Refrigerator _____
         Piped water   _____

9. Does the family participate in:
         Food stamp program   Yes _____ No _____
         WIC program   Yes _____ No _____
   Does the child participate in:
         School breakfast   Yes _____ No _____
         School lunch   Yes _____ No _____
         Day care food program   Yes _____ No _____
         Summer food program   Yes _____ No _____

10. Please check which, if any, of the following foods the child eats and how often.

	Less than once a week	Not daily but at least once a week	Every day or nearly every day
Cheese, yogurt, ice cream, pudding	_____	_____	_____
Milk	_____	_____	_____
Eggs	_____	_____	_____
Dried beans, peas, peanut butter, nuts	_____	_____	_____
Meat, fish, poultry, wild game	_____	_____	_____
Bread, rice, grits, cereal, tortillas, noodles, spaghetti	_____	_____	_____
Fruits or fruit juices	_____	_____	_____
Vegetables (including potatoes)	_____	_____	_____
Candy, desserts, sweets	_____	_____	_____

11. If the child eats fruits or drinks fruit juices every day or nearly every day, which ones does he or she eat or drink most often (not more than three)?

_____   _____   _____

12. If the child eats vegetables every day or nearly every day, which ones does he or she eat most often (not more than three)?

_____   _____   _____

13. Does the child usually eat between meals?   Yes _____ No _____
If yes, name the two or three snacks (including bedtime snacks) that the child has most often.

_____   _____   _____

14. Does the child eat:
    Sticky or sweet foods   Yes _____ No _____
    Salty foods   Yes _____ No _____
If yes, what are the foods? _____

_____

Is salt added to the child's food?   Yes _____ No _____

15. Below list the foods and beverages the child has had in the last 24 hours.

Time	Food eaten	Amount	How is this food prepared?

Questionnaire III—School-Age Child and Teenager

Date _____   Age _____

Name _____   Birth date _____

Please answer the following questions by checking the appropriate box or filling in the blank. Answer only those questions that apply to you or your child. All information is confidential.

1. Do you drink milk?   Yes _____ No _____
   If yes: Whole milk   _____
            2% milk   _____
            Skim milk   _____
            Other _____
   How often? _____
   Are there other beverages you often drink?
   Yes _____ No _____
   If yes, what? _____

2. How many times a day do you eat, including snacks?
   _____

3. Do you take vitamins or iron?   Yes _____ No _____
   If yes, how often? _____ What kind? _____

4. Are you on a special diet?   Yes _____ No _____
   If yes: Allergy   _____
            Weight reduction _____
            Other _____
   Who recommended the diet? _____

5. Do you eat clay, paint chips, dirt, paper, or anything else not usually considered food?   Yes _____ No _____
   If yes, what? _____ How often? _____

6. Does anyone in your household participate in:
       Food stamp program   Yes _____ No _____
       WIC program   Yes _____ No _____
   Do you participate in:
       School breakfast   Yes _____ No _____
       School lunch   Yes _____ No _____
       Summer food program   Yes _____ No _____

7. Who usually prepares your meals? _____
   Does this person have use of:
       Working stove   _____
       Refrigerator   _____
       Piped water   _____

8. Do you eat any:
       Sticky or sweet foods   Yes _____ No _____
       Salty foods   Yes _____ No _____
   Do you add salt to your food?   Yes _____ No _____

9. Please check which of the following foods you eat and how often.

	Less than once a week	Not daily but at least once a week	Every day or nearly every day
Cheese, yogurt, ice cream, pudding	_____	_____	_____
Milk	_____	_____	_____
Eggs	_____	_____	_____
Dried beans, peas, peanut butter, nuts	_____	_____	_____
Meat, fish, poultry, wild game	_____	_____	_____
Bread, rice, grits, cereal, tortillas, noodles, spaghetti	_____	_____	_____
Fruits or fruit juices	_____	_____	_____
Vegetables (including potatoes)	_____	_____	_____
Candy, desserts, sweets	_____	_____	_____

10. If you eat fruits or drink fruit juices every day or nearly every day, which ones do you eat or drink most often (not more than three)?

_____   _____   _____

11. If you eat vegetables every day or nearly every day, which ones do you eat most often (not more than three)?

_____   _____   _____

12. Do you usually eat anything between meals?

Yes _____ No _____

If yes, name the two or three snacks (including bedtime snacks) that you have most often.

_____   _____   _____

13. Below list the foods and beverages you have had in the last 24 hours.

Time	Food eaten	Amount	How is this food prepared?

Guidelines for Feeding During the First Year

Age/type of feeding	Specific recommendations
Birth to 6 months	
Breast-feeding	Most desirable complete diet for first half of year
	Requires supplements of fluoride (0.25 mg), regardless of the fluoride content of the local water supply, and iron by 6 months of age
	Requires supplements of vitamin D (400 units) if mother's diet is inadequate or if infant is not exposed to sufficient sunlight
Formula	Iron-fortified commercial formula is a complete food for the first half of the year*
	Requires fluoride supplements (0.25 mg) when the concentration of fluoride in the drinking water is below 0.3 parts per million (ppm)
	Evaporated milk formula requires supplements of vitamin C, iron, and fluoride (in accordance with the fluoride content of the local water supply)
6 to 12 months	
Solid foods	May begin to add solids by 5 to 6 months of age; earlier introduction tends to contribute to overfeeding
	First foods are strained, pureed, or finely mashed
	"Finger foods," such as teething crackers, raw fruit, or vegetables, can be introduced by 6 to 7 months
	Chopped table food or commercially prepared junior foods can be started by 9 to 12 months
	With the exception of cereal, the order of introducing foods is variable; a recommended sequence is weekly introduction of other foods, beginning with fruit, then vegetables, and then meat
	Breast-fed infants require more high-protein foods than formula-fed children
	As the quantity of solids increases, the amount of formula should be limited to approximately 900 ml (30 oz) daily

Method of introduction

Introduce solids when infant is hungry

Begin spoon feeding by pushing food to back of tongue because of infant's natural tendency to thrust tongue forward

Use small spoon with straight handle; begin with 1 or 2 teaspoons of food; gradually increase to 2 to 3 table-spoons per feeding

Introduce one food at a time, usually at intervals of 4 to 7 days, identify food allergies

As the amount of solid food increases, decrease the quantity of milk to prevent overfeeding

Never introduce foods by mixing them with the formula in the bottle

Cereal

Introduce commercially prepared iron-fortified infant cereals and administer daily until 18 months

Rice cereal is usually introduced first because of its low allergenic potential

Can discontinue supplemental iron once cereal is given

Fruits and vegetables

Applesauce, bananas, and pears are usually well tolerated

Avoid fruits and vegetables marketed in cans that are not specifically designed for infants because of variable and sometimes high lead content and addition of salt, sugar, or preservatives

Offer fruit juice only from a cup, not a bottle, to reduce the development of "nursing bottle caries"

Meat, fish, and poultry

Avoid fatty meats

Prepare by baking, broiling, steaming, or poaching

Include organ meats such as liver, which has a high iron, vitamin A, and vitamin B complex content

If soup is given, be sure all ingredients are familiar to child's diet

Avoid commercial meat/vegetable combinations because protein is low

Eggs and cheese

Serve egg yolk hard-boiled and mashed, soft cooked, or poached

Introduce egg white in small quantities (1 tsp) toward end of first year to detect an allergy

Use cheese as a substitute for meat and as "finger food"

From Wong D, Whaley L: *Clinical manual of pediatric nursing*, ed 3, St Louis, 1990, Mosby.
*The Academy of Pediatrics recommends breast-feeding or commercial formula-feeding for up to 12 months of age. After 1 year whole cow's milk can be given.
This section may be photocopied and distributed to families.

Guidelines for Formula-Feeding

Age	Average quantity taken in individual feedings	Average number of feedings per 24 hours
Birth to 3 weeks	2-3 oz	6-10
2 weeks to 2 months	5 oz	5-8
2 to 3 months	5-7 oz	5-6
3 to 4 months	6-8 oz	4-6
5 to 12 months	8 oz	3-4

From Bobak IM, Jensen MD: *Maternity and gynecologic care: the nurse and family,* ed 3, St Louis, 1993, Mosby.

Notes

Normal and Special Infant Formulas

Formula (manufacturer)	Protein source	Carbohydrate source	Fat source	Indications for use	Comments (nutritional considerations)
Human and cow's milk formulas					
Human breast milk	Mature human milk; whey/casein ratio: 60:40	Lactose	Mature human milk	For all full-term infants except those with galactosemia; may be used with low-birth-weight infants	Recommended sole form of feeding for the first 5 to 6 months; nutritionally complete except for fluoride
Evaporated cow's milk formulas	Milk protein; whey/casein ratio: 18:82	Lactose, sucrose	Butterfat	For full-term infants with no special nutritional requirements; use of undiluted cow's milk after 6 to 12 months controversial	Supplement with iron and vitamin C; A and D if not fortified; fluoride if fluoridated water is not used for formula preparation

From Wong D, Whaley L: *Clinical manual of pediatric nursing*, ed 3, St Louis, 1990, Mosby; modified from Kempe C e: al, editors: *Current pediatric diagnosis and treatment*, ed 9, Los Altos, Calif, 1987, Lange Medical Publications. Modifications based on product information from Carnation, 1988; Loma Linda, 1988; Mead Johnson Nutritionals, 1988; Ross Laboratories, 1988; Wyeth Laboratories, 1989. For the most current information, consult product labels or package enclosures. *Continued.*

Normal and Special Infant Formulas—cont'd

Formula (manufacturer)	Protein source	Carbohydrate source	Fat source	Indications for use	Comments (nutritional considerations)
Commercial infant formulas					
SMA (Wyeth)	Nonfat cow's milk, reduced mineral whey; whey/casein ratio: 60:40	Lactose	Oleo, coconut, oleic (safflower), and soy oils	For full-term and premature infants with no special nutritional requirements	Supplemented with iron, 12 mg/L
Enfamil (Mead Johnson)	Nonfat cow's milk, demineralized whey; whey/casein ratio: 60:40	Lactose	Soy, coconut oils	For full-term and premature infants with no special nutritional requirements	Available fortified with iron, 12 mg/L
Similac (Ross)	Nonfat cow's milk; whey/casein ratio: 18:82	Lactose	Soy and coconut oils, mono- and diglycerides	For full-term and premature infants with no special nutritional requirements	Available fortified with iron, 12 mg/L
Advance (Ross)	Nonfat cow's milk, soy protein isolate	Corn syrup	Corn and soy oils	For feeding of older infants	Lower caloric content (16 cal/oz), fortified with iron, 12 mg/L
Good Start H.A. (Carnation)	Hydrolyzed whey	Lactose, maltodextrin	Palm, oleic, and coconut oils	For full-term infants	Manufacturer's claim regarding hypoallergenicity has been withdrawn

Good Nature (Carnation)	Nonfat cow's milk	Corn syrup solids	Palm, corn, and oleic oils	For feeding older infants	Contains more protein and calcium than "starter" formulas
Baby Formula (Gerber)	Nonfat cow's milk; whey/casein ratio: 18:82	Lactose	Soy	For full-term and premature infants with no special nutritional requirements	Available fortified with iron, 11.5 mg/L
Similac Natural Care (Ross)	Nonfat cow's milk; whey protein concentrate	Hydrolyzed corn starch, lactose	MCT,* coconut, and soy oils	For low-birth-weight infants. Fed mixed with human milk or fed alternately with human milk. Improves vitamin/mineral content of human milk	Protein, 2.7 g/100 kcal. Osmolality 24 cal/oz; 300 mOsm/kg water
Enfamil Human Milk Modifier (Mead Johnson)	Whey protein concentrate, casein	Corn syrup solids		For low-birth-weight infants; fed mixed with human milk; increases protein, calorie, calcium, phosphorus, and other nutrients	Used only as human milk fortifier, not as separate formula. One packet of powder supplies 3.5 kcal

*MCT, medium chain triglycerides.

Continued.

Normal and Special Infant Formulas—cont'd

For milk protein–sensitive infants ("milk allergy"), lactose intolerance

Formula (manufacturer)	Protein source	Carbohydrate source	Fat source	Indications for use	Comments (nutritional considerations)
Prosobee (Mead Johnson)	Soy protein isolate	Corn syrup solids	Soy and coconut oils	With milk protein allergy, lactose intolerance, lactase deficiency; galactosemia	Hypoallergenic, zero band antigen; lactose and sucrose free
Isomil (Ross)	Soy protein isolate	Corn syrup, sucrose	Soy and coconut oils	With milk protein allergy, lactose intolerance, lactase deficiency; galactosemia	Lactose free
Isomil SF (Ross)	Soy protein isolate	Hydrolyzed corn starch	Soy and coconut oils	With milk protein allergy or sucrose intolerance	Sucrose and lactose free
Nursoy (Wyeth)	Soy protein isolate	Sucrose (liquid formula) Corn syrup solids (powdered formula)	Oleo, coconut, oleic, and soy oils	With milk protein allergy, lactose intolerance, lactase deficiency; galactosemia	Lactose free
Soyalac (Loma Linda)	Soybean solids	Sucrose, corn syrup	Soy oil	With milk protein allergy, lactose intolerance, lactase deficiency; galactosemia	Lactose free

I-Soyalac (Loma Linda)	Soy protein isolate	Sucrose tapioca dextrin	Soy oil	With milk protein allergy, lactose intolerance, lactase deficiency, galactosemia	Lactose and corn free

For infants with malabsorption syndromes, milk allergy (hydrolysate formulas)

RCF (Ross Carbohydrate Free) (Ross)	Soy protein isolate		Soy and coconut oils	With carbohydrate intolerance	Carbohydrate is added according to amount infant will tolerate
Portagen (Mead Johnson)	Sodium caseinate	Corn syrup solids, sucrose lactose	MCT (coconut source) and corn oil	For impaired fat absorption secondary to pancreatic insufficiency, bile acid deficiency, intestinal resection, lymphatic anomalies	Nutritionally complete
Nutramigen (Mead Johnson)	Casein hydrolysate and L-amino acids†	Corn syrup solids, modified corn starch	Corn oil	For infants and children sensitive to food proteins; use in galactosemic clients	Nutritionally complete hypoallergenic formula; lactose and sucrose free
Pregestimil (Mead Johnson)	Casein hydrolysate and L-amino acids	Corn syrup solids, modified tapioca starch	Corn oil, MCT	Disaccharidase deficiencies, malabsorption syndromes, cystic fibrosis	Nutritionally complete, easily digestible protein, carbohydrate, and fat; lactose and sucrose free

Continued.

†L-Amino acids include L-cystine, L-tyrosine, and L-tryptophan, which are reduced in hydrolyzed, charcoal-treated casein.

Normal and Special Infant Formulas—cont'd

Formula (manufacturer)	Protein source	Carbohydrate source	Fat source	Indications for use	Comments (nutritional considerations)
For infants with malabsorption syndromes, milk allergy (hydrolysate formulas)—cont'd					
Allinentum (Ross)	Casein hydrolysate and L-amino acids	Sucrose, modified tapioca starch	MCT, oleic, and soy oils	For infants and children sensitive to food proteins or with cystic fibrosis	Nutritionally complete; hypoallergenic formula, lactose free
Specialty formulas					
Lonalac (Mead Johnson)	Casein	Lactose	Coconut	For children with congestive cardiac failure, who require reduced sodium intake	For long-term management, additional sodium must be given; supplement with vitamins C and D and iron; Na = 1 mEq/L
Similac PM 60/40 (Ross)	Whey protein concentrate, sodium caseinate (60:40 ratio)	Lactose	Coconut, corn oils	For newborns predisposed to hypocalcemia and infants with impaired renal, digestive, and cardiovascular functions	Low calcium, potassium, and phosphorus; relatively low solute load; Na = 7 mEq/L

Diet modifiers

Product	Protein	Carbohydrate	Fat	Uses	Comments
Polycose (Ross)		Glucose polymers (corn syrup solids)		Used to increase calorie intake, as in failure-to thrive infants	Carbohydrate only; a powdered or liquid calorie supplement; powder 23 kcal/tbsp
Moducal (Mead Johnson)		Hydrolyzed corn starch		Used to increase carbohydrate intake	Carbohydrate only; a powdered calorie supplement: 30 kcal/tbsp
Casec (Mead Johnson)	Calcium caseinate			Used to increase protein intake	Protein only; negligible fat and no carbohydrate
MCT Oil (Mead Johnson)			90% MCT (coconut source)	Supplement in fat malabsorption conditions	Fat only; 8.3 kcal/g; 115 kcal/tbsp

Infants with phenylketonuria[‡]

Product	Protein	Carbohydrate	Fat	Uses	Comments
Lofenalac (Mead Johnson)	Casein hydrolysate, L-amino acids	Corn syrup solids, modified tapioca starch	Corn oil	For infants and children with phenylketonuria	111 mg phenylalanine per quart of formula (20 cal/qt); must be supplemented with other foods to provide minimal phenylalanine

Continued.

[‡]Ross Laboratories and Mead Johnson manufacture several specialty formulas for metabolic disorders for infants.

Normal and Special Infant Formulas—cont'd

Formula (manufacturer)	Protein source	Carbohydrate source	Fat source	Indications for use	Comments (nutritional considerations)
Infants with phenylketonuria—cont'd					
Phenyl-free (Mead Johnson)	L-Amino acids	Sucrose, corn syrup solids, modified tapioca starch	Corn oil, coconut oil	For children over 1 year of age with phenylketonuria	Phenylalanine free; permits increased supplementation with normal foods
PKU 1 (Milupa)	L-Amino acids	Sucrose		For infants with phenylketonuria (available as PKU 2 for children over 1 year of age)	Phenylalanine free and fat free; contains vitamins, minerals, and trace elements; must be supplemented with phenylalanine/protein, carbohydrate, and fat

Nutrition Guidelines for Children with Diabetes

Description

Diabetes during the pediatric years requires a balance of insulin, diet, and exercise. The major goal of nutrition therapy in insulin-dependent diabetes mellitus is to ensure a pattern of growth and maturation that simulates the pattern of healthy children without diabetes.

Indications

These guidelines should be considered in the nutrition therapy of a child or adolescent with insulin-dependent diabetes mellitus.

How to Order Diet

No concentrated sweets, low fat, three between-meal feedings.

General Guidelines

1. Three regular meals and between-meal feedings, as necessary, are provided. No specific distribution of carbohydrate, protein, and fat is designated.
2. Measurement of food is not required, but meals should consist of about the same amount of food each day and should be consumed at about the same time each day.
3. Concentrated sweets, such as sugar, candy, honey, and sweetened beverages, should be avoided unless required for the treatment of hypoglycemia.
4. Protein foods should be included in each meal and between-meal feedings to aid in stabilizing blood glucose level.
5. Limit intake of saturated fat and cholesterol. Use of skim and low-fat milk products and corn or vegetable oil margarine is encouraged. Egg yolks should be limited to three per week and intake of high-fat meats should be limited.
6. Intake of foods high in fiber and complex carbohydrates is encouraged.
7. Artificial sweeteners are routinely provided. Unrestricted use of these sweeteners should be discouraged.
8. Calories are not restricted unless the individual is overweight.

From *Diet manual,* 1994, Department of Dietetics and Nutrition, University of Kentucky Hospital Chandler Medical Center, Lexington, Ky.

Nutritional Adequacy

This diet is planned to meet nutrient requirements in accordance with the Recommended Dietary Allowances. Individual food choices and intake will determine actual nutritional adequacy.

Nutrition Guidelines for Children with Hypoglycemia

Treat hypoglycemia with one of the following: sugar, fruit juice with sugar, candy, jelly, honey, Monogel, or sweetened beverages. Follow with a small snack to stabilize blood glucose. An extra snack should be eaten before and after strenuous exercise to prevent hypoglycemia.

Meal Pattern
Breakfast

Juice, unsweetened
Cereal
Toast
Margarine
Milk, low fat
Sugar substitute

Lunch

Soup
Sandwich
Fruit, fresh or unsweetened
Milk, low fat

All between-meal feedings

Meat or substitute
Bread or substitute
Milk, low fat

Supper

Meat or substitute
Potato or substitute
Vegetable or salad
Bread
Fruit, fresh or unsweetened
Margarine
Milk, low fat

From *Diet manual,* 1994, Department of Dietetics and Nutrition, University of Kentucky Hospital Chandler Medical Center, Lexington, Ky.

References

Arky RA: Nutrition therapy for the child and adolescent with type I diabetes mellitus, *Pediatr Clin North Am* 31:711-719, 1984.

Krieger I: *Pediatric disorders of feeding, nutrition, and metabolism,* New York, 1982, Wiley.

Walker WA, Watkins JB, editors: *Nutrition in pediatrics—basic science and clinical application,* Boston, 1985, Little, Brown.

Nutrition Guidelines for Children with Cystic Fibrosis

Description

Maintenance of nutritional status is of primary importance in clients with cystic fibrosis. Inadequate growth occurs in the majority of clients with cystic fibrosis because of increased energy needs imposed by malabsorption, chronic pulmonary disease, and infection.

Indications

These guidelines should be considered in the individual with cystic fibrosis.

How to Order Diet

High-calorie, high-protein diet with between-meal feedings.

General Guidelines

1. The diet should be individualized based on nutritional status, growth velocity, and degree of malabsorption.
2. Pancreatic enzymes are necessary to improve absorption of dietary fat.
3. Fat should be included in the diet to increase calorie intake, but the amount is determined by individual tolerance. Indications for fat restriction include excessive steatorrhea in spite of pancreatic enzyme supplementation, prolapse of the rectum, and abdominal distention.

Nutritional Adequacy

This diet is planned to meet nutrient requirements in accordance with the Recommended Dietary Allowances. Individual food choice and intake will determine actual nutritional adequacy. A multivitamin supplement at double the normal dosage is routinely recommended.

From *Diet manual,* 1994, Department of Dietetics and Nutrition, University of Kentucky Hospital Chandler Medical Center, Lexington, Ky.

In the presence of malabsorption additional vitamin supplementation may be indicated.

Calorie Requirements

An intake of one and one half to two times the normal requirement is recommended.

Infants: 150-200 kcal/kg/day
Older children (1-9 years): 130-180 kcal/kg/day
Males (≥10 years): 100-130 kcal/kg/day
Females (≥10 years): 80-110 kcal/kg/day

Protein Requirements

An intake of two to two and one half times the normal requirement is recommended.

Infants: 4 g/kg/day
Older children (1-9 years): 3 g/kg/day
Young adults (≥10 years): 2.5-3 g/kg/day

References

Lloyd-Still JD, editor: *Textbook of cystic fibrosis,* Boston, 1983, Wright.

Pencharz PB: Energy intakes and low-fat diets in children with cystic fibrosis, *J Pediatr Gastroenterol Nutr* 2:400-401, 1983.

Suskind RM, editor: *Textbook of pediatric nutrition,* New York, 1981, Raven Press.

Walker WA, Watkins JB, editors: *Nutrition in pediatrics—basic science and clinical application,* Boston, 1985, Little, Brown.

Nutrition Guidelines for
Children with Phenylketonuria

Description

Phenylketonuria (PKU) is one of a group of inherited disorders of phenylalanine metabolism, some of which are associated with mental retardation. Each newborn in the state of Kentucky is screened for PKU, and those with elevated serum phenylalanine levels are referred for confirmation of diagnosis. The only known treatment for PKU is dietary restriction of phenylalanine. Diet therapy should be instituted before the third week of life to prevent permanent brain damage.

From *Diet manual,* 1994, Department of Dietetics and Nutrition, University of Kentucky Hospital Chandler Medical Center, Lexington, Ky.

Indications

These nutrition guidelines should be implemented for the individual with phenylketonuria.

How to Order Diet

Consult the dietitian before ordering a diet restricted in phenylalanine.

General Guidelines

1. Phenylalanine is found in large amounts in all protein-rich foods, such as commercial infant formula, meat, milk, eggs, and cheese. These foods are eliminated from the diet.
2. Limited amounts of starches, vegetables, and fruits are allowed.
3. Lofenalac and Phenyl-Free are two specially prepared commercial formulas from which the majority of phenylalanine has been removed. These products are the basis of the diet and provide for nitrogen and amino acid requirements.
4. The low-phenylalanine diet should be continued throughout life. Recent studies indicate that deterioration in intellectual function occurs in children with PKU who have discontinued the phenylalanine-restricted diet. Adults that discontinue the phenylalanine-restricted diet experience short-term memory deficits. Continua-

Recommended Nutrient and Energy Intake for Phenylketonuria

Age	Phenylalanine mg/kg	Protein	Calories
<3 months	40-70	2.5 g/kg	120 kcal/kg
3 to 6 months	25-50	2.5 g/kg	115 kcal/kg
6 to 9 months	25-40	2.25 g/kg	110 kcal/kg
9 to 12 months	20-35	2.25 g/kg	105 kcal/kg
1 to 4 years	15-30	25 g	1300 kcal
4 to 7 years	12-25	35 g	1700 kcal
7 to 11 years	10-20	45 g	2400 kcal
Females			
11 to 15 years	10-20	50 g	2200 kcal
15 to 19 years	8-20	50 g	2100 kcal
19 to 23 years	8-15	46 g	2100 kcal
>23 years	8-15	46 g	1800 kcal
Males			
11 to 15 years	10-20	50 g	2700 kcal
15 to 19 years	10-20	60 g	2800 kcal
>19 years	8-15	60 g	2700 kcal

tion of the diet is even more critical for women with PKU during their childbearing years to prevent problems such as mental retardation, microcephaly, and birth defects in their offspring.

Nutritional Adequacy

This diet is planned to meet nutrient requirements in accordance with the Recommended Dietary Allowances. Individual food choice and intake will determine actual nutritional adequacy. Regular monitoring and adjustments in the meal plan are necessary.

References

Florida State University: *Microcomputers in nutrition support of genetic disease,* Tallahassee, 1984, Florida State University.

Hunt MM, Berry JK, White PP: Phenylketonuria, adolescence, and diet, *J Am Diet Assoc* 85(10):1328-1334, 1985.

Seashore MR et al: Loss of intellectual function in children with phenylketonuria after relaxation of dietary phenylalanine restriction, *Pediatrics* 75:226-232, 1985.

"BRAT" Diet

Description

The "BRAT" diet is low in residue and high in carbohydrate.

Indications

The "BRAT" diet is used for short periods of time for children with diarrhea. It has not been shown to be clinically effective in controlled studies.

How to Order Diet

"BRAT" diet.

General Guidelines

1. Allowed foods are served often and in small amounts. Only one or two items per meal may be given to small children.
2. Other foods may be gradually added until a general diet is tolerated.
3. Milk and milk products should be the last foods to be resumed.

From *Diet manual,* 1994, Department of Dietetics and Nutrition, University of Kentucky Hospital Chandler Medical Center, Lexington, Ky.

Nutritional Adequacy

This diet is inadequate in all nutrients and should be used only for a limited period of time.

Meal Pattern
Breakfast

Banana, ½
Rice cereal or Cream of Wheat
Toast, white
Jelly
Fruit-flavored beverage

Between-meal feedings

Applesauce
Crackers, saltines
Fruit ice
Popsicle

Lunch/supper

Broth
Toast, white or rice
Banana, ½
Gelatin or Popsicle
Jelly
Fruit-flavored beverage

References

American Dietetic Association: *Manual of clinical dietetics,* Chicago, 1988, American Dietetic Association.
Self TW: Pitfalls of the "BRAT" diet, *Nutr MD* 12(4):1-2, 1986.

Diet for Pregnant Teenagers

Purpose

The following patterns are for pregnant teenagers under 18 years of age.

Principles

- Nutritional needs of pregnant teenagers are higher than that for pregnancies in women older than 18 years of age.
- The weight gain of slightly more than the usual 25 to 35 pounds is acceptable.
- Minimal daily intake should be 35 kcal/kg.
- Snacks are offered for pregnant and lactating teenagers midmorning, midafternoon, and bedtime to increase calorie intake.
- Vitamin supplements including 30 to 60 mg of ferrous iron and 400 mg of folic acid per day are recommended.
- If milk and milk products are not consumed, 500 mg b.i.d. of calcium gluconate or lactate should be given during the first and second trimester, and t.i.d. during the third trimester and lactation.

Adequacy

The teenage pregnancy and lactating food guides, including snacks, meet the 1980 Recommended Dietary Allowances. Approximately 76 g of protein and 2500 calories are recommended for 11- to 14-year-olds and 76 g of protein and 2400 calories are recommended for 15- to 18-year-olds.

Minimum Suggested Daily Food Guide

Food group	Pregnancy	Lactation
Milk	4 or more	4 or more
Meat or substitute	2 large servings (liver once/week)	2 large servings (liver once/week)
Eggs	3 to 5/week	3 to 5/week
Fruit and vegetables	5 servings (include 1 citrus daily and a dark green or leafy vegetable 3/week)	5 servings (include 2 citrus daily and a dark green or leafy vegetable 3/week)
Bread and cereals	5 servings	5 servings
Fat	2 tablespoons	2 tablespoons

Modified from University of Kentucky Medical Center: *Hospital diet manual,* Lexington, Ky, 1991.

♦ Guides for Adults

Clinical Signs of Nutritional Status

Body area	Signs of good nutrition	Signs of poor nutrition
General appearance	Alert, responsive	Listless, apathetic, cachectic
Weight	Normal for height; age, body build	Overweight or underweight (special concern for underweight)
Posture	Erect, arms and legs straight	Sagging shoulders, sunken chest, humped back
Muscles	Well developed, firm, good tone, some fat under skin	Flaccid, poor tone, undeveloped, tender, "wasted" appearance, cannot walk properly
Nervous control	Good attention span, not irritable or restless, normal reflexes, psychological stability	Inattentive, irritable, confused, burning and tingling of hands and feet (paresthesia), loss of position and vibratory sense, weakness and tenderness of muscles (may result in inability to walk), decrease or loss of ankle and knee reflexes
Gastrointestinal function	Good appetite and digestion, normal regular elimination, no palpable (perceptible to touch) organs or masses	Anorexia, indigestion, constipation or diarrhea, liver or spleen enlargement
Cardiovascular function	Normal heart rate and rhythm, no murmurs, normal blood pressure for age	Rapid heart rate (above 100 beats/minute tachycardia), enlarged heart, abnormal rhythm, elevated blood pressure

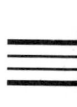

Williams SR: Nutritional guidance in prenatal care. In Worthington-Roberts BS, Vermeersch J, Williams SR, editors: *Nutrition in pregnancy and lactation*, St Louis, 1993, Mosby.

Continued.

Clinical Signs of Nutritional Status—cont'd

Body area	Signs of good nutrition	Signs of poor nutrition
General vitality	Endurance, energetic, sleeps well, vigorous	Easily fatigued, no energy, falls asleep easily, looks tired, apathetic
Hair	Shiny, lustrous, firm, not easily plucked, healthy scalp	Stringy, dull, brittle, dry, thin and sparse, depigmented, can be easily plucked
Skin (general)	Smooth, slightly moist, good color	Rough, dry, scaly, pale, pigmented, irritated, bruises, petechiae
Face and neck	Skin color uniform, smooth, pink, healthy appearance, not swollen	Greasy, discolored, scaly, swollen, skin dark over cheeks and under eyes, lumpiness or flakiness of skin around nose and mouth
Lips	Smooth, good color, moist, not chapped or swollen	Dry, scaly, swollen, redness and swelling (cheilosis), or angular lesions at corners of the mouth
Mouth, oral membranes	Reddish pink mucous membranes in oral cavity	Swollen, boggy oral mucous membranes
Gums	Good pink color, healthy, red, no swelling or bleeding	Spongy, bleed easily, marginal redness, inflamed, gums receding

Tongue	Good pink color or deep reddish in appearance, not swollen or smooth, surface papillae present, no lesion	Swelling, scarlet and raw, magenta color, beefy (glossitis), hyperemic and hypertrophic papillae, atrophic papillae
Teeth	No cavities, no pain, bright, straight, no crowding, well-shaped jaw, clean, no discoloration	Unfilled caries, absent teeth, worn surfaces mottled (fluorosis), malpositioned
Eyes	Bright, clear, shiny, no sores at corner of eyelids, membranes moist and healthy pink color, no prominent blood vessels or mount of tissue or sclera, no fatigue circles beneath	Eye membranes pale (pale conjunctivae), redness or membrane (conjunctival injection), dryness of infection (Bitot's spots), redness and fissuring of eye membrane (conjunctival xerosis), dull appearance of cornea (corneal xerosis), soft cornea (keratomalacia)
Neck (glands)	No enlargement	Thyroid enlarged
Nails	Firm, pink	Spoon-shaped (koilonychia), brittle, ridged
Legs, feet	No tenderness, weakness, or swelling, good color	Edema, tender calf, tingling weakness
Skeleton	No malformations	Bowlegs, knock-knees, chest deformity at diaphragm, beaded ribs, prominent scapulas

Diet History for Adults: Sample Form

Name _____   Date _____
Age _____
Family composition _____
Present weight _____   Usual weight _____
Height _____   Recent changes in weight _____
Number of meals per day _____   Number of snacks per day _____
Meals prepared by _____

Food preferences	Food allergies	Food aversions	Nonfavored but acceptable foods

List any foods that cause indigestion.

List any foods that cause diarrhea.

List any foods that cause flatulence (gas).

Any difficulty chewing or swallowing?

Dentures?

Usual bowel movements.

History of dietary problems.

History of diseases, surgical procedures, or weight problems.

Physical activity.

From Bodinski LH: *The nurse's guide to diet therapy,* New York, 1982, Delmar. Reprinted by permission.

Appetite _____   Recent changes in appetite ____
Breakfast at _____ AM   With _____
Usual breakfast   Serving size

_____   _____
_____   _____
_____   _____
_____   _____

Occasional breakfasts _____
Weekends _____   Holidays _____   Special _____
Eats lunch/dinner at _____ PM   With _____
At home _____   At work _____
Usual lunch/dinner   Serving size

_____   _____
_____   _____
_____   _____
_____   _____

Occasional lunch/dinners _____
Weekends _____   Holidays _____   Special _____
Eats supper/dinner at _____ PM   With _____
Usual supper/dinner   Serving size

_____   _____
_____   _____
_____   _____
_____   _____

Occasional supper/dinner _____
Weekends _____   Holidays _____   Special _____
Snacks   Time   Serving size

_____   _____   _____
_____   _____   _____
_____   _____   _____
_____   _____   _____

Nutrition Guidelines for Diabetes

Description

Guidelines for diabetes are based on recommendations by the American Diabetes Association and the American Dietetic Association. The diet for diabetes is modified in carbohydrate, meal volume, and meal frequency.

Indications

The Nutrition Guidelines for Diabetes are used for insulin-dependent diabetes mellitus (IDDM), non–insulin-dependent diabetes mellitus (NIDDM), and secondary diabetes.

How to Order Diet

Diabetic diet—specify calorie level.

General Guidelines

1. Overall recommendations for macronutrients and other components of the diet are the same for IDDM and NIDDM whether treated with insulin, with oral hypoglycemic agents, or by diet alone.
2. A decrease in calories is recommended when diabetes is associated with obesity.

Nutritional Adequacy

This diet is planned to meet nutrient requirements in accordance with the Recommended Dietary Allowances. Individual food choice and intake will determine actual nutritional adequacy. Generally diets providing 1200 calories or more are adequate.

Macronutrients and Dietary Components
Calories

Calories should be provided for weight loss, weight gain, or maintenance, as appropriate. Even a modest reduction in weight in the obese/overweight person can improve glycemic control.

Carbohydrate

Up to 55% to 60% of total calories. Lower calorie levels require a reduction in carbohydrate to allow for an increased percentage of calories from protein to meet protein needs and make the diet more

From *Diet manual,* 1994, Department of Dietetics and Nutrition, University of Kentucky Hospital Chandler Medical Center, Lexington, Ky.

Nutrition Strategies

Strategy	NIDDM (obese)	NIDDM (nonobese)	IDDM and NIDDM with insulin
Calories	Decrease	Maintenance	Maintenance
Regular meal times	Not crucial	Not crucial	Important
Equal carbohydrate distribution	Not crucial	Not crucial	Desirable
Consistency of day-to-day intake	Not critical if average daily calorie intake remains the same	Not critical if average daily calorie intake remains the same	Important
Increased number and frequency of feedings	Not usually necessary	Not usually necessary	Yes
Extra food for exercise	Not usually necessary	Not usually necessary	Important
Modification of amount and type of fat	Yes	Yes	Yes
Use of food to treat hypoglycemia	Not usually necessary	Not usually necessary	Important

NIDDM, non–insulin-dependent diabetes mellitus; *IDDM*, insulin-dependent diabetes.

acceptable to the individual. Emphasis is on complex, unrefined carbohydrate, which results in an increase in fiber intake. Sucrose and other refined sugars may be allowed in small quantities dependent on blood glucose control and weight.

Exchange Lists for Meal Planning

Food Values for Exchange Lists

Exchange list	Amount	Protein (g)	Fat (g)	Carbohydrate (g)	Fiber (g)	Calories
Bread and Starch	Varies	3	0.9*	15	2-8	80
Meat	1 oz					
Lean		7	3	0	0	55
Medium fat†		7	5	0	0	73
High fat		7	8	0	0	100
Vegetable	½ cup	2	0	5	2-3	28
Fruit	Varies	0	0	15	2	60
Milk	1 cup					
Skim		8	0	12	0	80
Low fat (1%)		8	1	12	0	89
Low fat (2%)		8	5	12	0	125
Whole		8	10	12	0	152
Fat	1 tsp	0	5	0	0	45

*For calculation purposes, 0 grams of fat per bread exchange.
†For calculation purposes, use medium fat meat values.

Exchange Lists

Bread and Starch
Cereals/grains/pasta

Bran cereals, concentrated	⅓ cup
Bran cereals, flaked	½ cup
Bulgur, cooked	½ cup
Cooked cereals	½ cup
Cornmeal, dry	2½ tbsp
Grape-Nuts	3 tbsp
Grits, cooked	½ cup
Other ready-to-eat unsweetened cereals	¾ cup
Pasta, cooked	½ cup
Puffed cereal	1½ cup
Rice, white or brown, cooked	⅓ cup
Shredded wheat	½ cup
Wheat germ	3 tbsp

Starch foods prepared with fat
Count as 1 bread and starch exchange plus 1 fat exchange unless
    otherwise specified.

Biscuit, 2½-inch diameter	1
Chow mein noodles	½ cup
Corn bread, 2-inch cube	1 (2 oz)
Crackers, round butter type	6
French fried potatoes, 2 × 3½ inch	10 (1½ oz)
Muffin, plain, small	1
Pancake, 4-inch diameter	2
Potato chips (plus 2 fat exchanges)	1 oz
Stuffing, bread, prepared	¼ cup
Taco shell, 6-inch diameter	2
Waffle, 4½-inch square	1
Whole-wheat crackers, fat added	4 to 6 (1 oz)

Meat

One exchange is equal to any one of the following items.

Lean meat and substitutes

Beef	USDA Select or Choice grades of lean beef, such as round, sirloin, and flank steak; tenderloin; and chipped beef	1 oz
Pork	Lean pork, such as fresh ham; canned, cured, or boiled ham; Canadian bacon, tenderloin	1 oz
Veal	All cuts are lean except veal cutlets, ground or cubed; examples of lean veal are chops and roasts	1 oz
Poultry	Chicken, turkey, Cornish hen, without skin	1 oz
Fish	All fresh and frozen fish	1 oz
	Crab, lobster, scallops, shrimp, clams fresh or canned in water	2 oz
	Oysters	6 medium
	Tuna, fresh or canned in water	¼ cup
	Herring, uncreamed or smoked	1 oz
	Sardines, canned	2 medium
Wild game	Venison, rabbit, squirrel	1 oz
	Pheasant, duck, goose, without skin	1 oz

High-fat meat and substitutes

Lamb	Patties, ground lamb	1 oz
Fish	Any fried fish product	1 oz
Cheese	All regular cheeses, such as American, Blue, Cheddar, Monterey Jack, Swiss	1 oz
Other	Luncheon meat, such as bologna, salami, pimento loaf	1 oz
	Sausage, such as Polish, Italian smoked	1 oz
	Knockwurst	1 oz

	Bratwurst	1 oz
	Frankfurter, turkey or chicken	1 frank (10/lb)
	Peanut butter (contains unsaturated fat)	1 tbsp

Count as one high-fat meat exchange plus one fat exchange.

Other	Frankfurter, beef, pork, or combination	1 frank (10/lb)

Vegetables

One exchange is equal to ½ cup of cooked vegetables or vegetable juice and 1 cup of raw vegetables.

Artichoke (½ medium)
Asparagus
Beans, green, wax, Italian
Bean sprouts
Beets
Broccoli
Brussels sprouts
Cabbage, cooked
Carrots
Cauliflower
Eggplant
Greens, collard, mustard, turnip
Kohlrabi
Leeks

Mushrooms, cooked
Okra
Onions
Pea pods
Peppers, green
Rutabaga
Sauerkraut
Spinach, cooked
Summer squash, crookneck
Tomato (1 large)
Tomato/vegetable juice
Turnips
Water chestnuts
Zucchini, cooked

Fruit Juice

Apple juice/cider	½ cup
Cranberry juice cocktail	⅓ cup
Grapefruit juice	½ cup
Grape juice	⅓ cup
Orange juice	½ cup
Pineapple juice	½ cup
Prune juice	⅓ cup

Milk

One exchange is equal to any one of the following items.

Skim and very-low-fat milk

Skim milk	1 cup
Milk, ½%	1 cup
Milk, 2%	1 cup
Buttermilk, low fat	1 cup
Skim milk, evaporated	½ cup
Dry milk, nonfat	⅓ cup
Yogurt, plain, nonfat	8 oz

Low-fat milk

Milk, 2%	1 cup
Yogurt, plain, low fat, with added nonfat milk solids	8 oz

Whole milk

Whole milk	1 cup
Whole milk, evaporated	½ cup
Yogurt, plain, whole	8 oz

Fat

Unsaturated fats

Avocado, medium	⅛ avocado
Margarine	1 tsp
Margarine, diet	1 tbsp
Mayonnaise	1 tsp
Mayonnaise, reduced calorie	1 tbsp

Free Foods

Drinks

Bouillon or broth, without fat
Bouillon, low sodium
Carbonated beverages, sugar free
Carbonated water
Club soda
Cocoa powder, unsweetened, 1 tbsp
Coffee and tea
Drink mixes, sugar free
Tonic water, sugar free

Fruits

Cranberries, unsweetened, ½ cup
Rhubarb, unsweetened, ½ cup

Vegetables (Raw, 1 cup)

Cabbage
Celery
Chinese cabbage
Cucumber
Green onion
Hot peppers
Mushrooms
Radishes
Zucchini

Seasonings, herbs, and spices

Flavoring extracts
Herbs and spices
Hot pepper sauce
Lemon and lemon juice
Lime and lime juice
Soy sauce, regular and low sodium
Wine, used in cooking, ¼ cup
Worcestershire sauce

Salad greens
Endive
Escarole
Lettuce
Romaine
Spinach

Sweet substitutes
Candy, hard, sugar free
Gelatin, sugar free
Gum, sugar free
Jam/jelly, sugar free
Pancake syrup, sugar free, 1 to 2 tbsp
Sugar substitutes
Whipped topping, 2 tbsp

Condiments
Catsup, 1 tbsp
Horseradish
Mustard
Pickles, dill, unsweetened
Salad dressing, low calorie, 2 tbsp
Taco sauce, 3 tbsp
Vinegar

Fat substitutes
Butter flavoring
Butter flakes, imitation
Nonstick pan spray

Food Pattern

Refer to the Exchange Lists for Meal Planning on pp. 336-340.

References

American Diabetes Association: Position statement: clinical practice recommendations, *Diabetes Care* 14(suppl 2), 1991.

Anderson J et al: New perspectives in nutrition management of diabetes mellitus, *Am J Med* 85:159-165, 1988.

Bantle JP: The dietary treatment of diabetes mellitus, *Med Clin North Am* 27, 1988.

Nutrition Guidelines for Diabetes During Pregnancy

Description
This diet is based on the Exchange List for Meal Planning (see pp. 336-340) with modification in the frequency of meals and an increase in calcium-containing foods to meet nutritional needs during pregnancy.

Indications
The Nutrition Guidelines for Diabetes during Pregnancy are used for gestational diabetes and preexisting diabetes and pregnancy.

How to Order Diet
Diabetic diet for pregnancy—specify calorie level.

General Guidelines
1. Calorie intake should be sufficient to achieve desired weight gain without promoting ketonuria.
2. The diet should consist of approximately 50% to 55% carbohydrate, 15% to 20% protein, and 25% to 30% fat as a percentage of total calories.
3. Emphasis is on complex, unrefined carbohydrate sources, which results in an increase in fiber intake.
4. The meal pattern provides three meals and three between-meal feedings. The bedtime feeding should contain a protein source.
5. Additional milk or calcium sources are included to meet increased calcium requirements.
6. Reduced intake of artificial sweeteners is encouraged, but they are not expressly prohibited. Aspartame is preferred over saccharin.
7. Supplementation with a prenatal vitamin is recommended because food intake may not supply adequate levels of nutrients such as folic acid and iron. Additional iron supplementation may be recommended. Individuals should be counseled about food sources of nutrients with particular attention to folic acid and iron.

Nutritional Adequacy
This diet is planned to meet nutrient requirements in accordance with the Recommended Dietary Allowances. Iron and folic acid intake may be inadequate without supplementation. Individual food choice and intake will determine actual nutritional adequacy.

From *Diet manual,* 1994, Department of Dietetics and Nutrition, University of Kentucky Hospital Chandler Medical Center, Lexington, Ky.

Calorie Requirements for Diabetes During Pregnancy

First trimester: 30-32 kcal/kg ideal body weight
Second/third trimester: 38 kcal/kg ideal body weight
Greater than 120% ideal body weight: 24 kcal/kg present body weight

High-Carbohydrate, High-Fiber Diet

Description

A diet high in fiber and complex carbohydrate and low in fat improves glycemic control, lowers insulin requirements, and decreases serum cholesterol in comparison with traditional diets for individuals with diabetes. This diet emphasizes increased consumption of plant foods. The diet was developed by Dr. James Anderson and associates in 1974 at the Veterans Affairs Medical Center, Lexington, Kentucky.

Indications

The high-carbohydrate, high-fiber (HCF) diet is used for individuals with diabetes who can implement the more stringent standards of this diet.

How to Order Diet

High-carbohydrate, high-fiber diet—specify calorie level.

General Guidelines

1. The high-carbohydrate, high-fiber diet is based on eight exchange groups: starches, garden vegetables, fruits, cereals, beans, milk, protein, and fats.
2. Except for the fat exchange list, the HCF exchanges include only low-fat or high-fiber foods.
3. The diet is designed to provide 20 to 30 g of fiber per 1000 calories and 200 mg or less of cholesterol daily.

Nutritional Adequacy

This diet is planned to meet nutrient requirements in accordance with the Recommended Dietary Allowances. Individual food choice and intake will determine actual nutritional adequacy. Because of the high fiber content a multivitamin with iron is recommended.

From *Diet manual,* 1994, Department of Dietetics and Nutrition, University of Kentucky Hospital Chandler Medical Center, Lexington, Ky.

Macronutrients and Dietary Components

Calories	Calories should be provided for weight loss, weight gain, or maintenance, as appropriate.
Carbohydrate	55% to 60% of total calories with approximately two thirds being complex carbohydrate.
Protein	15% to 20% of total calories or a minimum of 45 g per day.
Fat	20% to 25% of total calories with 10% or less as saturated fat.

High-Carbohydrate, High-Fiber Exchange Lists

Starches
Breads and flour
Bagel, whole grain	½ bagel
Bread crumbs, whole grain	¾ cup
Bread, pita	½ pocket
Bread, pumpernickel, rye	1 slice (1 oz)
Bread, whole grain	1 slice (1 oz)
Cornmeal, dry	2½ tbsp
English muffin, whole grain	½ muffin
Flour, oat, wheat, rye, buckwheat	2½ tbsp
Oat bran muffin	½ muffin
Roll, rye or wheat	1 small (1 oz)
Tortilla, corn or flour	1 small (1 oz)

Grains
Barley, dry	1½ tbsp
Bulgur, dry	1½ tbsp
Pasta, cooked	½ cup
Rice, cooked	⅓ cup

Starchy vegetables
Corn	½ cup or 4-inch ear
Parsnips, cooked	½ cup
Peas, green	½ cup
Potato, with peel	1 small (2½ oz)
Pumpkin	1 cup
Squash, winter, cooked	¾ cup
Sweet potato, cooked	⅓ cup or ½ small
Yam, cooked	⅓ cup or ½ small

Crackers/snacks

Graham crackers, 2½-inch square	2
Popcorn, popped, no oil	3 cups
Rice cakes	2
Rye crackers	6 small squares
Soda crackers (lower in fiber)	6 squares
Melba toast (lower in fiber)	4 slices
Crispbreads	2 slices
Flatbreads	4 slices

Fruits

Apple, raw, small	1 apple
Apple slices	1 cup
Applesauce, unsweetened	½ cup
Apricots, fresh	3 apricots
Apricots, canned, water-pack	8 halves
Apricots, canned, juice-pack	4 halves
Banana, 9 inches long	½
Blackberries	¾ cup
Blueberries	¾ cup
Boysenberries	¾ cup
Cantaloupe	⅓ melon
Cantaloupe, cubed	1 cup
Casaba melon	⅛ melon
Casaba melon, cubed	1 cup
Cherries, sweet	12
Cranberries	1¼ cup
Dates	2½
Figs, large	1 fig
Fruit cocktail, canned, water-pack	¾ cup
Fruit cocktail, canned, juice-pack	½ cup
Fruit salad, canned, water-pack	¾ cup
Fruit salad, canned, juice-pack	½ cup
Grapes	15
Grapefruit	½
Grapefruit sections	¾ cup
Honeydew melon	⅛ melon
Honeydew melon, cubed	1 cup
Kiwi, large	1 kiwi
Mango	½ mango
Melon balls	1 cup
Nectarine	1 nectarine
Orange	1 orange
Orange sections	¾ cup
Papaya	½ papaya or 1 cup
Peach, medium	1 peach
Peaches, canned, water-pack	1 cup
Peaches, canned, juice-pack	½ cup
Pear	½
Pears, canned, water-pack	3 halves
Pears, canned, juice-pack	½ cup
Pineapple	¾ cup
Pineapple, canned, water-pack	¾ cup

Pineapple, canned, juice-pack	½ cup
Plums, medium	2 plums
Pomegranate	½ pomegranate
Prunes	3 prunes
Raisins	2 tbsp
Raspberries	1 cup

Cereals

Cereals that are lower in fiber may be chosen occasionally. These include Corn Chex, Corn Flakes, Cream of Rice, Cream of Wheat, Rice Chex, Product 19, Puffed Rice, Rice Krispies, and Special K. Choose cereals that contain less than 2 g of fat and 5 g of sugar per serving.

Beans

Black-eyed peas (cowpeas)	½ cup
Butter beans	½ cup
Chick-peas (garbanzo beans)	⅓ cup
Kidney beans	½ cup
Lentils	½ cup
Lima beans	½ cup
Other beans and peas	½ cup
Peas, split	½ cup
Pinto beans	½ cup
Soybeans	½ cup plus 1 fat exchange
White beans	½ cup

Milk

Skim milk	1 cup
Milk, ½%	1 cup
Milk, 1%	1 cup plus ½ fat exchange
Milk, 2%	1 cup plus 1 fat exchange
Buttermilk, low fat	1 cup
Skim milk, evaporated	½ cup
Dry milk, nonfat	5 tbsp
Yogurt, plain, nonfat	5 oz

Protein

Amounts listed are for raw meat, fish, and poultry.

Fish	Abalone, bass, cod, flounder, grouper, halibut, mackerel, monkfish, orange roughy, pompano, sole, snapper, and other varieties of whitefish	2 oz
	Crab, lobster, scallops, shrimp, clams	2 oz
	Herring, in tomato sauce	1 oz
	Salmon	1 oz
	Swordfish	1½ oz
	Tuna, fresh or frozen	1 oz
	Tuna, canned in water	¼ cup
Cheese	Cottage, dry curd	½ cup
	Cottage, 1% fat	¼ cup
	Mozzarella, part skim	½ oz
	Parmesan	2 tbsp
	Low calorie, less than 50 calories/oz	1 oz

Eggs	Egg substitute, less than 200 calories/cup	¼ cup
	Egg whites	3 whites
Poultry	Chicken, without skin	1 oz
	Turkey, without skin	1 oz
Meats	Beef, round, flank, sirloin, tenderloin	1 oz
	Lamb	1 oz
	Pork, lean; chops, tenderloin; fresh, canned, boiled, or cured ham	1 oz
	Veal, lean; chops, roast	1 oz
Other	Tofu	2½ oz

Fats

Avocado, medium	⅛ avocado
Margarine	1 tsp
Margarine, reduced-calorie	1 tbsp
Mayonnaise	1 tsp
Mayonnaise, reduced-calorie	1 tbsp
Nuts	
Almonds	6 whole (¼ oz)
Cashews	4 whole (¼ oz)
Chopped	1 tbsp (¼ oz)
Peanuts	10 large (¼ oz)
	20 small
Pecans	5 halves (¼ oz)
Pistachios	15 whole (¼ oz)
Walnuts	5 halves (¼ oz)
Oil, corn, cottonseed, olive, safflower, soybean, sunflower	1 tsp
Olives, black	8 small
Olives, green	6 medium
Peanut butter	1½ tsp
Salad dressing, mayonnaise type	2 tsp
Salad dressing, mayonnaise type, reduced-calorie	1 tbsp
Seeds	
Sunflower	1 tbsp (¼ oz)
Pumpkin	2 tsp (⅓ oz)
Squash	2 tsp (⅓ oz)
Soybean kernels	1½ tbsp (⅓ oz)

Free Vegetables

Each serving is equal to ½ cup raw. If more than 2 cups of free vegetables are eaten per day, count each additional serving as ½ garden vegetable exchange.

Alfalfa sprouts	Lettuce
Cabbage, Chinese	Mushrooms
Cabbage	Parsley
Cabbage, red	Radishes
Celery	Romaine
Cucumbers	Spinach
Endive	Swiss chard
Escarole	Watercress
Hot peppers	

Free Foods

Artificial sweetener
Bouillon, low fat
Broth, low fat
Butter flavorings
Carbonated water
Club soda
Coffee and tea
Gelatin, sugar free
Herbs and spices
Horseradish

Lemon and lemon juice
Lime and lime juice
Mineral water
Mustard
Nonstick pan spray
Pickles, dill
Salad dressing, with less than
    10 calories/tbsp
Sugar-free beverages
Vinegar

References

Anderson JW: *HCF exchanges: a sensible plan for healthy eating,* Lexington, Ky, 1987, HCF Diabetes Foundation.

Anderson JW, Bryant CA: Dietary fiber: diabetes and obesity, *Am J Gastroenterol* 81:898-906, 1986.

Anderson JW, Chew WL: Plant fiber: carbohydrate and lipid metabolism, *Am J Clin Nutr* 32:346-363, 1979.

Anderson JW et al: Dietary fiber and diabetes: a comprehensive review and practical application, *J Am Diet Assoc* 87:1189-1197, 1987.

Anderson JW, Smith BM, Geil PB: High-fiber diet for diabetes: safe and effective treatment, *Postgrad Med* 88:157-168, 1990.

No Concentrated-Sweets Diet

Description

Liberalized carbohydrate intake and portions may be appropriate for individuals with diabetes who cannot fully implement the standard diabetic diet. Decreased calorie intake as a result of anorexia may also necessitate a liberalization of diet.

Indications

This diet may be used for individuals with diabetes who do not require insulin or who cannot fully understand or implement the diabetic diet. It may also be used for individuals with diabetes who have a decreased appetite.

How to Order Diet

No concentrated-sweets diet.

From *Diet manual,* 1994, Department of Dietetics and Nutrition, University of Kentucky Hospital Chandler Medical Center, Lexington, Ky.

General Guidelines

1. This diet is adapted from the basic meal pattern.
2. Foods containing simple sugar are omitted.
3. Moderate fat intake is encourage with an emphasis on reducing saturated fat.

Nutritional Adequacy

This diet is planned to meet nutrient requirements in accordance with the Recommended Dietary Allowances. Individual food choice and intake will determine actual nutritional adequacy.

Meal Pattern
Breakfast

Fruit or juice
Cereal
Egg
Toast
Milk
Margarine
Beverage, sugar free
Diet jelly
Sugar substitute/salt/pepper

Lunch/supper

Meat or substitute
Potato or substitute
Vegetable or salad
Fruit
Bread
Margarine
Milk (supper)
Beverage, sugar free
Sugar substitute/salt/pepper

Nutrition Guidelines for Reactive Hypoglycemia

Description
A diet modified in carbohydrate and meal frequency may improve symptoms of hypoglycemia.

Indications
The nutrition guidelines are used for reactive hypoglycemia.

How to Order Diet
Hypoglycemia diet—specify calorie level and number of feedings.

General Guidelines
1. Simple carbohydrates, milk, and fruit are limited. Fruit may be initially excluded, then gradually added based on tolerance.
2. Concentrated sweets are omitted because of the potential for rapid absorption of glucose.
3. Adequate protein, fat, and fiber are encouraged with each meal.
4. Three meals and either one or three between-meal feedings are provided depending on individual need.
5. The diet should be adapted to individual tolerance.
6. The Exchange Lists for Meal Planning are used for meal planning.

Nutritional Adequacy
This diet is planned to meet nutrient requirements in accordance with the Recommended Dietary Allowances. Individual food choice and intake will determine actual nutritional adequacy. The diet may be inadequate in vitamin C until fruits are included and low in calcium, phosphorous, and vitamin D if milk is eliminated.

Food Pattern
Refer to the Exchange Lists for Meal Planning on pp. 336-340.

From *Diet manual*, 1994, Department of Dietetics and Nutrition, University of Kentucky Hospital Chandler Medical Center, Lexington, Ky.

Nutrition Guidelines for
Pregnancy and Lactation

Description
Additional nutrients in the form of food and vitamins are required during pregnancy and lactation.

Indications
The diet for pregnancy and lactation provides adequate nutrition to support maternal weight gain and lactation and in the adolescent to support continued growth and development.

How to Order Diet
Regular diet for pregnancy/lactation; regular diet for pregnancy/lactation (adolescent).

General Guidelines
1. Calorie intake should be sufficient to achieve recommended weight gain during pregnancy. Intentional weight loss is contraindicated.
2. If milk and milk products are not consumed, calcium supplementation may be indicated.
3. Between-meal feedings are offered three times per day at midmorning, midafternoon, and bedtime to increase calorie intake.
4. A sodium restriction is not indicated during pregnancy.

Minimum Recommended Daily Food Intake During Pregnancy and Lactation

Food group	Adult	Adolescent
Milk and dairy products	4 servings	5 servings
Meat or protein substitute	2 to 3 servings	3 servings
Fruits and vegetables	5 servings Include a vitamin C source daily Include a vitamin A source at least three times per week	5 servings
Breads and cereals	6 servings	6 servings
Fluids, other than milk	6 to 8 cups	6 to 8 cups

From *Diet manual,* 1994, Department of Dietetics and Nutrition, University of Kentucky Hospital Chandler Medical Center, Lexington, Ky.

Nutritional Adequacy

The diet is planned to meet nutrient requirements in accordance with the Recommended Dietary Allowances. Individual food choice and intake will determine actual nutritional adequacy. Supplementation with a prenatal vitamin is recommended because food intake may not supply adequate levels of folic acid and iron.

Meal Pattern
Breakfast

Fruit or juice
Cereal
Egg or substitute
Bread
Margarine
Milk
Jelly
Sugar/salt/pepper

Midmorning

Fruit

Lunch/supper

Meat or substitute
Starch or substitute
Vegetable or salad
Margarine
Fruit or dessert
Bread
Milk
Sugar/salt/pepper

Midafternoon

Bread or starch
Milk

Bedtime

Meat or substitute
Bread or starch

Calorie Requirements During Pregnancy

Normal weight	13-16 kcal/lb or 29-25 kcal/kg
Underweight	17 kcal/lb or 37 kcal/kg
Overweight	11 kcal/lb or 24 kcal/kg
Adolescents	18-21 kcal/lb or 40-46 kcal/kg

Use current pregnancy weight to assess calorie needs; in morbid obesity, adjusted weight should be used.

Protein Requirements During Pregnancy and Lactation

Pregnancy 18+ years	60 g/day
Lactation	
First 6 months	65 g/day
Second 6 months	62 g/day

Recommended Weight Gain During Pregnancy

Normal weight	25-35 lb
Underweight	28-40 lb
Overweight	15-35 lb
Obese	15 lb
Twins	44 lb
Adolescents	35 lb

References

American Dietetic Association: *Manual of clinical dietetics,* 1988.

Food and Nutrition Board: *Recommended dietary allowances,* ed 10, Washington, DC, 1989, National Academy of Sciences.

Pemberton CM et al: Normal nutrition. In *Mayo Clinic diet manual,* ed 6, Philadelphia, 1988, BC Decker.

Worthington-Roberts B, Williams SR: *Nutrition in pregnancy and lactation,* St Louis, 1993, Times Mirror/Mosby College.

Zeman FJ: *Clinical nutrition and dietetics,* ed 2, New York, 1991, Macmillan.

Adult Diets for Vomiting and Diarrhea

Diet for Diarrhea

If bowel movements are frequent (more than once an hour) take sips of ginger ale, 7-Up, or other similar drinks. Do not consume milk or milk products.

Increase amount of fluid intake as bowel movements slow down.

Do not consume foods until frequency of bowel is down to one every 8 hours, then start on soft foods, such as crackers, toast, jello, and soup.

Assume a regular diet when bowel movements begin to have some consistency.

If no relief is felt in 24 hours, call your physician.

Diet for Vomiting

As long as you are vomiting, consume just ice chips or sips of ginger ale, 7-Up, or other similar drinks. Do not consume milk or milk products.

When you haven't vomited for 2 to 3 hours, increase fluid intake by 2 to 3 oz at a time.

When you haven't vomited for 6 to 8 hours, consume soft foods, such as crackers, toast, jello, soup, soft boiled egg, etc., then assume regular diet when you are hungry.

If no relief is felt in 24 hours, call your physician.

From Lexington-Fayette County Health Department, Division of Nutrition and Health Education, Lexington, Ky, 1992.

Vegetarian Diet

Description

Vegetarian diets are designed to use combinations of vegetable and plant proteins to meet essential protein needs. They are classified according to the extent animal foods are excluded.

Indications

The vegetarian diet is used for clients who choose to restrict animal products in the diet.

How to Order Diet

Vegetarian diet; lacto-ovo vegetarian diet, if known; lacto vegetarian diet, if known.

General Guidelines

1. Adequate calories are provided to meet energy needs and spare protein to promote efficient protein utilization.
2. A variety of vegetable and plant proteins are included in each vegetarian diet.
3. A variety of meat substitutes (cheese, peanut butter, nuts, dried beans/peas) are included in each vegetarian diet.
4. The vegetarian, or vegan, diet is not recommended without nutrition counseling. Nutrition counseling should include a discussion of nutrients and their sources.
5. Food preferences will be obtained to determine individual client practices and will be incorporated into the meal pattern.

Nutritional Adequacy

Individual food choice and intake will determine actual nutritional adequacy. More nutrients are deficient with progressive levels of restriction. Nutrients that may be deficient are high biological value protein, vitamin B_{12}, vitamin D, riboflavin, calcium, iron, and zinc. Specific nutrients are listed by classification of vegetarian diet.

From *Diet manual,* 1994, Department of Dietetics and Nutrition, University of Kentucky Hospital Chandler Medical Center, Lexington, Ky.

Meal Pattern
Breakfast
Fruit or juice
Cereal, cooked
Meat substitute
Bread
Margarine
Jelly
Sugar/salt/pepper

Lunch/supper
Vegetarian soup
Meat substitute
Starch or substitute
Vegetable or salad
Bread
Fruit or juice
Margarine
Sugar/salt/pepper

Classification of Vegetarian Diets

Classification	Foods allowed	Foods omitted	Limiting nutrients
Lacto-ovo	Fruits, grains, legumes, nuts, seeds, eggs, vegetables, milk/milk products	Animal meat	Iron
Lacto	Fruits, grains, legumes, nuts, seeds, vegetables, milk/milk products	Animal meat Eggs	Iron Vitamin D Calcium Riboflavin
Vegan	Fruits, grains, legumes, nuts, seeds, vegetables	All animal products	HBV protein Iron Calcium Vitamin D Riboflavin Vitamin B_{12}

*HBV, high biological value.

Protein Complement Guide

Food Group	Limiting essential amino acid	Protein complementation
Eggs	None	Complete protein
Grains	Lysine, isoleucine	Grains and legumes Grains and milk or eggs
Legumes	Methionine, cystine, tryptophan (except when soy protein is included in diet)	Legumes and grains Legumes and seeds or nuts
Milk products	None	Complete protein
Nuts and seeds	Lysine, isoleucine (except when cashews and pumpkin seeds are included in diet)	Nuts, seeds, and legumes
Other vegetables	Cystine, methionine, isoleucine (except spinach)	Vegetable and nuts, seeds, and legumes Vegetable and grain Vegetable and eggs or milk/milk products

References

Pemberton CM et al: Normal nutrition. In Mayo Clinic: *Diet manual,* ed 6, Philadelphia, 1988, BC Decker.

American Dietetic Association: *Manual of clinical dietetics,* 1988.

University of Alabama Birmingham: *Manual for nutritional management,* Birmingham, 1986, University of Alabama.

Zeman FJ: *Clinical nutrition and dietetics,* ed 2, New York, 1991, Macmillan.

Vegetarian Varieties

The Institute of Food Technologists, in the July 1991 issue of its journal, *Food Technology,* describes six types of vegetarians. They are listed here by degree of exclusion of animal foods and by the foods included in the diet:

- *Semi-vegetarian*—dairy foods, eggs, chicken, and fish, but no other animal flesh
- *Pesco-vegetarian*—dairy foods, eggs, and fish, but no other animal flesh
- *Lacto-ovo-vegetarian*—dairy foods and eggs, but no animal flesh
- *Lacto-vegetarian*—dairy foods, but no animal flesh or eggs
- *Ovo-vegetarian*—eggs, but no dairy foods or animal flesh
- *Vegan*—no animal foods of any type

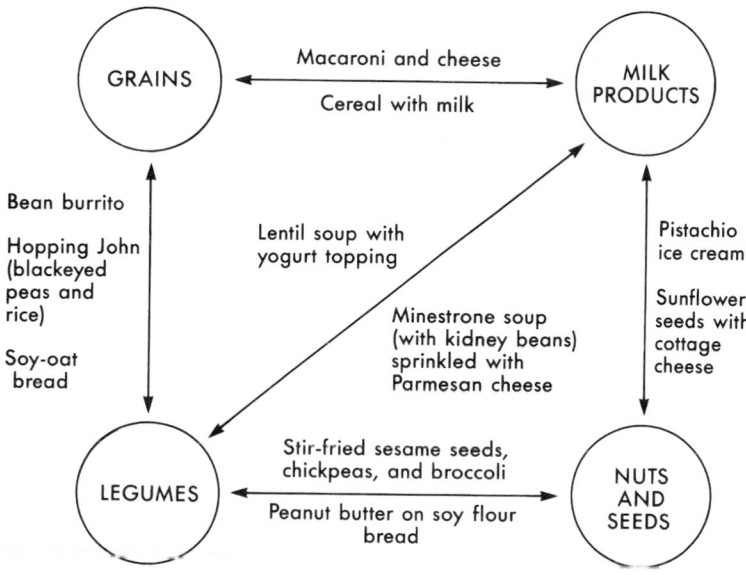

Complementary proteins. The circled items are major types of protein in many vegetarian diets. Items connected by arrows are complementary. Examples of dishes providing complementary proteins are given beside the arrows. (From Bobak IM, Jensen MD: *Maternity and gynecologic care: the nurse and the family,* ed 5, St Louis, 1993, Mosby.)

Fat in Selected Vegetarian Foods

Food	Fat (g)
Butter, 1 pat	4
Margarine, 1 pat	4
Salad dressing, creamy, 2 tbsp	16
Vegetable oil, 1 tbsp	14
Nuts and seeds, 1 oz	14
Peanut butter, 1 tbsp	8
Tofu, 4 oz	5
Cooked dried beans, 1 cup	1
Eggs, 1 large	6
Skim milk, 1 cup	Trace
Soy milk, 1 cup	7
Whole milk, 1 cup	8
Cheese, 3 oz	27
Ice cream, 1 cup	14
Tofu ice cream, 1 cup	2-17
Fruit, 1 medium	0
Grains, cooked, 1 cup	1
Vegetables, 1 cup	0-1
Crackers, 4	1-4
Cookies, 4	4-12
Bread, 1 slice	1
Chips, 10	7
French fries, 10	8
Olives, 4 medium	2
Avocado, half	15
Coconut, 2 tbsp	3
For comparison:	
Hamburger on bun	20

From The Vegetarian Resource Group, Baltimore, Md.

Use this table and food labels to make choices so the total amount of fat in your diet is low. A low-fat diet does not mean never eating salad dressing again. It does mean taking a minute to think about all the food you eat in a day and deciding if you would rather use 2 tablespoons of salad dressing or get about the same amount of fat from a tablespoon of peanut butter and 16 crackers.

The vegetarian's protein intake should be assessed especially carefully. Plant proteins tend to be "incomplete," or lacking in one or more amino acids required for growth and maintenance of body tissues. However, combinations of different types of complementary incomplete proteins, in which one protein source will be rich in an amino acid that the other protein source lacks, and vice versa, can provide sufficient amounts of complete protein. The Fig. on p. 357 demonstrates complementary protein combinations. It is probably not essential that complementary proteins be consumed at the same meal. It is an excellent practice to become accustomed to planning meals around complementary proteins to ensure that the diet is balanced and that all types of protein foods are included.

Notes

General Guidelines

Suggested Weights for Adults

Height*	Weight (in pounds)[†] 19 to 34	35 and over
5'0"	97-128[‡]	108-138
5'1"	101-132	111-143
5'2"	104-137	115-148
5'3"	107-141	119-152
5'4"	111-146	122-157
5'5"	114-150	126-162
5'6"	118-155	130-167
5'7"	121-160	134-172
5'8"	125-164	138-178
5'9"	129-169	142-183
5'10"	132-174	146-188
5'11"	136-179	151-194
6'0"	140-184	155-199
6'1"	144-189	159-205
6'2"	148-195	165-210
6'3"	152-200	168-216
6'4"	156-205	173-222
6'5"	160-211	177-228
6'6"	164-216	182-234

*Without shoes.
†Without clothes.
‡The higher weights in the ranges generally apply to men, who tend to have larger body frames and more muscle; the lower weights more often apply to women, who have smaller body frames and less muscle. Weights even below the range may be appropriate for some small-boned people. (Source: National Research Council, 1989.)

Determine Your Nutritional Health

The Warning Signs of poor nutritional health are often overlooked. Use this checklist to find out if you or someone you know is at nutritional risk.

Nutrition Checklist

Read the statements below. Circle the number in the yes column for those that apply to you or someone you know. For each yes answer, score the number in the box. Total your nutritional score.

	YES
I have an illness or condition that made me change the kind and/or amount of food I eat.	2
I eat fewer than 2 meals per day.	3
I eat few fruits, vegetables, or milk products.	2
I have 3 or more drinks of beer, liquor, or wine almost every day.	2
I have tooth or mouth problems that make it hard for me to eat.	2
I don't always have enough money to buy the food I need.	4
I eat alone most of the time.	1
I take 3 or more different prescribed or over-the-counter drugs a day.	1
Without wanting to, I have lost or gained 20 pounds in the last 6 months.	2
I am not always physically able to shop, cook, and/or feed myself.	2
Total	

Total Your Nutritional Score. If it's—

0-2   Good! Recheck your nutritional score in 6 months.

3-5   You are at moderate nutritional risk. See what can be done to improve your eating habits and life-style. Your office on aging, senior nutrition program, senior citizens center, or health department can help. Recheck your nutritional score in 3 months.

6 or more   You are at high nutritional risk. Bring this checklist the next time you see your doctor, dietitian or other qualified health or social service professional. Talk with them about any problems you may have. Ask for help to improve your nutritional health.

Remember that warning signs suggest risk but do not represent diagnosis of any condition. To learn more about the Warning Signs of poor nutritional health, see the following table.

The Nutrition Screening Initiative is a project of the American Academy of Family Physicians, the American Dietetic Association, the National Council on the Aging, Inc, and funded in part by Ross Products Division, Abbott Laboratories.

The Nutrition Checklist is based on the Warning Signs described below; use the word DETERMINE to remind you of the Warning Signs

---

Disease

Any disease, illness, or chronic condition that causes you to change the way you eat, or makes it hard for you to eat, puts your nutritional health at risk. Four out of five adults with chronic diseases are affected by diet. Confusion or memory loss that keeps getting worse is estimated to affect one out of five older adults. This can make it hard to remember what, when, or if you've eaten. Feeling sad or depressed, which happens to about one in eight older adults, can cause big changes in appetite, digestion, energy level, weight, and well-being.

Eating poorly

Eating too little and eating too much both lead to poor health. Eating the same foods day after day or not eating fruit, vegetables, and milk products daily will also cause poor nutritional health. One in five adults skip meals daily. Only 23% of adults eat the minimum amount of fruit and vegetables needed. One in four older adults drink too much alcohol. Many health problems become worse if you drink more than one or two alcoholic beverages per day.

Tooth loss/mouth pain

A healthy mouth, teeth, and gums are needed to eat. Missing, loose, or rotten teeth or dentures that don't fit well or cause mouth sores, make it hard to eat.

Economic hardship

As many as 40% of older Americans have incomes of less than $6000 per year. Having less—or choosing to spend less—than $25 to $30 per week for food makes it hard to get the foods you need to stay healthy.

Reduced social contact

One third of all older people live alone. Being with people daily has a positive effect on morale, well-being, and eating.

Multiple medicines

Many older Americans must take medicines for health problems. Almost half of older Americans take multiple medicines daily. Growing old may change the way we respond to drugs. The more medicines you take, the greater the chance for side effects such as increased or decreased appetite, change in taste, constipation, weakness, drowsiness, diarrhea, nausea, and others. Vitamins or minerals when taken in large doses act like drugs and can cause harm. Alert your doctor to everything you take.

Involuntary weight loss/gain

Losing or gaining a lot of weight when you are not trying to do so is an important warning sign that must not be ignored. Being overweight or underweight also increases your chance of poor health.

Needs assistance in self-care

Although most older people are able to eat, one of every five has trouble walking, shopping, buying, and cooking food, especially as they get older.

Elder years above age 80

Most older people lead full and productive lives. But as age increases, risk of frailty and health problems increase. Checking your nutritional health regularly makes good sense.

Notes

Family Nutritional Assessment Tool

Family members	Age	Educational level	Developmental stage
1.			
2.			
3.			
4.			
5.			
6.			

Family's perception of health status (describe)

Nutritional practices

Who decides on the menu?
Who does the grocery shopping?
Who prepares the meals?
Number of meals consumed per day?
Describe mealtime (who is present, when, where, and atmosphere).
Does mealtime serve a particular function? (For example, are the day's activities planned? Are problems discussed?)
Snacks consumed and frequency
Knows food sources from the basic four food groups
24-hour food recall

Dietary fat

Use of red meat, fish, and poultry (once a week, three times, etc.)
How often do you eat cheese? What kinds do you purchase?
How often do you use cold cuts?
How often do you use fish/chicken? (Describe preparation.)
How often do you use processed foods such as bakery products, frozen dinners?
How much milk or other dairy products do you consume? What types?

Cholesterol and saturated fat

How many eggs does the family eat per week?
What kind of fat do you use in cooking?
What kind of vegetable oil do you use?

Complex carbohydrates and fiber

How often do you eat fruit? How do you eat it (juices, fresh, canned)?
What kind of vegetables do you eat (canned, frozen, fresh)?
What kind of bread do you eat (whole grain, white)?

Sugar consumption

Do you use sugar in cooking? Do you buy candy, pastries, sweetened cereals?

James K: Family nutrition and weight control. In Bomar P, editor: *Nurses and family health promotion: concepts, assessment and interventions,* Baltimore, 1989, Williams & Wilkins.

Sodium

How often do you use processed foods (canned or packaged, such as macaroni and cheese)?

Do you add salt to food?

Alcohol consumption

How often do you use alcohol?

Caffeine

How much coffee and tea do you drink per day?

Supplements

Do you take vitamins or mineral supplements? What and how much? Why?

Cultural influences

"Special" foods

Eating habits unique to culture

Family food preferences or restrictions

Economics

Do you receive any supplementary income to purchase food items?

Eating problems

Do you have problems with indigestion, vomiting, nausea, sore mouth?

Do you have any difficulty swallowing liquids or solids or chewing and feeding yourselves?

Medications

Are you on any medications? Do they affect your appetite or weight?

Weight

Has weight changed in the last 6 months? How much? Describe events associated with the change.

Elimination pattern

Describe bowel and urinary patterns.

Activity and exercise patterns

Usual daily/weekly activities of family members

Source of nutrition information

Magazines, family member, schools, health food store

Family work patterns

Do family members work outside of the home? Type of work and hours?

Physical assessment

Describe appearance of the family

Height

Weight

Blood pressure

Pulse/respirations

Percent body fat

$$\text{Relative weight} = \frac{\text{Actual weight} \times 100}{\text{Ideal weight}}$$

Example:

160 (actual weight) × 100 = 16,000

16,000 divided by ideal weight of 140 = 114%

The closer relative weight is to 100%, the better.

   120 to 139 mild obesity

   140 to 159 moderate obesity

160+ severe obesity

Family strengths/weaknesses

Identify nutritional concerns of the family

Barrier to change? Are there reasons why the family cannot change the problem area?

Assessment summary

Check problem area or potential problems

1. Dietary fat
2. Cholesterol and saturated fat
3. Complex carbohydrates and fiber
4. Sugar
5. Sodium
6. Alcohol
7. Caffeine
8. Supplements
9. Cultural influences
10. Economics
11. Eating problems
12. Medications
13. Weight changes
14. Elimination pattern
15. Activity and exercise
16. Nutrition resources
17. Work patterns
18. Notes of concern

Nursing diagnosis
Plan and intervention
Evaluation

Nutritional History Guidelines
for Home Care Clients

Client name _____   Marital status _____
Age _____   Family or significant
Gender _____   others _____
                                _____

Primary medical diagnosis   _____
_____

Height _____   _____
Weight _____   Recent weight change (note
                                amount, time period, and cause)
Frame (small, medium, large)   _____
_____   _____

Allergies (food or drug)   Smoking (packs per day) _____
_____   _____

Medications _____   _____
_____   _____

Describe dosage schedule for medications, that is, are they taken
with meals or on an empty stomach?
_____

Food preferences _____
_____

Food intolerances or restrictions _____
_____

Therapeutic diet or nutritional support prescription _____
_____

What do the client or family find to be the easiest and most difficult parts of the therapeutic diet or nutritional support plan?
_____
_____

What, if anything, would the client or family like to change about
the therapeutic diet or nutritional support plan?
_____
_____

Usual daily dietary intake (including fluids)
_____
_____

From Sebastian T: Nutrition in home care. In Martinson I, Widmer J, editors: *Home
health care nursing,* Philadelphia, 1989, Saunders.   *Continued.*

Nutritional History Guidelines
for Home Care Clients—cont'd

Availability of foodstuffs:
  Who does the shopping? _____
  Where do you shop? _____
  Do you have transportation problems with regard to shopping?
  _____
  Are you limited by seasonal availability of foods? (Explain) ____
  _____

Financial concerns regarding diet _____
Cultural/religious concerns _____
What is the meaning of food to this family (e.g., social or suste-
nance only)? _____
Food storage:
  Refrigeration: _____
  Hygiene: _____
Food preparation:
  Electricity, gas: _____
  Functioning stove, oven: _____
  Sufficient utensils: _____
  Who prepares the food? _____
  Who makes food decisions? _____
Health problems (describe in terms of onset, chronology, quality,
associated factors, aggravating factors, alleviating factors, how the
problem is managed, whether the intervention is effective) _____
_____
_____
_____
_____

  Indigestion (pre- or post-prandial) _____
  Dysphagia _____
  Difficulty chewing _____
  Diabetes _____
  Cardiovascular disease _____
  Hypertension _____
  Condition of teeth/gums _____
  Dentures (full, partial) _____

Guidelines for Teaching Breast-Feeding

Here are some things to know before you start.

About Yourself

You can assume any comfortable position. Let the breast fall forward without tension. Leave one hand free to guide the nipple into the child's mouth.

The nipple can be made more prominent by gently rolling it between your fingers. The areolar area will be put in the baby's mouth with the nipple. This prevents bruising the nipple.

Colostrum is the yellow fluid you can express from your breasts now. It is good for the baby. It contains some fat and protein and helps baby resist infections.

Milk may be expected to appear 48 to 96 hours after delivery. Before the milk comes in, the breasts feel soft to the touch. After the milk comes in, the breasts feel full and hard.

The Breast-Feeding Technique

Hold the baby so that the infant's cheek touches the breasts. The pressure against the outer angle of the lip begins the rooting reflex. The baby will turn toward the nipple. The baby can smell the colostrum and milk, which also will cause turning toward the nipple.

Put the baby to the breast by guiding the nipple and areolar tissue into the infant's mouth and over the tongue. Compress the breast with thumb above and fingers below areola to permit the infant to latch on effectively.

Expected Infant Responses and Maternal Sensations

At first the baby sucks in short bursts of three to five sucks followed by single swallows. In 1 to 2 days a sucking pattern evolves. This consists of 10 to 30 sucks followed by swallowing. The infant's lips and jaws exert pressure on the areola, and the tongue "cradles" the nipple so that the tip is not retracted. The pressure, combined with negative intraoral pressure, brings milk into the mouth.

When the baby is sucking properly, there is no "clicking" noise. This clicking noise means the infant is sucking on her or his own tongue in the back of the throat, past the nipple. You should hear the rhythmic suck-swallow breathing pattern that indicates milk is flowing. Some mothers can sense if the infant has drawn the areolar tissue into the mouth along with the nipple.

From Bobak IM, Jensen MD: *Maternity and gynecologic care: the nurse and the family,* ed 5, St Louis, 1993, Mosby.

Breast-Feeding the Baby

Get the baby ready to put to the breast by first making sure the infant is awake. If necessary, waken the baby by stroking the cheek, rubbing the feet, and talking to her or him. The nurse may help you position the baby so that the head is directly facing the breast and the nipple is not pulled to one side.

Now put the infant to breast by bringing the baby to the breast, not the breast to the baby. The baby's face, chest, genitals, and knees should all be facing your body. Touch the infant's upper lip with your nipple, and watch how the baby will turn toward you with an open mouth. Pull the baby as close to you as you can.

Feel how the baby's jaws fit behind the nipple and the nipple is deep in the infant's mouth.

If infant needs more breathing space, lift your breast, or make a "dimple" in your breast for breathing space.

CAUTION: Making a "dimple" may be done too vigorously, which may dislodge the nipple.

You may need to hold your nipple throughout the entire feeding for a few weeks.

It is a good idea to use both breasts at each feeding. You need to empty both breasts because an empty breast signals the woman's body to produce more milk. Once the milk has come in, you can tell which breast to start with next time by feeling the weight. The heaviest one has the most milk, so start with that one. In the meantime, put a safety pin on your bra on the side that you finished, so you will know which side to start out with next time.

To remove the baby from the breast, place a finger in the corner of the baby's mouth until the suction is broken. The breast can then be comfortably removed.

Before putting the baby to the other breast, burp the infant. Some babies never burp; others do so frequently. Gently rub or pat the baby's back.

After feeding, place the baby on the right side. This allows air in the stomach to come up and not bring the milk with it.

How to Have a Totally Breast-Fed Baby and Work Too!

(Going Back to Work at 6 Weeks Postpartum)

Starting out:

First 3 to 4 weeks breast-feed only to establish your milk supply.

Nurse your baby every 2 to 3 hours to build up your milk supply.

Relax and enjoy 6 weeks of nursing totally.

Establishing a home milk supply by pumping your breasts:

Do NOT attempt to pump until the fifth week home from the hospital.

Weeks 5 and 6 when baby doesn't nurse every 3 hours, pump. This will mean you are either feeding or pumping every 3 hours.

In the beginning you will only be able to pump approximately ½ to 1 ounce of breast milk. Don't panic. After practicing *and* believing, you will be able to pump 1 to 3 ounces or more!

How to pump at home:

Relax and drink plenty of fluids.

Take a warm shower or use warm compresses on your breasts.

Pump 15 minutes on each side while nursing the baby by propping the baby on your lap with pillows on one side and pumping the other side. Baby feeding facilitates milk "let-down" and you will be able to obtain more breast milk while pumping. The baby will be well fed from one-sided nursing.

Pump at every first morning feeding; you'll get a good amount of breast milk for a reserve supply as baby has gone longer between feedings.

Pumping at work:

Pump every 3 to 4 hours (or more often) to increase your milk supply.

Pump after 6 to 8 hours away from the baby or when engorgement is felt. This will give you 4 to 12 ounces of milk, enough to feed your baby the next day when added to your supply at home.

Storage:

Freeze immediately after pumping even at work. You can carry home the milk pumped at work in a small ice cooler. Remember that breast milk is now more precious than gold.

Freeze in 1 to 2 ounces amounts in plastic baby bottle liners sealed with twist ties. Sit plastic bags in glass to freeze any spillage.

Date milk and use oldest first.

From Fountain Valley Community Hospital: *Childbirth education,* Fountain Valley, Calif, 1983.

Equipment:
    Breast pads—Evenflo or Sears.
    Handpump—Kaneson.
    Electric pump—Eggnell (suggested that the equipment be rented).
        The cost is 80% to 100% covered by insurance if prescribed by
        your doctor. Have your doctor prescribe the pump in the hospital.
    Plastic baby bottles and nipples. Always use the same brand.
Preparation of frozen breast milk for feeding baby:
    Hold plastic bag under hot running water until thawed and warm.
    Pour into plastic bottle and feed the baby.

Guidelines for Teaching
Formula-Feeding

Baby needs to be wide awake.

The hospital bottles of formula can be stored at room temperature. You may use this brand or the one your pediatrician recommends. They contain 4 oz of formula (120 ml). Your baby will probably drink 2 to 3 oz (60 to 90 ml) at a feeding for a few days and then increase. If you do not use all the formula, throw the remainder away because it spoils once opened.

You can keep track of how many ounces the baby drinks in 1 day by writing it down. When you take the baby for a checkup, your physician or nurse will ask you the amount of intake.

Your baby will probably be hungry every 2½ to 3 hours. If your baby fusses or cries in between feedings, check the diaper or the infant's need to be picked up and cuddled. As the baby gets older, thirst may occur. Check with the pediatrician concerning water supplementation.

Test the temperature of the formula by letting a few drops fall on the inside of your wrist. If the formula feels comfortably warm to you, it is the correct temperature. If the formula is refrigerated, warm it by placing the bottle in a pan of hot water. Check it often for correct temperature.

Test the size of the nipple hole by holding the bottle and nipple upside down. The formula should drip from the nipple. If it runs in a stream, the hole is too big. If it has to be shaken for the formula to come out, the hole is too small. To correct this, you can try a softer nipple or enlarge the hole in the nipple or both. To enlarge the hole, heat a needle stuck into a cork (used as a handle) and insert the hot

From Bobak IM, Jensen MD: *Maternity and gynecologic care: the nurse and the family,* ed 5, St Louis, 1993, Mosby.

needle into the nipple. New nipples may be softened by boiling for 5 minutes before using. If the nipple collapses, unscrew the bottle lid to let air in.

Some newborns need burping. They tend to swallow air when sucking. Burp the baby who has been crying before feeding, then after every ounce of formula. As the infant gets older and you get more experienced, you will know when to burp the baby.

To feed the baby, place the nipple in the infant's mouth over the tongue. It should rest against the roof of the mouth. This stimulates the sucking reflex.

Hold the bottle like a pencil. Keep nipple filled with milk so the infant does not suck air.

Start out with the baby held away from you until the nipple is in the mouth. The baby who is too close will turn toward you and not the nipple; this is the rooting reflex.

After the baby starts feeding, you can hold the infant close.

Some newborns take longer to feed than others. Slow, patient feeding, keeping the baby awake, and encouraging the infant to take more may be necessary.

The stools of a formula-fed newborn are soft but formed. They will be a yellow with a characteristic odor. The baby probably will defecate either during the feeding or after. Change the diaper immediately because the composition of the stool is irritating to the skin.

Safety Tips

Do not prop the bottle. The nipple may fall against the throat and block the air, or the baby could drown in the formula or aspirate any that was regurgitated.

Newborns should never be left alone while feeding until they are old enough to remove the bottle from their mouth.

Bottles taken to bed can lead to early dental problems in young children (nursing bottle caries or baby bottle syndrome).

Practice how to hold the newborn, and use the bulb syringe in case the baby should choke.

After the baby is finished, place the infant in the crib on the right side so air can come up easily.

Dietary Guidelines Directed at Problems of Obesity

- Avoid becoming overweight by controlling caloric intake and increasing exercise.
- Increase intake of complex carbohydrates and naturally occurring sugars to 50% to 60% of the energy intake.
- Reduce intake of refined sugars to 6 or fewer teaspoons per day.
- Reduce fat intake to less than 30% of energy intake.
- Reduce saturated fat intake to 10% and receive the rest of fat intake from 10% each of unsaturated and polyunsaturated fats.
- Reduce cholesterol to less than 300 mg per day.
- Reduce salt intake to 3 g (1+ teaspoonfuls).
- Eat a variety of foods.
- Maintain ideal body weight.
- Include adequate starch and fiber in the diet.
- Consume alcohol in moderation if at all.

Notes

From US Department of Agriculture and the Department of Health and Human Services: *Dietary guidelines for Americans,* Washington, DC, 1992.

Controlling Fat in the Diet

Healthy Substitutes for Fatty Foods

Choose these . . .	Instead of these . . .
Breads	
French bread, pita bread, water bagels, Italian bread, English muffins, plain bread sticks, whole grain breads, or corn tortillas (unfried)	Croissants, "butter-topped" bread, challah, crescent rolls, biscuits, toaster cakes, pastries, and other prepared rolls
Crackers	
Melba toast, oyster crackers, saltines, soda crackers, matzo, Swedish flat breads	"Snack" crackers with ingredients that include butter, hydrogenated oils, palm oil, coconut oil, lard, and other saturated fats
Starches	
Potatoes, dried beans, peas and legumes, plain rice, pasta, most cereals	Pancake, waffle, biscuit, quick bread mixes, muffin mixes, flavored rice and pasta mixes, granola cereal
Oatmeal may actually help reduce your cholesterol	
Fruits and vegetables	
Enjoy all except . . .	Coconut, avocado, olives, frozen vegetables with sauces
Processed meat	
Lean boiled ham, turkey, or chicken products	Hot dogs, bologna, salami, sausage, bacon
Baked desserts/cookies	
Angel food cake, animal crackers, ginger snaps, plain graham crackers	Those with ingredients that include beef fat, lard, hydrogenated vegetable oils, chocolate, eggs (or "add eggs"), coconut oil, palm oil. Also, frostings with hydrogenated vegetable or animal fats
Snack foods	
Pretzels, plain popped corn	Potato chips, corn chips
Frozen desserts	
Sherbet, fruit juice bars, low-fat frozen yogurt, ice milk	Ice cream

Modified from Culligan D: *The Pawtucket heart health program,* Hamden, Conn, 1988, Quinnipiack Valley Health District.

Fat and Cholesterol Content of Selected Foods

Make a habit of reading nutrient labels on foods. They'll give information similar to that shown on the food table below, which gives examples of some commonly eaten foods and their fat, cholesterol, and caloric contents.

Food	Serving size	Calories	Fat (g)	Saturated fat (g)	Cholesterol (mg)	Sodium (mg)
Dairy products						
Milk						
Fluid whole	1 cup	150	8.2	5.1	33	120
Skim	1 cup	86	0.4	0.3	4	126
Cheese						
Cheddar	1 oz	114	9.4	6.0	30	176
Cottage—creamed	½ cup	109	4.7	3.0	16	425
Cottage—low fat, 1% fat	½ cup	82	1.2	0.7	5	459
Mozzarella, part skim	1 oz	72	4.5	2.9	16	132
Eggs (whole, raw)	1 med	79	5.6	1.7	213	69
Fats and oils						
Peanut butter (smooth)	2 tsp	63	5.5	0.9	0	52
Butter	1 tsp	36	4.1	2.5	11	41
Tub margarine						
Safflower oil	1 tsp	34	3.8	0.4	0	51
Corn oil	1 tsp	34	3.8	0.7	0	51

Meat, poultry, fish

Lean beef, average all grades, cooked	1 oz	63	2.9	1.1	25	18
Beef liver, braised	1 oz	46	1.4	0.5	110	30
Lean pork, center loin, fresh, broiled	1 oz	65	3.0	1.0	28	22
Bacon, pan-fried, 4½ slices	1 oz	163	14	5.0	24	452
Frankfurters (beef and pork)	1 oz	91	8.3	3.1	14	318
Chicken, flesh without skin (stewed)					
Light meat	1 oz	45	1.1	0.3	22	18
Dark meat	1 oz	54	2.5	0.7	25	21
Fish					
Flounder, cooked, dry heat	1 oz	33	0.4	0.1	19	30
Salmon, coho, cooked, moist heat	1 oz	52	2.1	0.4	14	17
Tuna, light, canned in water drained solids	1 oz	37	0.1	0.1	—	101
Shellfish					
Lobster, Northern, cooked, moist heat	1 oz	28	0.2	Trace	20	108
Shrimp (cooked)	1 oz	28	0.3	0.1	55	63

Modified from American Heart Association: *Cholesterol and your heart*, AHA National Center, Dallas, Tex, 1989, The Association.

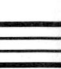

Suggestions for a Low-Fat Diet

For a Diet Low in Fat, Saturated Fat, and Cholesterol
Fats and oils

- Use fats and oils sparingly in cooking.
- Use small amounts of salad dressings and spreads, such as butter, margarine, and mayonnaise. One tablespoon of most of these spreads provides 10 to 11 g of fat.
- Choose liquid vegetable oils most often because they are lower in saturated fat.
- Check labels on foods to see how much fat and saturated fat are in a serving.

Meat, poultry, fish, dry beans, and eggs

- Have two or three servings, with a daily total of about 6 oz. Three oz of cooked lean beef or chicken without skin—the size of a deck of cards—provides about 6 g of fat.
- Trim fat from meat; take skin off poultry.
- Have cooked dry beans and peas instead of meat occasionally.
- Moderate the use of egg yolks and organ meats.

Milk and milk products

- Have two or three servings daily. (Count as a serving: 1 cup of milk or yogurt or about 1½ oz of cheese.)
- Choose skim or low-fat milk and fat-free or low-fat yogurt and cheese most of the time. One cup of skim milk has only a trace of fat, 1 cup of 2%-fat milk has 5 g of fat, and 1 cup of whole milk has 8 g of fat.

From US Department of Agriculture and the Department of Health and Human Services: *Dietary guidelines for Americans,* Washington, DC, 1990.

Figure Out Your Fat

The recommendation is that no more than 30% of total calories come from fat. Food labels list fat in grams. To find out what *your* total intake of fats in grams should be limited to, multiply your daily calories by 0.30 (30%) and divide by 9 (the number of calories in a gram of fat).

Example: 2200 calories × 0.30 = 660 calories from fat
660 calories ÷ 9 = 73 g of fat

Getting a Variety of Foods

The Dietary Guidelines say that the many nutrients you need should come from a variety of foods, not from a few highly fortified foods or supplements. A good way to ensure variety is to choose foods each day from the five major food groups. USDA has developed a daily food guide for a well-balanced diet that suggests the following:

- Vegetables—3 to 5 servings
- Fruits—2 to 4 servings
- Breads, cereals, rice, pasta—6 to 11 servings
- Milk, yogurt, cheese—2 to 3 servings
- Meat, poultry, fish, dried beans and peas, eggs, nuts—2 to 3 servings

From Food and Drug Administration, DHHS pub # 91-2247, HFI-40, 1991, Rockville, Md.

Eating Disorders

Eating Disorder Definitions

According to the American Psychiatric Association, a person diagnosed as bulimic or anorectic must have all of that disorder's specific symptoms:

Bulimia nervosa

- Recurrent episodes of binge eating (minimum average of two binge-eating episodes a week for at least 3 months)
- A feeling of lack of control over eating during the binges
- Regular use of one or more of the following to prevent weight gain: self-induced vomiting, use of laxatives or diuretics, strict dieting or fasting, or vigorous exercise
- Persistent overconcern with body shape and weight

Anorexia nervosa

- Refusal to maintain weight that's over the lowest weight considered normal for age and height
- Intense fear of gaining weight or becoming fat, even though underweight
- Distorted body image
- In women, three consecutive missed menstrual periods without pregnancy

---

From Food and Drug Administration, DHHS pub # 92-1194, HFI-40, 1994, Rockville, Md.

Clinical Manifestations
of Bulimia and Anorexia

1. Loss of tooth enamel
2. Tooth decay
3. Infection of the mouth
4. Gastrointestinal bleeding
5. Gastritis or esophagitis

⎫ associated with vomiting of food and gastric acid ⎬ (items 1–5)

6. Malnutrition
7. Loss of rectal tone
8. Loss of minerals and bone mass
9. Diarrhea

⎫ associated with purging ⎬ (items 7–9)

10. Amenorrhea
11. Hyperactivity without fatigue
12. Agitated behavior
13. Disorganized thinking
14. Excessive weight loss
15. Sleep disorder
16. Epigastric pain

From Phipps WJ, Sands J, Lehman MK, Cassmeyer V: *Medical-surgical nursing: concepts and clinical practice,* ed 5, St Louis, 1995, Mosby.

Guidelines for Teaching the Client
with an Eating Disorder

Educating the client about the eating disorder is important. Elements of the teaching include the following:

1. Disease concept of eating disorders
2. Medical aspects of the disease
3. The need for an adequate and prudent diet
4. The importance of finding healthy ways to cope with life
5. The awareness of an increased tendency to transfer obsessions
6. Signs and symptoms of relapse
7. Importance of aftercare
8. Importance of a stable support system

Expected Client Outcomes for the Client with an Eating Disorder

Expected client outcomes for the client with bulimia or anorexia include but are not limited to the following:

1. Maintains optimal nutrition.
2. Maintains adequate hydration.
3. Remains free of infection.
4. Demonstrates improved activity tolerance.
5. Maintains positive body image.
6. Verbalizes improved self-esteem.
7. Demonstrates improved management of anxiety.
8. Demonstrates improved and effective coping mechanisms.
9. Admits that bulimia or anorexia is a problem in his or her life.
10. Verbalizes a plan to carry out desired health related behavior.
11. Verbalizes knowledge of disease and treatment.
12. Demonstrates increased ability to cope with interpersonal encounters and social isolation.

Evaluation

To evaluate the effectiveness of nursing interventions, compare client behaviors with those stated in the expected client outcomes. Successful achievement of client outcomes for the client with anorexia or bulimia is indicated by the following:

1. Sustains weight gain.
2. Has good skin turgor with moist and pink mucous membranes.
3. Does not have nosocomial infection.
4. Able to be up and about without assistance and able to do own activities of daily living.
5. Speaks positively about own body image, and exhibits pleasure at change in appearance.
6. Demonstrates improved self-esteem by speaking positively about self.
7. Appears less anxious and sits or lies quietly without exhibiting nervousness.
8. Demonstrates improved coping mechanisms by being less angry and frustrated and not withdrawing when things do not go as planned.

From Phipps WJ, Sands J, Lehman MK, Cassmeyer V: *Medical-surgical nursing: concepts and clinical practice,* ed 5, St Louis, 1995, Mosby.

9. Verbalizes that bulimia or anorexia is a problem that is affecting his or her life and needs to be addressed.
10. Discusses how to maintain weight at desired level, participates in moderate exercise, and attends Overeaters Anonymous (OA) meetings regularly.
11. Discusses his or her disease, how to care for self, how to avoid complications, and the need for regular follow-up.
12. Interacts more comfortably with a variety of persons.

PART FIVE
INTERVENTION GUIDES

Often the nurse, in addition to teaching, must carry out clinical procedures in the home. The following guides will help the nurse establish and execute needed care. This list is not considered to be exhaustive but is to be used as a reference for common activities of the community health nurse.

Techniques for the Nurse

Hand Washing Technique

1. Use a sink with warm running water, soap, and paper towels.
2. Push wristwatch and long uniform sleeves up above wrists. Remove jewelry, except a plain band, from fingers and arms.
3. Keep fingernails short and filed.
4. Inspect the surface of the hands and fingers for breaks or cuts in the skin and cuticles. Report such lesions when caring for highly susceptible clients.
5. Stand in front of the sink, keeping hands and uniform away from the sink surface. (If hands touch the sink during hand washing, repeat the process.) Use a sink where it is comfortable to reach the faucet.
6. Turn on the water. Turn on hand-operated faucets by covering the faucet with a paper towel.
7. Avoid splashing water against your uniform or clothes.
8. Regulate flow of water so the temperature is warm.

Modified from Potter PA, Perry AG: *Fundamentals of nursing: concepts, process, and practice,* ed 3, St Louis, 1993, Mosby.

9. Wet hands and lower arms thoroughly under running water. Keep the hands and forearms lower than the elbows during washing.
10. Apply 1 ml of regular or 3 ml of antiseptic liquid soap to the hands, lathering thoroughly. If bar soap is used, hold it throughout the lathering period. Soap granules and leaflet preparations may be used.
11. Wash the hands, using plenty of lather and friction for at least 10 to 15 seconds. Interlace the fingers and rub the palms and back of hands with a circular motion at least 5 times each.
12. If areas underlying fingernails are soiled, clean them with fingernails of the other hand and additional soap or a clean orangewood stick. Do not tear or cut the skin under or around the nail.
13. Rinse hands and wrists thoroughly, keeping hands down and elbows up.
14. Repeat steps 10 through 12 but extend the actual period of washing for 1-, 2-, and 3-minute hand washings.
15. Dry the hands thoroughly from the fingers up to the wrists and forearms.
16. Discard paper towel in proper receptacle.
17. To turn off a hand faucet, use a clean, dry paper towel.

Remember to treat the inside of your "black bag" as clean. Always wash hands before removing supplies and equipment from bag or putting clean supplies in the bag. Carry soap and paper towels in outside packets of your bag or at inner top.

Sterilizing Equipment in the Home

Moist-Heat Sterilization
1. When boiling equipment, have a large pan with handles on both sides and a lid and use wide-mouth jars.
2. It is best to boil equipment about 1 hour before use. It will then be sterile and cool enough to handle.
3. Always boil equipment immersed in water in a covered pan. Start timing after water begins to boil and boil for 10 minutes.
4. If equipment won't be used for a while, keep the lid on the pan until ready for use.

Dry-Heat Sterilization
1. You can use any metal pan, such as a cake or pie pan to sterilize dressings in the oven.

Modified from Humphrey C: *Home care nursing handbook,* Baltimore, 1994, Aspen.

2. Place the clean dressings, wrapped in a clean cloth, into the pie tin and bake in a preheated oven at 350°F for 1 hour. Wrap the cloth so that you will not contaminate the dressings upon unwrapping. Let cool slightly before using.

Solutions

Solutions Used as Disinfectants

Bleach—undiluted is used for spillage of body fluids, that is, blood, vomitus, and excreta for clients with hepatitis.

Bleach—diluted in a mixture of 1:10 can be used for cleaning contaminated surfaces when caring for clients with AIDS.

Lysol solution should be mixed as directed on bottle. Never use anywhere near food. All items in contact with solution should be rinsed well.

White vinegar in a mixture of 1:3 can be used to disinfect respiratory and tracheostomy equipment. First, wash equipment well with friction and soap and water. Place in vinegar solution and store in a closed container. Allow to air dry before using.

Solutions for Wounds and Irrigations

Although solutions used for dressing changes and some irrigation procedures can be purchased already prepared and sterilized, often client situations demand that these solutions be made in the home. High cost, lack of financial resources, long-term use, and lack of transportation to purchase supplies often mean that the nurse can best ensure that procedures are complied with by teaching families how to make their own solutions in the home.

In the following section, procedures for making and storing solutions in the home are given in a simple format that can be easily taught to clients. Once a procedure is established, solutions can be made in the home easily and without danger to the client and will save a great deal of money. Things to remember when using solutions in the home are as follows:

- Teach the family the difference between sterile and clean technique.
- Use safe containers, such as canning jars, mayonnaise jars, and such.
- Label all solutions with name and date prepared.
- Keep solutions out of reach of small children and pets.

Modified from Humphrey C: *Home care nursing handbook,* Baltimore, 1994, Aspen; Modified Dakin's solution: Yale New Haven Hospital Drug Information Center, New Haven, 1993.

Sterile water: A new container of sterile water should be made daily, and the solution in the jar should be stored in a cool place.

Equipment

Large pan with a lid, small-mouth glass jar with a lid (1 quart size, a mayonnaise jar is a good choice), tap water

Procedure

1. Fill the jar to the top with tap water.
2. Stand jar up in the pan and fill up the pan with enough water to cover the jar. Drop the jar lid into the pan and be sure it sinks to the bottom.
3. Cover the pan, bring the water to a boil, and boil for 20 minutes.
4. After the 20 minutes, remove from heat, cool, and pour off enough water from the pan that you can handle the jar comfortably or use tongs that have also been boiled. Touching only the outside of the jar, take the jar out of the pan and set it on a counter.
5. Pour off the remaining water in the pan, remove the jar lid, touching only the outside of the rim and place it on the jar. *Note:* This procedure can be followed to prepare an empty sterile jar and lid. Water can be boiled in another container and poured into the sterile empty jar, the lid attached and water stored.

Normal saline: Normal saline is simply water that has a certain amount of salt in it that is compatible with all body fluids. If you are using the normal saline for a bladder irrigation or other sterile procedure, make a new supply every day. If it is used for a clean dressing or other clean procedure, it will keep refrigerated for 1 week.

Equipment

Table salt—iodized or noniodized—tap water, teaspoon, measuring cup, quart jar with lid, and pan

Strength

Normal saline: 0.9%

Procedure

1. Wash teaspoon, measuring cup, jar, and lid in hot soapy water and rinse well in hot water.
2. Boil at least 6 cups of tap water in a pan for 20 minutes and let cool.
3. Pour 4 cups of the boiled water into a clean jar.
4. Add 2 teaspoons of salt and mix well with the water.
5. Put the lid on the jar, write the date you made the solution on the outside of the jar, and put in the refrigerator.

Modified Dakin's solution: Dakin's solution can be made from bleach. Bleach is 5.25% sodium hypochlorite, and full strength Dakin's solution is 0.5% sodium hypochlorite. The solution is good only for 3 days because it deteriorates.

Equipment
Bleach, sterile water, a liter glass jar with cover, and a teaspoon that has been sterilized

Strength
30 ml bleach
1000 ml sterile water
2 teaspoons baking soda (a buffer)

Procedure
1. Into the sterile jar, put the amount of bleach desired to achieve the strength ordered.
2. Add enough sterile water to fill to the top. The water does not have to be cooled before adding to the bleach if the solution is to be used immediately. If the solution is to be stored, it is preferable to cool the water before adding to the bleach.
3. Cover with a sterile lid and store at room temperature.

Both Dakin's solution and chlorpactin (bleach) use hypochlorite and water as a mixture. However, Dakin's is less expensive to use, less irritating to the tissue (if buffered), and works equally as well as chlorpactin. Chlorpactin is a brand name for hypochlorite (bleach). It must be purchased in a packet or vial and mixed according to the directions on the product.

Chloramine T (Chlorazene): This solution is similar to Dakin's solution in terms of activity. It is more stable and lasts longer but should not be used in place of Dakin's solution without the permission of the physician. It is used in 1% or 2% solutions applied in the same manner as Dakin's solution. You must have Chlorazene tablets (purchased by prescription) to make this solution.

Equipment
Chlorazene tablets, sterile water, and a small container

Strength
1% Chlorazene-1 tablet to 1 oz water
2% Chlorazene-2 tablets to 1 oz water

Procedure
Mix together in small, clean container.

Acetic acid: Acetic acid can be made with white vinegar because vinegar contains 5% acetic acid. Acetic acid may be used for dressings but should not be used for bladder irrigations because the acid can cause a negative effect on kidney functioning. Even though the solution can be kept in the refrigerator up to 1 week, a fresh solution made every day is best.

Equipment
White distilled vinegar, sterile water, 1.5 quart jar or glass bowl, jar with cover, tablespoon, measuring cup, and large pan

Strength
0.25 acetic acid = 4 tablespoons vinegar in 5 cups of boiled water

Procedure
1. Wash tablespoon, measuring cup, jar, and lid in hot, soapy water. Rinse well in hot water.
2. Boil at least 6 cups of water in the pan for 20 minutes and let it cool.
3. Add 4 tablespoons of white, distilled vinegar, and mix well.
4. Put the lid on the jar and write the date you made it on a label on the outside of the jar.

Notes

Improvising Equipment

Bed Cradle

To alleviate the pressure of the covers over the feet of a bedbound client try:

- Laying a lightweight walker on the bed to support the covers.
- Putting a small, open-legged television table under the covers with the tabletop facing the foot of the bed. This can also be used as a footboard.
- Using an empty cardboard box with the top cut off to allow the client room to move feet.

Bed Table

- A bed table can be improvised by placing the longer end of an adjustable-height ironing board across the bed.
- A bed table/tray can be improvised with a cardboard or wooden box that has had the two wide sides cut out and then placed over the client's lap.

Footboards

When footboards are unavailable, high-topped canvas basketball sneakers work well at keeping the client's feet aligned to prevent foot drop. They should be worn with cotton socks and rotated with a schedule of on 4 hours, off 4 hours to keep feet dry and healthy.

Bed Rails

A card table can be used as a bed rail for clients. Simply open two legs and slip them under the mattress. Make a soft cushion against the card table with pillows or blankets. This should not be used with a client who is very active, but it can be extremely helpful when used to ensure safety of the elderly or sedated client.

Ice Collar

A wet dish towel frozen around a large cylinder (that is, a can) makes an effective ice collar. Wrap a cloth around a frozen juice can or put a frozen juice can in a sock and roll the can over a muscle in spasm.

Leg- or Arm-Lift Exerciser

To make an inexpensive leg-lift or arm-lift exerciser, sew together the waistband of a man's cotton brief. Then slip the amount of weight ordered (can be 5 pounds of sugar, plastic bag filled with rice or flour,

Modified from Humphrey C: *Home care nursing handbook,* Baltimore, 1994, Aspen.

and so on) into the brief through one leg hole. The client puts the extremity to be exercised through one leg hole and out the other and moves the extremity up and down in the manner desired.

Making a Temporary Eye Shield*

Many serious eye injuries seen in offices and clinics call for a metal eye shield to protect the eye while the client travels to a hospital or to another physician's office. If one is not available, create a disposable shield by cutting a circle with a 5- to 6-inch diameter out of a client folder. Remove a 1-in "pie slice" and then pull the sides together with tape to form a slightly conical shape. This makes a sturdy, lightweight eye shield (see figure below).

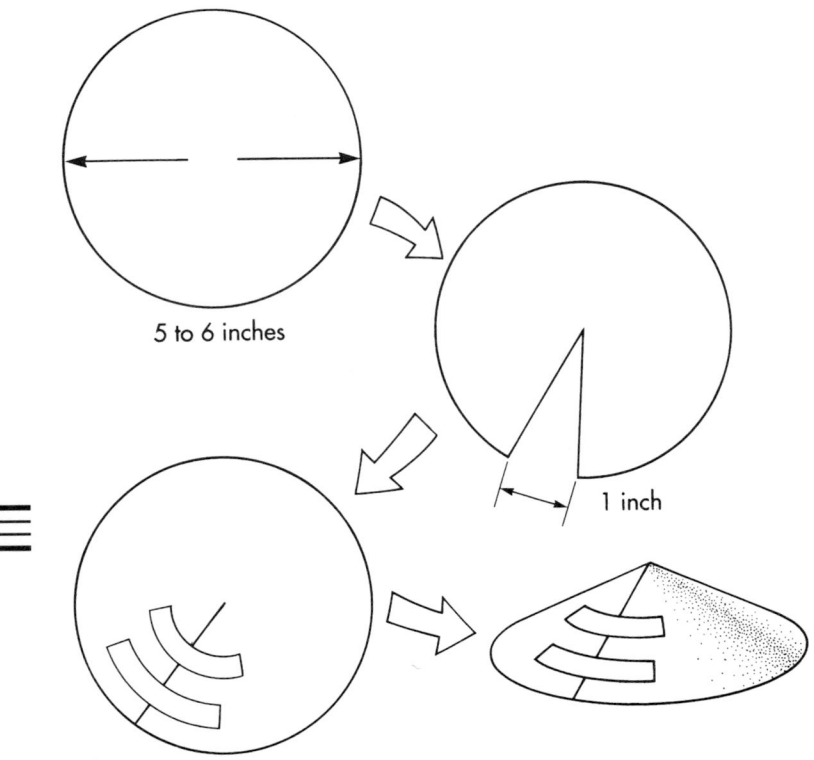

5 to 6 inches

1 inch

*Modified from Brewer T: Making a temporary eye shield, *Consultant* 78(12):53, 1988.

Specimen Collection Techniques

Specimen source	Amount needed*	Collection device*	Specimen collection and transfer
Wound	As much as possible (after cleaning skin to remove flora)	Cotton-tipped swab or syringe	Have clean test tube or culturette tube on clean paper towel. After swabbing center of wound site, grasp collection tube by holding it with paper towel. Carefully insert swab without touching outside of tube. After washing hands and securing tube's top, transfer tube into bag held by nurse outside room.
Blood	10 ml per culture bottle, from two different venipuncture sites	Syringe and culture media bottles	Perform venipuncture at two different sites to decrease likelihood of both specimens being contaminated by skin flora. Have second nurse at client's door holding culture bottles and swabing off bottletops with alcohol. Change needles after venipuncture. Inject 10 ml of blood into each bottle. Nurse at doorway secures tops of bottles, labels specimens, and sends to laboratory.

Continued.

From Potter PA, Perry AG: *Fundamentals of nursing: concepts, process, and practice,* ed 3, St Louis, 1993, Mosby.
*Agency policies may differ on type of containers and amount of specimen material required.

Specimen Collection Techniques—cont'd

Specimen source	Amount needed*	Collection device*	Specimen collection and transfer
Stool	Small amount, approximate size of a walnut	Clean cup with seal top (not necessary to be sterile) and tongue blade	Place cup on clean paper towel in client's bathroom. Using tongue blade, collect needed amount of feces from client's bedpan. Transfer feces to cup without touching cup's outside surface. Wash hands and place seal on cup. Transfer specimen into clean bag held by nurse outside room.
Urine	1 to 5 ml	Syringe and sterile cup	Place cup or tube on clean towel in client's bathroom. Use syringe to collect specimen if client has a Foley catheter. Have client follow procedure to obtain a clean voided specimen if not catheterized. Transfer urine into sterile container either by injecting urine from syringe or pouring it from used container. Wash hands and secure top of container. Transfer specimen into clean bag held by nurse outside room.

Peritoneal Dialysis and
Continuous Ambulatory Dialysis

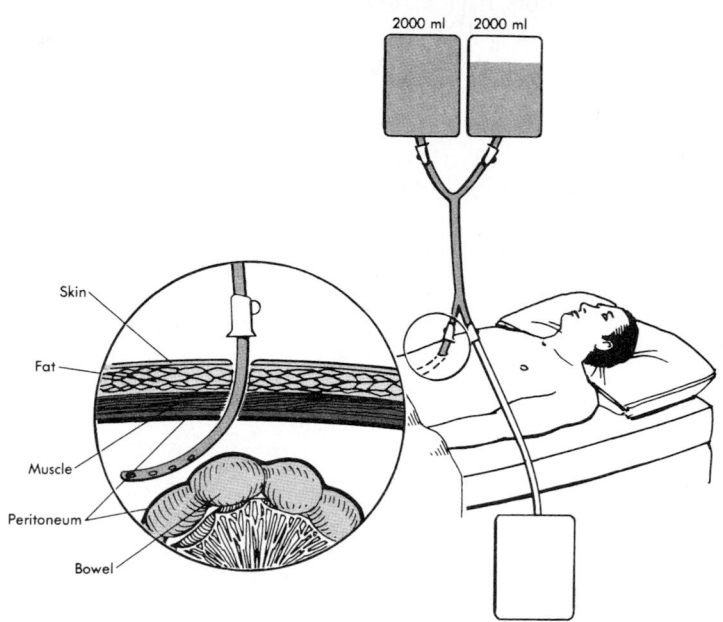

Client receiving peritoneal dialysis. Dialysis fluid is being inserted into peritoneal cavity. (From Phipps WJ, Sands J, Lehman MK, Cassmeyer V: *Medical-surgical nursing,* ed 5, St Louis, 1995, Mosby.)

Assessment

1. Obtain client's weight.
2. Obtain vital signs.
3. Measure abdominal girth.
   a. Mark midpoint of client's abdomen. Keep mark as reference for future measurements.
4. Inspect catheter site for erythema, tenderness, drainage.
5. Measure body temperature.
6. Review dialysis procedure for PD or CAPD.
7. Review physician's orders:
   a. PD: usually include 24 exchanges with specific dialysate volume and composition, as well as specific dwell time, which is commonly 20 minutes.

From Perry A, Potter P: *Clinical nursing skills and techniques,* ed 2, St Louis, 1990, Mosby.

   b. CAPD: usually include three to five exchanges with specific dialysate volume and composition, as well as specific dwell time, which can range from 4 to 8 hours.

8. Obtain laboratory data as ordered:

   a. PD: every 12 to 24 hours.

   b. CAPD: can vary depending on individual needs.

Evaluation

1. Obtain weight.
2. Obtain dialysis fluid balance.
3. Obtain vital signs.
4. Measure abdominal girth.
5. Inspect catheter site for erythema, tenderness, drainage.
6. Obtain body temperature.
7. Inspect returned dialysate solution.

Expected outcomes

1. Decreased weight.
2. Positive fluid balance.
3. Stable vital signs.
4. Decreased abdominal girth.
5. No erythema, tenderness, drainage at catheter site.
6. No fever.
7. Dialysate return is clear or slightly light yellow.

Unexpected outcomes

1. Increased weight or no weight change.
2. Negative fluid balance.
3. Decreased blood pressure and tachycardia.
4. Increased abdominal girth.
5. Erythema, tenderness, drainage at catheter site.
6. Fever.
7. Dialysate drainage abnormal:
   a. Cloudy.
   b. Bright red blood.
   c. Brown color or presence of stool.
8. Cramps.
9. Sudden respiratory distress.
10. Poor instillation flow.
11. Poor drainage.
12. Scrotal swelling.
13. Leak at catheter site.

Recording and Reporting

1. Document client's weight, abdominal girth, dialysis fluid balance before and after PD.
2. Document client's vital signs before, during, after dialysis.
3. Document temperature and status of catheter site.
4. Record color of drainage.
5. Record condition of catheter dressing or if new dressing applied.
6. Note any unexpected outcomes and action taken by nurse and physician.

Follow-up Activities

1. Remove catheter if the following occur:
   a. Signs of local infection.
   b. Catheter displacement.
2. Stop dialysis and notify physician for:
   a. Change in vital signs.
   b. Respiratory distress.
   c. Bright red blood.
   d. Fecal contents in drainage.
   e. Scrotal swelling.
   f. Complaints of cramps.

Special Considerations

- Fever is early sign of catheter-induced peritonitis.
- Changes in blood pressure and increased respiratory rate may signal intolerance to amount of fluid instilled in peritoneal cavity.
- A 1-kg weight gain in 24 to 48 hours can be correlated with 1 L of retained fluid.
- Large volume of dialysate instilled may give client urge to defecate.
- Client receiving PD should be encouraged to move around in bed. However, movements should avoid stressing catheter or tubing.
- CAPD clients have increased abdominal girth during dwell time of exchange.
- Clients on CAPD may experience fresh weight gain caused by dextrose absorption.

Teaching Considerations

- Teach CAPD clients scrub and exchange procedures according to policy.
- Review teaching plan with client before discharge and during each clinic visit.
- Ask client to correctly demonstrate scrub and exchange procedure.
- Periodically review potential complications and signs and symptoms.

- Review medications and dietary and fluid restrictions.
- Instruct client when and who to contact in emergency.
- Instruct client to correctly take blood pressure.
- Instruct client to correctly weigh self.
- Instruct client about common symptoms associated with peritonitis.

Home Care Considerations

- CAPD clients must do the following to correctly complete CAPD exchanges:
  a. Achieve goals under Planning.
  b. Demonstrate CAPD scrub and aseptic exchange.
  c. State signs of infection.
  d. Adhere to fluid, dietary, medication therapies.
  e. Perform activities of daily living. CAPD is designed so client can maintain normal daily activities.

Cast Care

1. Client education
   a. Before cast application, explain why and how the cast will be applied.
   b. Advise the client that the plaster cast will feel warm as it dries.
   c. Explain the extent to which the client will be immobilized.
   d. Following cast application, explain care of the cast and expectations after discharge.
   e. Instruct client not to insert sharp objects (coat hangers or pencils) under the cast, because these may abrade the skin and lead to infection.
2. Handling the new cast
   a. Support wet cast with the flat of the hands or on pillows to avoid indentations that will cause pressure on underlying skin.
   b. Place cotton blankets or other absorbent material under the cast to aid the drying process.
   c. Expose the cast to air as much as possible to aid the drying process.
   d. Turn the client frequently to aid the drying process.
   e. Use a fan to circulate air over the cast.
   f. *Do not apply paint, varnish, or shellac to the cast; plaster is a porous material that allows air to circulate to the skin.*

From Phipps WJ, Sands J, Lehman MK, Cassmeyer V: *Medical-surgical nursing: concepts and clinical practice,* ed 5, St Louis, 1995, Mosby; Perry A, Potter P: *Clinical nursing skills and techniques,* ed 2, St Louis, 1990, Mosby.

3. Skin care
   a. Inspect skin at edges of cast and underlying the cast for redness or irritation; apply petal-shaped strips of adhesive tape or moleskin around rough edges of cast.
   b. Remove plaster crumbs from skin with a washcloth moistened with warm water.
   c. Use creams and lotions sparingly because they may soften the skin and cause the cast to stick to the skin.
   d. Apply waterproof material around perineal area to prevent soiling of and damage to cast and irritation of the skin.
   e. Attend to complaint of pain under the cast, particularly over bony prominences, because this may indicate pressure on the skin. If discomfort is not relieved by repositioning, report to physician. Cast pressure may need to be relieved by windowing or bivalving (cutting cast into two halves).

4. Turning
   a. Turning to any position is generally permitted, as long as the integrity of the cast is not compromised and the client is comfortable.

5. Toileting (for a long leg or hip spica cast)
   a. Use a fracture pan with blanket roll or padding as support under the small of the back.
   b. Elevate the head of the bed, if permitted, or place the bed in reverse Trendelenburg's position.

6. Abdominal discomfort
   a. Cast may be "windowed" (an opening cut into it) to provide relief of abdominal distention or a port for checking bladder distention.

7. Mobilization
   a. Weight bearing is at the discretion of the physician, and the amount of weight bearing will be prescribed.
   b. A cast shoe or a walking heel incorporated into a lower extremity cast will permit weight bearing without damaging the cast.

8. Prevention of neurocirculatory problems
   a. Perform neurocirculatory checks every hour for at least 24 hours after cast application to detect difficulty from swelling or pressure of cast on nerves or vessels. Notify physician of color changes, alterations in sensation, or motion unrelieved by position change; cast may need to be bivalved to relieve pressure.
   b. Elevate affected extremity on pillows until danger of swelling is over (usually 24 to 48 hours).

   c. After mobilization of client with lower extremity or upper extremity cast, avoid keeping extremity in dependent position for prolonged periods.

   d. After lower extremity cast is removed, encourage client to wear elastic stocking and elevate affected leg at rest until full mobility is regained.

Special Considerations

- Casts are removed earlier in babies, children, and older persons to facilitate muscle and joint function.
- If cast is applied for clubfoot, person applying cast can usually mold cast in desired position.
- Plaster of paris casts on babies or children and older persons may have less plaster to aid in moving or lifting.
- Clients in casts may be more comfortable than when not in cast if deformity or crepitation (ends rubbing against each other with fracture) is present.
- Client with wet large limb or wet spica cast requires three people to assist in turning. Proper assistance prevents undue pressure on cast.
- Realign pillows to promote cast drying when client is repositioned.

Teaching Considerations

- Clients must be taught to care for casts in home to protect it from moisture and unnecessary wear.
- If child has clubfoot, parents and child should be taught that frequent cast changes are necessary. Cast changes accommodate normal bone and tissue growth and correction of abnormality.
- Babies in casts for treatment of clubfoot have limited maneuverability.
- Teach client about effects of pressure from cast on underlying skin and tissue.
- Prepare client for itching sensations under cast. Client should avoid sticking objects down or in casts to scratch because these objects can cause break in underlying skin and subsequent infections.
- If client must use crutches instruct in crutch-walking techniques.
- Teach client proper range of joint motion (ROJM) and isometric exercises for affected extremity.

Home Care Considerations

- Client must inspect cast and petal rough edges to reduce risk of trauma to underlying skin and need for cast changes.
- Client must inspect cast daily for foul odor, which indicates skin excoriation or infection under cast.

- Client must inspect skin daily for pressure or friction areas.
- Client must inspect cast daily for cracks or changes in alignment.
- Client must keep plaster of paris cast dry. When bathing, casted extremity must not be submerged because cast absorbs water. If cast becomes wet, dry immediately.
- Synthetic casts may be cleaned with warm water and mild soap.
- Some synthetic casts, those applied with polypropylene stockinette, may be emersed in water. Thorough drying with blow dryer on cool or warm is essential. Complete drying prevents skin maceration.

Application of Male External Catheter

The external application of a urinary drainage device is a convenient, safe method of draining urine in male clients. The condom catheter is suitable for incontinent or comatose clients who still have complete and spontaneous bladder emptying. The condom is a soft, pliable rubber sheath that slips over the penis. A strip of elastic adhesive is placed around the top of the condom to secure it. The catheter may be attached to a leg drainage bag or a standard urinary drainage bag.

A condom catheter may remain in place 1 to 2 days. With each catheter change, the nurse cleanses the urethral meatus and penis thoroughly and looks for signs of skin irritation.

Assessment

1. Assess urinary elimination patterns, ability to voluntarily urinate, and continence.
2. Assess mental status of client so appropriate teaching related to condom can be implemented.
3. Assess condition of penis.
4. Assess client's knowledge of the purpose of a condom catheter.

Evaluation

1. Observe urinary drainage.
2. Remove condom and inspect skin on penile shaft for signs of breakdown or irritation at least daily during hygiene and when condom is reapplied.

Expected outcomes are based on goals of care:

1. Client is continent with condom catheter intact.
2. Penile shaft is free of skin irritation or breakdown.

From Perry A, Potter P: *Clinical nursing skills and techniques,* ed 3, St Louis, 1994, Mosby.

Unexpected outcomes that may occur include the following:

1. Skin around penis is reddened and excoriated.
2. Urination is reduced or infrequent.
3. Urine leaks from tubing.
4. Penile swelling.

Special Considerations

- Condom catheter is suitable for incontinent or comatose male clients with complete and spontaneous bladder emptying.
- Check policy to determine if physician's order is required to apply condom.
- Procedure should be explained, even if client is comatose, because client may be able to hear.
- Some apply thin layer of plasticized skin spray to skin of penile shaft to protect skin from ulceration and irritation caused by rubber condom and adhesive holding it in place.
- Never use adhesive tape because it is too constrictive.

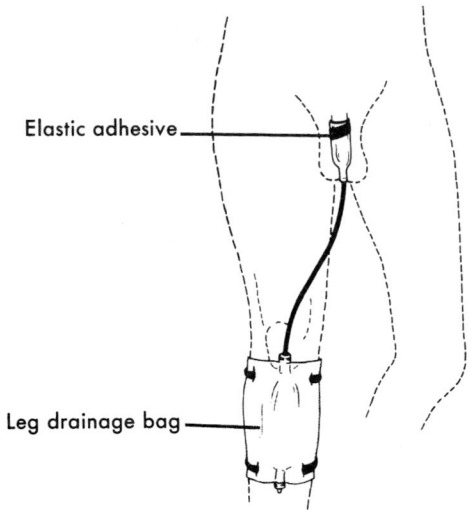

Emergency Procedures

Sequence of CPR in Adults

Step 1: Assess level of consciousness

1. Shake victim's shoulder and shout, "Are you OK?"
2. If no response, summon help.
3. Place victim supine on *firm* surface.

Step 2: Open airway

1. Hyperextend neck by head-tilt or neck-lift methods.
2. Place ear over victim's nose and mouth.
   a. Look to see if chest is moving.
   b. Listen for air escaping during exhalation.
   c. Feel for air movement against face.
3. If victim is not breathing, proceed to step 3.

Step 3: Initiate artificial ventilation

1. Give four quick mouth-to-mouth breaths without allowing victim to exhale completely after each ventilation.

Step 4: Assess circulation

1. Palpate carotid pulse.
2. If carotid pulse not palpable, proceed to step 5.

Step 5: Initiate external cardiac compressions

1. If only one rescuer:
   a. Do 15 cardiac compressions at a rate of 80/min.
   b. Follow with two artificial ventilations.
   c. Repeat sequence.
2. If two rescuers:
   a. One person does cardiac compressions, at a rate of 80/min without pause
   b. Second rescuer ventilates victim quickly after every five compressions.
3. Palpate carotid pulse after first minute of CPR to assess effectiveness, and subsequently every few minutes to check for return of spontaneous circulation.

Modified from Perry A, Potter P: *Clinical nursing skills and techniques,* ed 2, St Louis, 1990, Mosby.

Mouth-to-Mouth Ventilation

Mouth-to-mouth ventilation is performed as follows:

1. Maintain victim in head-tilt position.
2. Pinch nostrils.
3. Take a deep breath and place mouth around outside of victim's mouth, forming a tight seal.
4. Blow into victim's mouth—two full breaths.
5. Adequate ventilation is demonstrated by:
   a. Rise and fall of chest (1 to 2 in).
   b. Hearing and feeling air escape as victim passively exhales.
   c. Feeling in own airway the resistance of victim's lungs expanding.

External Cardiac Compressions

1. Position yourself close to victim's sternum.
2. Place heel of one hand on sternum two finger widths above xiphoid process of sternum, second hand on top of first hand with fingers parallel and pointing away from body. Place fingers between each other in an interlocking position.
3. Position shoulders directly over victim's sternum.
4. Keep elbows locked in a straight position.
5. Depress lower sternum $1\frac{1}{2}$ to 2 in.
6. Keeping hands in position, release pressure on sternum to allow heart to fill.
7. Repeat, depressing and releasing sternum.
8. Perform compressions regularly and smoothly.

Sequence of CPR in Infants and Children

Infant (1-12 Months)

A. Proper hand position (see Fig. on p. 405):
   (1) Draw an imaginary line between the nipples, over the breast bone (sternum).
   (2) Place the index finger of the hand farthest from the infant's head just under the intermammary line where it intersects the sternum. The area of compression is one finger's width below this intersection at the location of the middle and ring fingers.

Modified from Potter PA, Perry AG: *Fundamentals of nursing,* ed 2, St Louis, 1989, Mosby.

B. Using two fingers, compress 1.3 to 2.5 cm (½ to 1 in) at least 100 times per minute.
C. At the end of every fifth compression a pause should be allowed for a ventilation (1½ seconds).
D. Reassess victim after 10 cycles (5 compressions: 1 ventilation each cycle) to determine return of pulse and respiration and the need to continue CPR.

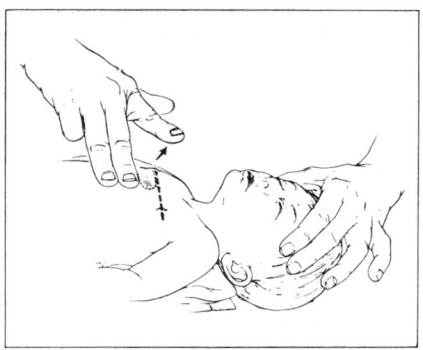

Locating finger position for chest compression in infant.

Child (1-7 Years)

A. Proper hand position:
   (1) Locate lower margin of the victim's rib cage on the side next to the rescuer with the middle and index fingers.
   (2) Follow the margin of the rib cage with the middle finger to the notch where the ribs and sternum meet.
   (3) Place index finger next to middle finger.
   (4) Place heel of other hand next to the index finger with long axis of the heel parallel to sternum.
B. Compress sternum with one hand 2.5 to 3.8 cm (1 to 1½ in) at a rate of 100 times per minute.
C. At the end of every fifth compression a pause should be allowed for a ventilation (1 to 1½ seconds).
D. Reassess victim after 10 cycles (5 compressions: 1 ventilation each cycle) to determine return of pulse and respiration and need to continue CPR.

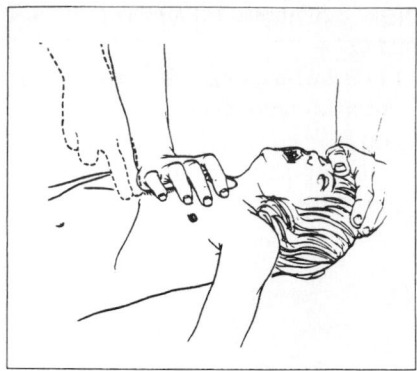

Locating hand position for chest compression in child.

Note: Infants (up to 1 year) and children (1 to 8 years) should be administered mouth-to-mouth resuscitation as described starting on p. 404 except for the following:

- Do not tilt the head as far back as an adult's head.
- Both the mouth and nose of the infant should be sealed by the mouth.
- Give breaths to a child once every 4 seconds.
- Blow into the infant's mouth and nose once every 3 seconds with less pressure and volume than for a child.

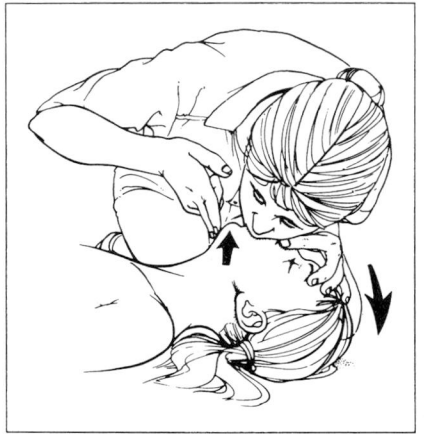

Mouth-to-mouth seal.

Heimlich Abdominal Thrust Maneuver

1. Stand behind victim.
2. Encircle arms around victim's waist.
3. Place one fist between umbilicus and sternum with thumb against abdomen.
4. Place second hand over fist.
5. Press on abdomen with quick upward thrusts.
6. For infants, the chest thrusts are delivered with two fingers over the breastbone between the nipples. The baby's head should be lower than the chest for thrusts.
7. Start mouth-to-mouth resuscitation if breathing stops.

Notes

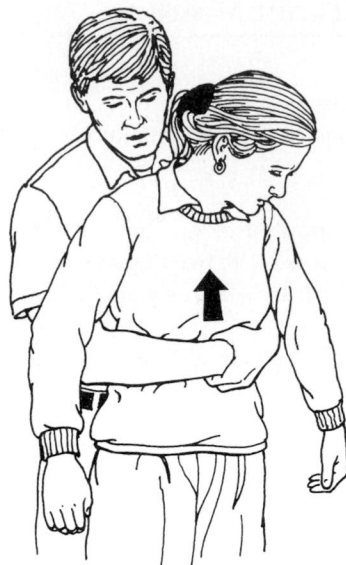

Heimlich abdominal thrust maneuver. Rescuer places fist between umbilicus and xiphoid process with the thumb pressed against the abdomen. Pressure is applied upward.

Heimlich maneuver in infants.

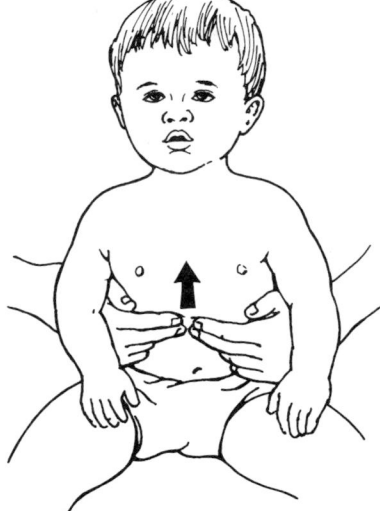

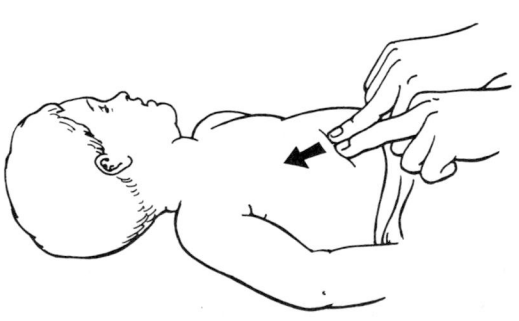

Signs and Symptoms in Early and Late Shock

	Early shock	Late shock
Respiratory system	Hyperventilation; ↑ minute volume; ↓ $Paco_2$; normal Pao_2	Respirations shallow; breath sounds may suggest congestion; ↑ $Paco_2$; ↓ Pao_2
Cardiovascular system	Blood pressure normal to slightly lowered; ↑ diastolic pressure; ↓ pulse pressure; tachycardia; cardiac output normal in hypovolemic shock, and increased in septic shock; mild vasoconstriction in hypovolemic and cardiogenic shock; vasodilation in septic shock	↓ Blood pressure; ↓ cardiac output; tachycardia continues; vasoconstriction worsens in hypovolemic, cardiogenic, and septic shock
Renal system	Decreased urine output; ↑ urine osmolality; ↓ urine sodium concentration; hypokalemia	Oliguria or complete renal shutdown; hyperkalemia; buildup of waste products
Acid-base balance	Respiratory alkalosis	Metabolic acidosis; respiratory acidosis

From Phipps WJ, Sands J, Lehman MK, Cassmeyer V: *Medical-surgical nursing: concepts and clinical practice,* ed 5, St Louis, 1995, Mosby. *$Paco_2$,* carbon dioxide pressure; *Pao_2,* oxygen pressure.

Continued.

Signs and Symptoms in Early and Late Shock—cont'd

	Early shock	Late shock
Vascular compartment	Fluid shift from interstitial space to intravascular compartment; thirst	Fluid shift from intravascular space to interstitial and intracellular spaces, causing edema
Skin	Minimal to no changes in hypovolemic and cardiogenic shock; warm, flushed skin in septic shock	Cool, clammy skin in hypovolemic, cardiogenic, and septic shock; cool, mottled skin in neurogenic and vasogenic shock
Hematological system	Release of red blood cells (RBCs) from bone marrow to increase vascular volume; platelet aggregation	Disseminated intravascular coagulation (DIC)
Mental-neurological system	Restless; alert; confused	Lethargy; unconsciousness
GI-hepatic system	No obvious changes	Perfusion decreases; bowel sounds possibly diminished

Types of Shock

Hypovolemic	Shock from loss of fluid from vascular system (through blood loss or fluid loss)
Cardiogenic	Shock from inability of heart to pump blood to tissues (decreased cardiac output)
Distributive	Shock from massive vasodilation (from interference with sympathetic nervous system or effects of histamine or toxins)

Notes

Clinical Manifestations of Hypovolemic Shock

Parameter (for a 70-kg male)	Class I early	Class II moderate	Class III major or progressive	Class IV severe or profound
Approximate blood volume loss (ml)	Up to 750	750-1500	1500-2000	2000 or more
% of blood volume	Up to 15%	15%-30%	30%-40%	40% or more
Neurological/behavioral status	Slightly anxious	Mildly anxious, restless; muscle fatigue and weakness evident	Agitated, confused; progressive decrease in activity; progressive thirst evident	Stuporous, lethargic, unconscious; dilated pupils may be evident
Heart rate	<100	>100 Mild tachycardia	>120 Tachycardia	140 or higher Irregular pulse, decreased pulse amplitude
Blood pressure	Normal	Normal	Decreased	Severe hypotension
Pulse pressure (mm Hg)	Normal or increased	Decreased	Decreased	Decreased
Respirations	14-20, normal	20-30, normal	30-40, hyperpnea	>35, shallow, irregular
Urine output (ml/hr)	30 or more	20-30	5-15	Negligible
Capillary blanch test	Normal	Slight delay	Defined delay	No refilling observed
Skin	Pale flushed, slightly cool	Slightly cold, pale	Cold and moist	Cold and cyanotic, mottled

From McQuillian KA, Wiles CE: Initial management of traumatic shock. In Cardona DV et al, editors: *Trauma nursing from resuscitation through rehabilitation*, Philadelphia, 1988, WB Saunders. In Phipps WJ, Sands J, Lehman MK, Cassmeyer V: *Medical surgical nursing*, ed 5, St Louis, 1995, Mosby.

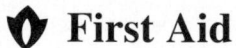 # First Aid

First Aid Tips

A physician should be called immediately for all serious injuries or suspected poisoning.

Bruises—Rest injured part. Apply cold compresses for half hour (no ice next to skin). If skin is broken, treat as a cut. For wringer injuries always consult physician without delay.

Scrapes—Use wet gauze or cotton to sponge off gently with clean water and soap.

Bleeding—To control most bleeding, apply a compress directly over a wound. Place the cleanest material available (sterile gauze is best) over the wound and press firmly until the bleeding stops or until a physician reaches the victim. A bandage can also be used to keep the material in place. If blood is spurting out of the wound, it is an indication that an artery has ruptured and, in addition to the direct pressure on the wound, you also should apply firm pressure with your finger at a point located about 2 inches above the wound. Tourniquets are used only when the bleeding cannot be controlled in any other way, such as in cases where a limb has been severed or severely mangled.

Cuts—Minor—Wash with clean water and soap. Hold under running water. Apply sterile gauze dressing. Major—Apply dressing. Press firmly to stop bleeding—use tourniquet only if necessary. Bandage. Secure medical care. *Do not* use iodine or other antiseptics before the physician arrives.

Puncture wounds—Consult physician immediately.

Slivers—Wash with clean water and soap. Remove with tweezers or forceps. Wash again. If large or deep, consult physician.

Nosebleeds—In sitting position blow out from the nose all clot and blood. Insert into the bleeding nostril a wedge of cotton moistened with any of the common nose drops. With the finger against the outside of that nostril apply firm pressure for 5 minutes. If bleeding stops remove packing (no rush, here). Check with a physician if bleeding persists.

From Chemical Specialties Manufacturers Association, Inc: *Your child and household safety,* Washington, DC, 1988, The Association.

These are basic first aid principles to be used in case of an emergency until professional help can be obtained or consulted. Any person relying solely upon this information does so at his or her own risk.

Fainting and unconsciousness—Keep in flat position. Loosen clothing around neck. Summon physician. Keep client warm. Keep mouth clear. Give nothing to swallow.

Convulsions—Contact physician. If caused by fever, sponge body with cool water, apply cold cloths to head. Lay on side with hips elevated. Biting of tongue is rare but be sure that the tongue is not blocking the passage of air to the lung.

Head injuries—*Do not* move unless additional danger would occur to injured person. Consult physician immediately.

Poisoning—See following First Aid for Poisoning Chart.

Bites or stings (A) Insect—Remove stinger *at base* if present. Do not squeeze stinger as it is removed. Cold compresses. Consult physician promptly if there is *any* reaction. (B) Animal—Wash with clean water and soap. Hold under running water for 2 or 3 minutes if not bleeding profusely. Apply sterile dressing. Consult physician. If possible, catch or retain the animal and maintain alive for observation regarding rabies. Notify police or health officer. (C) Human—(Can be serious) Wash thoroughly with soap and water. See physician for severe bites. (D) Snake—Nonpoisonous—No treatment necessary. If there is a question, treat as "Poisonous." Poisonous— (Keep calm and work fast.) Complete rest. Apply constricting band above the bite (not too tight). Get victim to physician or hospital immediately.

Burns and scalds—If caused by chemicals: Wash burned area thoroughly with water. Consult physician. Bring chemical container to physician or hospital. Extensive burns—Keep client in flat position. Remove clothing from burned area—*If adherent, leave alone.* Cover with clean cloth. Keep client warm. Take client to hospital or to a physician at once. *Do not* use ointments, greases, powder, etc. Application of cold water or compresses to minor burns relieves pain. Electric burns with shock may require artificial respiration.

Fractures—Any deformity of injured part usually means a fracture. *Do not* move person if fracture of leg or back is suspected. Summon physician at once. If person *must* be moved, immobilize with adequate splints.

Sprains—Elevate injured part. Apply cold compresses for half hour. If swelling is unusual, do not use injured part until seen by physician.

Eyes—To remove foreign bodies, *do not* use a moist cotton swab. Irrigate thoroughly with water. Immediate and copious irrigation with plain water is procedure for most chemicals splashed in eyes. Contact physician or hospital immediately.

Choking—The American Red Cross and the American Heart Association both agree that the recommended first aid for choking victims is the abdominal thrust, also known as the Heimlich maneuver. **Slaps on the back are no longer advised and may even prove detrimental in an attempt to assist a choking victim.**

First Aid Treatment for Poisoning

In all cases except poisonous bites, the principle of first aid is to get the poison **out** or **off**, or to **dilute** it. Always call a **physician, hospital, poison control center,** or **rescue unit promptly.** The following are safe first aid measures for various types of poisoning:

1. Swallowed Poison
   - Dilute chemical or household product poisons by giving water or milk, one or two glassfuls.
   - Make client vomit if so directed. *But not if:*
     Client is unconscious or having seizures.
     Swallowed poison was a strong corrosive (lye, strong acid, drain cleaner, etc.).
     Swallowed poison contains kerosene, gasoline or other petroleum distillates (unless directed otherwise or containing a dangerous pesticide or chemical which must be removed).

To Induce Vomiting
   - Give one tablespoonful (½ ounce) of Syrup of Ipecac for a child 1 year of age or older, plus at least 1 cup of water. *Never substitute milk or carbonated fluids.* If no vomiting occurs in 20 minutes, this dose may be repeated once only. Older children and adults can be given 2 tablespoonsful (1 ounce) at one time. After vomiting has ceased, offer a mixture of activated charcoal (2 to 4 tablespoonsful) in a glass of water. Palatable suspensions are available.
   - If no Ipecac syrup is available, try to induce vomiting by tickling back of throat with a spoon handle or other blunt object, after giving water.
   - *Do not* give salt or mustard to children.
   - *Do not* waste time waiting for vomiting, but transport victim promptly to a medical facility. Bring package or container with intact label.

2. Fumes or gases—for example, fuel gases, auto exhaust, dense smoke from fires or fumes from poisonous chemical.
   A. Get victim into fresh, clean air.
   B. Loosen clothing.

From Chemical Specialties Manufacturers Association, Inc: *Your child and household safety,* Washington, DC, 1988, The Association.

    C. If victim is not breathing, start artificial respiration promptly. *Do not* stop until victim is breathing well, or help arrives.

    D. Have *someone else* call a physician, hospital, poison control center, or rescue unit.

    E. Transport victim to a medical facility promptly.

3. Eye

    A. Gently wash eye out immediately, using plenty of water (or milk in an emergency), for 5 minutes with eyelids held open.

    B. Remove contact lenses if worn; *never* permit the eye to be rubbed.

    C. Call physician, hospital, poison control center, or rescue unit and transport victim to a medical facility promptly.

4. Skin (acids, lye, other caustics, pesticides, etc.)

    A. Wash off skin immediately with a large amount of water; use soap if available.

    B. Remove any contaminated clothing.

    C. Call physician, hospital, poison control center, or rescue unit and transport victim to a medical facility if necessary.

5. Poisonous bites

    A. Snakes

        1. Don't let victim walk; keep victim as quiet as possible.

        2. Do not give alcohol.

        3. Call physician, hospital, poison control center, or rescue unit, and transport victim promptly to a medical facility.
        En route, or while awaiting transportation

        4. Apply suction to bite wound with mouth or suction cup.

        5. If victim stops breathing, use artificial respiration.

    B. Insects (spiders, scorpions, or unusual reaction to other stinging insects such as bees, wasps, hornets, etc.)

        1. Do not let victim walk or exercise.

        2. Place any available cold substance on bite area to relieve pain.

        3. A paste of Adolph's Meat Tenderizer or baking soda applied to the bite will often reduce the swelling and itching by its enzymatic action.

        4. If victim stops breathing, use artificial respiration.

        5. Call physician, hospital, poison control center, or rescue unit, and transport victim promptly to a medical facility. (Persons with known unusual reactions to insect stings should carry emergency treatment kits and an emergency identity card.)

    C. Animal bites
    Bat and skunk bites, and other unprovoked animal bites, may be from a rabid animal. Call physician or medical facility; wash

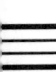

wound gently but thoroughly with soap and water. (Also see
First Aid—Bites.)

D. Poisonous marine animals

Apply any cold substance to relieve pain. (For "sting ray," heat
is better.) Call physician or medical facility if reaction is
severe.

Pediculosis

Identification. Infestation of the head, the hairy parts of the body or
clothing (especially along the seams of inner surfaces), with adult lice,
larvae, or nits (eggs), which results in severe itching and excoriation
of the scalp or body. Secondary infection may occur with ensuing
cervical lymphadenitis. Crab lice usually infest the pubic area; they
may infest facial hair (including eyelashes), axillae, and body surface.

Incubation period. Under optimal conditions the eggs of lice
hatch in a week, and sexual maturity is reached approximately 8 to
10 days after hatching.

Methods of Control

A. Preventive measures:
   (1) Avoid physical contact with infested individuals and their
       belongings, especially clothing and bedding.
   (2) Health education of the public in the value of laundering
       clothing and bedding in hot water (55°C or 131°F for 20
       minutes) or dry cleaning to destroy nits and lice.
   (3) Regular direct inspection of all primary school children for
       head lice and, when indicated, of body and clothing, par-
       ticularly of children in schools, institutions, nursing homes,
       and summer camps.

B. Control of infested persons, contacts, and the immediate environment:
   (1) Report to local health authority: Official report not ordinarily
       justifiable; school authorities should be informed.
   (2) Isolation: Contact isolation until 24 hours after application of
       effective insecticide.
   (3) Concurrent disinfection: With body lice in members of a
       family or group, to include clothing, bedding and other
       appropriate vehicles of transmission (e.g., cosmetic articles),
       treated by laundering in hot water, by dry cleaning, or by

application of an effective chemical insecticide and ovicide. After chemical treatment has been completed, clothes and laundry facilities should be rinsed adequately.

(4) Quarantine: None.

(5) Immunization of contacts: Does not apply.

(6) Investigation of contacts: Examination of household and other close personal contacts, with concurrent treatment as indicated.

(7) Specific treatment: For head and pubic lice, 1% gamma benzene hexachloride lotions (Lindane, Kwell) (not recommended for infants, young children, and pregnant or lactating women), pyrethrins synergized with piperonyl butoxide (A-200 Pyrinate, RID, and XXX), 0.5% malathion (Prioderm) carbaryl, and benzyl benzoate are effective. Retreatment after 7 to 10 days is recommended to ensure that no eggs have survived. For body lice: Clothing and bedding should be washed with the hot cycle of an automatic washing machine, or, if not available, dusted with powders containing 1% lindane or, preferably, in view of widespread resistance to lindane, 1% malathion or pyrethrins with piperonyl butoxide or carbaryl, and then laundered before using. Abate (temephos) as a 2% dusting powder is also effective and is recommended by WHO for use in areas where strains of body lice are resistant to malathion.

Removal of a Tick

1. Put on gloves.
2. Use curved forceps or tweezers to remove tick.
3. Grasp tick firmly as close to the skin as possible and pull upward with a steady, even pressure. Do not twist or jerk.
4. Try not to squeeze or crush the body of the tick because its fluids may contain infectious agents.
5. After removal, wash the site with soap and water. Clean with a disinfectant.
6. Contact a physician if signs of a reaction (or symptoms) occur within the next few weeks.

Checklist of Treatments for Animal Bites

1. Cleanse and flush wound immediately (first aid).
2. Thorough wound cleansing under medical supervision.
3. Rabies immune globulin or vaccine as indicated.
4. Tetanus prophylaxis and antibacterial treatment when required.
5. No sutures or wound closure advised unless unavoidable.

From Benenson A: *Control of communicable diseases in man,* ed 15, Washington, DC, 1990, American Public Health Association.

Rabies Postexposure Prophylaxis Guide

The following recommendations are only a guide. In applying them, take into account the animal species involved, the circumstances of the bite or other exposure, vaccination status of the animal, and presence of rabies in the region. Local or state health officials should be consulted if questions arise about the need for rabies prophylaxis.

Species	Condition of animal at time of attack	Treatment
Domestic dog and cat	Healthy and available for 10 days of observation	None, unless animal develops rabies
	Rabid or suspected rabid	RIG and HDCV
	Unknown (escaped)	Consult public health official. If treatment is indicated, give RIG and HDCV.
Wild carnivores skunk, fox, bat, coyote, bobcat, raccoon	Regard as rabid unless proven negative by laboratory tests	RIG and HDCV
Other livestock, rodents, and lagomorphs (hares and rabbits)	Consider individually. Local and state public health officials should be consulted on questions about the need for rabies prophylaxis. Bites of squirrels, hamsters, guinea pigs, gerbils, chipmunks, rats, mice, other rodents, rabbits, and hares almost never call for antirabies prophylaxis.	

From Benenson A: *Control of communicable diseases in man,* ed 15, Washington, DC, 1990, American Public Health Association.

Skin and Wound Care

Helpful Tips

- Remind clients they can use a hair dryer to dry skin thoroughly. This is especially important in obese clients and for any area that drying well with a towel might be difficult or painful. The heat setting should always be on low and the dryer always kept moving to facilitate air circulation.
- A small, 6-in hem gauge that is marked in centimeters can be used to measure the size of wounds, or the area of drainage, on a bandage. Carry one in your nursing bag.
- In females who need breast or sternal dressings, instead of using Montgomery straps, a binder, or tape, the client's bra may be used. This holds the dressing in place, is more comfortable, and reduces skin irritation.
- When immobilizers or binders are used, especially those with Velcro bindings or fasteners, a disposable baby diaper liner can be used for padding to prevent skin irritation and breakdown. They are well padded and serve the purpose perfectly.
- Vaseline gauze can be made by using roller gauze and regular petroleum jelly. Accordian pleat (fold back and forth) the gauze in a metal mixing bowl or a shallow glass pan. Put a generous amount of petroleum jelly on top of the gauze, cover with aluminum foil and bake at 375°F for 25 minutes. If sterile gauze is needed, individual aluminum foil packets can be made. Purchase unsterile dressings, wrap in aluminum foil and bake for 25 minutes at 375°F to sterilize.

Notes

Modified from Humphrey C: *Home care nursing,* Norwalk, Conn, 1994, Aspen.

Protocols for Pressure Ulcer Interventions

Once the assessment has been completed and the risk factors identified, specific protocols may be applied. Within the protocol, some interventions may be contraindicated in certain institutions, and many will undoubtedly require physician's orders or clinical privileges.

Stage I protocol

1. "At Risk" protocol	
2. Cleansing	Normal saline
	Neutral cleanser
3. Dressing and/or treatment	Open to air
	Skin barrier
	Transparent dressing
	Vasodilator spray
4. Additional	Massage around, but not over, site unless vasodilator is used.

Stage II protocol

1. "At Risk" protocol	
2. Cleansing	Normal saline
	Antiseptic solution
	Neutral cleanser
3. Rinsing	Normal saline
4. Dressing and/or treatment	

Clean—	Infected—
W → W normal saline	W → W with normal saline
Skin barrier	Antiseptic solution
Hydrocolloid	Antibiotic solution
Transparent	
Topical antibiotic	

Stages III, IV, and V protocols

1. "At Risk" protocol		
2. Cleansing	Normal saline	
	Antiseptic solution	
3. Rinsing	Normal saline	
4. Dressing and/or treatment	Clean— no necrosis	Infected—no necrosis
	W → W normal saline	W → W normal saline
	Hydrocolloid with granules	Antiseptic solution
	(Dressing used on III only)	Antibiotic solution
		Systemic antibiotic
	Necrosis	Necrosis
	W → W or W → D with normal saline	W → W or W → D with normal saline

From Thomason S: Protocols for pressure ulcer interventions, *Sci Nurs* 5(3), 1988.
NOTE: On all charts, W → W = Wet to Wet, W → D = Wet to Dry.

Continued.

Stages III, IV, and V protocols—cont'd

Enzymes	Antiseptic solution
Hydrocolloid with granules (Dressing used on III only)	Antibiotic solution
	Enzymes
	Systemic antibiotic
Whirlpool	Whirlpool
Surgical	Surgical
Debridement or excision	Debridement or excision
Drainage—	Hydrophilic Absorption

Closed pressure ulcer protocol
1. "At Risk" protocol
2. Cleansing

    Normal saline
    Antiseptic solution (not hydrogen peroxide)

3. Rinsing   Normal saline
4. Dressing and/or treatment   Infected—no necrosis

Clean—no necrosis   W → W normal saline

W → W normal saline   Antiseptic solution
    Antibiotic solution
    Systemic antibiotic

Necrosis   Necrosis

W → W or W → D with normal saline   W → W or W → D with normal saline

Drainage: Antiseptic solution

Drainable ostomy pouch   Antibiotic solution

Surgical excision   Systemic antibiotic

Performing Wound Irrigation

Steps
1. Assess client's level of pain.
2. Review record for physician's prescription for irrigation of open wound and type of solution to be used.
3. Identify recent recording of signs and symptoms related to client's open wound:
   a. Extent of impairment of skin integrity
   b. Elevation of body temperature
   c. Drainage from wound (amount, color)
   d. Odor
   e. Consistency of drainage
   f. Size of wounds, including depth, length, and width

From Perry A, Potter P: *Clinical nursing skills and techniques,* ed 2, St Louis, 1990, Mosby.

4. Administer prescribed analgesic 30 to 45 min before starting wound irrigation procedure.
5. Gather equipment at bedside:
   a. Sterile basin
   b. 150- to 500-ml prescribed sterile irrigating solution warmed to body temperature
   c. Sterile irrigation syringe, sterile soft catheter, if needed
   d. Clean basin
   e. Clean gloves (check policy of institution)
   f. Sterile gloves
   g. Waterproof underpad
   h. Sterile dressing tray and supplies for dressing change, including packing, if ordered
   i. Leakproof refuse bag
   j. Gown
6. Explain procedure.
7. Position client comfortably to permit gravitational flow of irrigating solution through wound and into collection basin. Position client so that wound is vertical to collection basin.
8. Warm sterile irrigating solution to approximate body temperature.
9. Form cuff on leakproof refuse bag and place it near bed.
10. Close room door or bed curtains.
11. Place waterproof underpad on bed surface in front of wound.
12. Place clean basin directly under wound.
13. Wash hands
14. If gown is needed, apply it now.
15. Prepare sterile field using sterile dressing set and supplies.
16. Add sterile basin and pour in estimated volume of warm sterile irrigating solution and set irrigating syringe in basin with solution.
17. Place several strips of adhesive tape within reach and *not* on sterile field.
18. Put on clean gloves and remove soiled dressing and discard in leakproof refuse bag.
19. Remove and discard gloves.
20. Inspect wound and make mental note of healing process, inflammation, drainage, or purulent matter.
21. Apply sterile gloves.
22. Irrigate wound with wide opening:
    a. Fill syringe with irrigating solution.
    b. Hold syringe tip 2.5 cm (1 in) above upper end of wound.
    c. Using slow, continuous pressure, flush wound.
    d. Repeat Steps 22a through 22c until solution draining into basin is clear.

23. Irrigate deep wound with very small opening:
    a. Attach soft catheter to filled irrigating syringe.
    b. Lubricate tip of catheter with irrigating solution. Gently insert tip of catheter until resistance is felt, and then pull out about 1.2 cm (½ in) to remove tip from fragile inner wall of wound.
    c. Using slow, continuous pressure, flush wound.
    d. Pinch off catheter just below syringe.
    e. Remove syringe, fill, and reattach to catheter. Repeat until return is clear.
24. Dry wound edges with sterile gauze.
25. Apply sterile dressing.
26. Remove and dispose of gloves.
27. Secure dressing with adhesive tape.
28. Assist client to comfortable position.
29. Dispose of equipment; retain remaining bottle of sterile solution.
30. Wash hands.
31. Inspect dressing periodically.
32. Evaluate skin integrity.
33. Record wound appearance, irrigation, and client response in nurses' notes.

Surgical Wound Classification

Wound classification	Description and example
Clean	Wounds in which the GI or respiratory tract is not entered; no inflammation or break in aseptic technique
	Cholecystectomy, hysterectomy
Clean contaminated	Clean operation in which the GI or respiratory tract is entered
	Colon resection
Contaminated	Nonpurulent inflammation, gross spillage from GI tract, fresh traumatic wounds, or major breaks in sterile technique
	Gunshot wound
Dirty or infected	Old traumatic with dead tissue, pus encountered, or perforated viscus found
	Ruptured abscess

From Phipps WJ, Sands J, Lehman MK, Cassmeyer V: *Medical-surgical nursing: concepts and clinical practice,* ed 5, St Louis, 1995, Mosby.

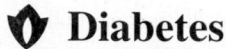 Diabetes

Obtaining Blood for Glucose Testing

To obtain a drop of blood to check glucose level, use a lancet or a mechanical device (Autoclix). Alcohol wipes are also needed.

1. Choose a site on the end of any fingertip. Wash and dry hands thoroughly. Or wipe the fingertip with alcohol, and let the alcohol evaporate.
2. Squeeze the fingertip with the thumb of the same hand. Place the fingertip (with thumb still pressed against it) on a firm surface, such as a table.
3. *If using a lancet,* twist off the protective cap. Then grasp the lancet and quickly pierce the fingertip.
   Remove thumb from the fingertip to release pressure and permit blood flow.
   If using the Autoclix, depress its plunger to insert a new lancet, and remove the lancet's cap. Then place the lancet at the puncture site and gently press the Autoclix to release the lancet into fingertip.
4. Milk the finger gently until there is a hanging drop of blood that looks large enough to cover the reagent area of the test strip. Be patient. If blood doesn't flow immediately from the puncture site, keep milking the finger before trying another site.

Modified from Lieberman A: *Community and home health nursing,* Springhouse, Pa, 1990, Springhouse Corp.

Testing Blood for Glucose

Two types of reagent strips are commonly used to test blood glucose levels visually: Chemstrip bG and Visidex II. Also a glucose meter can be used to measure levels electronically. Be sure to follow the manufacturer's directions precisely. The following instructions will help use reagent strips to check blood glucose levels. The procedure is identical for both types of strips. Here's what to do:

1. Begin by assembling the necessary equipment: a lancet, a vial with reagent strips, cotton balls, a watch or clock with a second hand, and a pen.

Modified from Lieberman A: *Community and home health nursing,* Springhouse, Pa, 1990, Springhouse.

2. Remove a reagent strip from its vial. Then replace the cap, making sure it's tight. Obtain a drop of blood from the end of any fingertip, following the directions. Wipe away first blood droplet with cotton ball. Lightly squeeze puncture site until large droplet of blood has formed. Carefully lift the strip to the drop of blood. (The strip has a shiny, slippery undersurface; the blood will roll off it if not placed on the strip correctly.) Let the blood completely cover the reagent area *without* rubbing or smearing it. If the blood smears, start over with a new strip.

3. As the drop of blood is placed on the reagent area, look at a watch or a clock. Wait exactly 60 seconds. Make sure to keep the strip level.

   After 60 seconds, gently wipe all the blood off the strip with a clean, dry cotton ball. Wipe the strip three times, using a clean side of the cotton ball each time. Then wait another 60 seconds.

4. Now determine the blood glucose level by holding the reagent strip next to the area of color blocks on the vial. Then match the colors that have appeared on the strip with the two color blocks (in the 2-minute row) on the vial. *Example:* If both colors match the block labeled 120, the blood glucose level is approximately 120 mg/dl. If the colors fall between two blocks, take the average of the two numbers. *Example:* If the colors fall between the two blocks labeled 120 and 180, the blood glucose level is approximately 150 mg/dl.

   If the reading exceeds 240 mg/dl, wait another 60 seconds. Then compare the reagent area with the blocks in the 3-minute row.

5. Write the date, time, and the client's initials on the reagent strip and store it in an empty vial. Make sure the cap is on on tight. The colors on the reagent area will last for up to a week.

Guidelines for Foot Care for the Client with Diabetes

1. Inspect feet daily for color changes, temperature changes, swelling, cuts, cracks, redness, blisters, or other signs of trauma; report changes immediately. (A mirror can be used to see bottom of feet.)
2. Wear well-fitting shoes and clean stockings when walking; never walk barefoot.
   a. Inspect shoes, before putting them on, for foreign objects, nail points, or wrinkles.
   b. There should be enough room in shoes to allow the toes to wiggle easily.
   c. Break in new shoes gradually.
3. Bathe feet daily and dry them well, paying particular attention to area between the toes.
4. Immediately after bathing, when toenails are soft, cut (or have someone else cut) nails straight across; smooth cut nails with an emery board.
5. If feet are dry, apply bland cream or petroleum jelly to heels and feet (but not toes).
6. Do not self-treat calluses, corns, or ingrown toenails; consult a podiatrist if these are present.
7. Bath water should be 30° to 32°C (84° to 90°F) and should be tested with a bath thermometer or elbow before immersing the feet.
8. Heating pads and hot-water bottles should not be used; wear socks if feet are cold.
9. Measures that increase circulation to the lower extremities should be instituted, including:
   a. Avoid smoking.
   b. Avoid crossing legs when sitting.
   c. Protect extremities when exposed to cold.
   d. Avoid immersing feet in cold water.
   e. Use socks or stockings that do not apply pressure to the legs at specific sites.
   f. Institute an exercise regimen.
10. Do not walk or jog in the dark; have a light source.
11. Obtain proper shoes before jogging.

From Phipps WJ, Sands J, Lehman MK, Cassmeyer V: *Medical-surgical nursing: concepts and clinical practice,* ed 5, St Louis, 1995, Mosby.

Assessment of Feet of the Client with Diabetes

Color: Compare one foot with the other.
Temperature: Compare both feet with upper legs; assess for line of demarcations.
Sensory function: Test for pinprick and vibratory sense (Semmes-Weinstein monofilament).
Reflexes: Test Achilles tendon reflex.
Pulses: Check dorsalis pedis and posterior tibialis.
Lesions: Examine for calluses, cuts, bruises, cracks, or infection.
Self-care: Discuss self-care regimen being used.

From Phipps WJ, Sands J, Lehman MK, Cassmeyer V: *Medical-surgical nursing: concepts and clinical practice,* ed 5, St Louis, 1995, Mosby.

Risk Categories and Associated Footwear Guidelines

	Clinical findings	Footwear changes
Category 0	Has protective sensation	Education on proper footwear
Category 1	Has lost protective sensation	Add soft insole to shoe of proper contour and fit
Category 2	Has lost protective sensation and has foot deformity	Depth footwear or custom shoe for severe deformity, molded insoles
Category 3	Has lost protective sensation and has history of foot ulcer	Inspect type and condition of footwear and insoles at every visit

From Coleman W: In Haire-Joshu D, editor: *Management of diabetes mellitus—perspective of care across the life span,* St Louis, 1992, Mosby.

Insulin Injection Sites

Rotate injection sites as numbered. Make injections 1 in apart. After sites in one area are used, move to the next area.

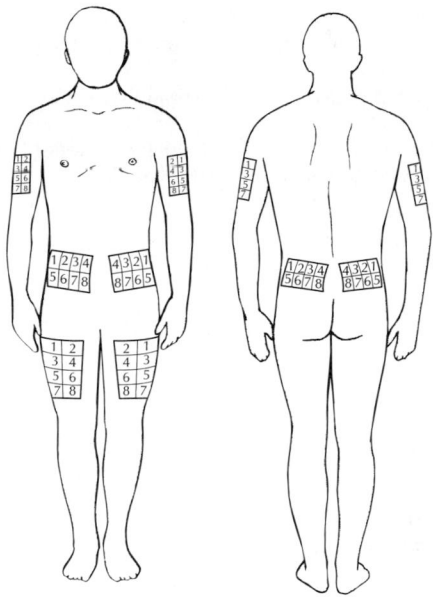

Subcutaneous injection site diagram.

From Potter PA, Perry AG: *Fundamentals of nursing: concepts, process, and practice,* ed 3, St Louis, 1993, Mosby.

Diabetic Emergencies

Hyperglycemia	Hypoglycemia
Symptoms	
Increased thirst and urination	Shakiness, pounding of heart
Large amounts of sugar and ketones in urine	Excessive sweating, faintness
Blood glucose levels over 300 mg/dl	Headache, impaired vision
Weakness, abdominal pains, generalized aches	Irritability, personality change
Deep breathing	Not able to wake
Loss of appetite, nausea, and vomiting	Hunger
Causes	
Too little insulin	Too much insulin
Failure to follow diet	Not eating enough food
Infection, fever	Unusual amount of exercise
Emotional stress	Delayed meal
Treatment	
Give fluids *without* sugar if able to swallow	Take food containing sugar (orange juice, milk, crackers)
Test blood frequently (if possible) for elevated glucose	Do not give fluids if client is not conscious
Test urine frequently for ketones	Get medical assistance immediately if not responsive to treatment
Call the doctor	Can give subcutaneous glucagon if available

From Bergenstal R: Acute and chronic complications of diabetes, *Caring* 3(11), 1988. Reprinted by permission of the National Association for Home Care.

Specimen Labeling and Transport

Purpose

- To identify laboratory specimen(s) with appropriate data.
- To safely deliver the specimens to the laboratory for analysis.

Equipment

1. Tape or specimen label; biohazard labels
2. Plastic bags
3. Laboratory requisition
4. Antiseptic wipes
5. Leak- and puncture-proof cooler or container with biohazard sign posted on the outside
6. Disposable nonsterile gloves

Procedure

1. Clarify with the physician the designated laboratory for the delivery of specimens.
2. Clarify with the designated laboratory, color of the test tubes, a specimen collection container, and the client data that is required to process the specimen.
3. Clean blood and body substances from outside of test tube(s) or speci-container(s) with antiseptic wipes as needed.
4. Label the specimen container in the following manner:
   a. Client's name
   b. Test to be performed by the laboratory
   c. Time and date specimen was collected
   d. Initials of the person who collects the specimen
5. Place test tubes or the specimen container in a plastic bag, and **seal** it to prevent possible leakage during transport. Place a biohazard label on the outside of the plastic bag. Double bag the specimen to prevent possible leakage when using ice to refrigerate the specimens or PRN as needed.
6. Place the specimen into a leak- and puncture-proof cooler or container.
7. Place cooler or container on the floorboard of the car during transport.
8. Fill out the laboratory requisition, and transport the specimen.
9. Call the physician with the lab results as soon as they are available.
10. Discard disposable items in a plastic trash bag, and secure.

From Rice R: *Handbook of home health nursing procedures,* St Louis, 1994, Mosby.

Nursing Considerations

- Many specimens **must** be delivered to the laboratory within 30 minutes to 1 hour after sampling.
- Consult with the laboratory concerning the type of container or test tube that should be used to collect the specimen and whether the specimen should be refrigerated by placing it on ice; also inquire about a time frame for deliveries. Many laboratories provide courier services to pick up specimens at the client's home.

Documentation Guidelines

- Document the following on the visit report: the type of laboratory test ordered by the physician, date and time the specimen was collected; designated laboratory for delivery; and other pertinent findings.
- Document physician notification of laboratory test results on the visit report or appropriate home health agency communique; and any subsequent orders.
- Update the client care plan.

♥ Orthopedic Care

Range of Motion

- Assess family/primary caregiver's ability, availability, and motivation to assist client with exercises client is unable to perform independently.
- Assist family/primary caregiver to arrange environment to promote exercise program, e.g., space allocation, lighting, temperature.
- Consult physical therapist for additional assistance or exercises and client's response to exercise program.
- Develop schedule for recording the performance of the exercise program.
- Instruct client or caregiver in performing exercise slowly.
- Teach caregiver how to provide adequate support to joint being exercised.
- Instruct to exercise only to point of resistance and to stop if client expresses pain.
- Each exercise should be repeated five times during exercise period.

Neck

- *Flexion:* Bring chin to rest on chest (ROM: 45*) (Fig. 12).
- *Extension:* Return head to erect position (ROM: 45) (Fig. 12).
- *Hyperextension:* Bend head as far back as possible (ROM: 10) (Fig. 12).
- *Lateral flexion:* Tilt head as far as possible toward each shoulder (ROM: 40-45) (Fig. 13).
- *Rotation:* Rotate head in circular motion (ROM: 360) (Fig. 14).

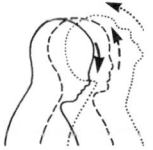 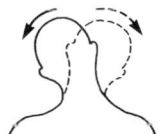 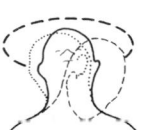

Fig. 12   Fig. 13   Fig. 14

Modified from Perry AG, Potter PA: *Clinical nursing skills and techniques,* ed 2, St Louis, 1990, Mosby.

*Ranges are measured in degrees using a goniometer.

Shoulder

- *Flexion:* Raise arm from side position forward to above head (ROM: 180) (Fig. 15).
- *Extension:* Return arm to position at side of body (ROM: 180) (Fig. 15).
- *Hyperextension:* Move arm behind body, keeping elbow straight (ROM: 45-60) (Fig. 15).
- *Abduction:* Raise arm to side to position above head with palm away from head (ROM: 180) (Fig. 16).
- *Adduction:* Lower arm sideways and across body as far as possible (ROM: 320) (Fig. 16).

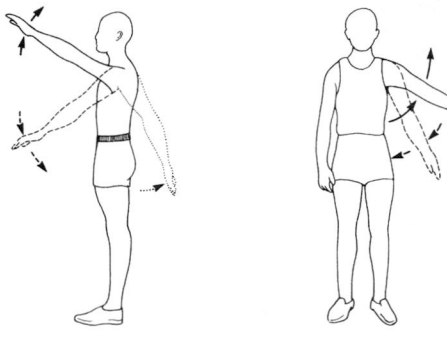

Fig. 15   Fig. 16

- *Internal rotation:* With elbow flexed, rotate shoulder by moving arm until thumb is turned inward and toward back (ROM: 90) (Fig. 17).
- *External rotation:* With elbow flexed, move arm until thumb is upward and lateral to head (ROM: 90) (Fig. 17).
- *Circumduction:* Move arm in full circle. Circumduction is a combination of all movements of ball-and-socket joint (ROM: 360) (Fig. 18).

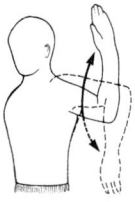
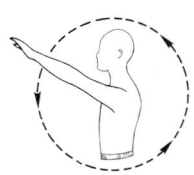

Fig. 17   Fig. 18

Elbow

- *Flexion:* Bend elbow so that lower arm moves toward its shoulder joint and hand is level with shoulder (ROM: 150) (Fig. 19).
- *Extension:* Straighten elbow by lowering hand (ROM: 150) (Fig. 19).
- *Hyperextension:* Bend lower arm back as far as possible (ROM: 10-20).

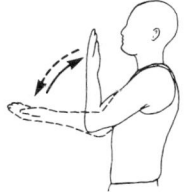

Fig. 19

Forearm

- *Supination:* Turn lower arm and hand so palm is up (ROM: 70-90) (Fig. 20).
- *Pronation:* Turn lower arm so palm is down (ROM: 70-90) (Fig. 20).

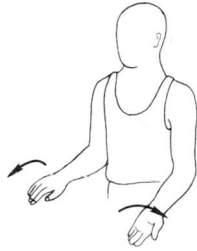

Fig. 20

Wrist

- *Flexion:* Move palm toward inner aspect of forearm (ROM: 80-90) (Fig. 21).
- *Extension:* Move fingers so fingers, hands, and forearm are in same plane (ROM: 80-90) (Fig. 21).
- *Hyperextension:* Bring dorsal surface of hand back as far as possible (ROM: 80-90) (Fig. 21).
- *Abduction (radial flexion):* Bend wrist medially toward thumb (ROM: Up to 30) (Fig. 22).
- *Adduction (ulnar flexion):* Bend wrist laterally toward fifth finger (ROM: 30-50) (Fig. 22).

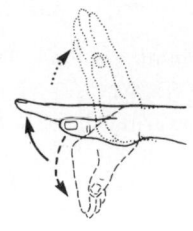 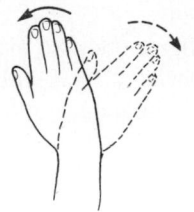

Fig. 21   Fig. 22

Fingers

- *Flexion:* Make fist (ROM: 90) (Fig. 23).
- *Extension:* Straighten fingers (ROM: 90) (Fig. 24).
- *Hyperextension:* Bend fingers back as far as possible (ROM: 30-60) (Fig. 24).
- *Abduction:* Spread fingers apart (ROM: 30) (Fig. 25).
- *Adduction:* Bring fingers together (ROM: 30) (Fig. 25).

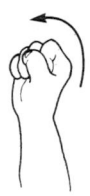 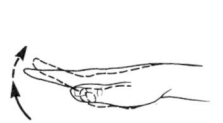 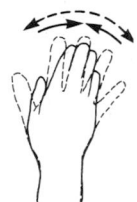

Fig. 23   Fig. 24   Fig. 25

Thumb

- *Flexion:* Move thumb across palmar surface of hand (ROM: 90) (Fig. 26).
- *Extension:* Move thumb straight away from hand (ROM: 90).
- *Abduction:* Extend thumb laterally (usually done when placing fingers in abduction and adduction) (ROM: 30).
- *Adduction:* Move thumb back toward hand (ROM: 30).
- *Opposition:* Touch thumb to each finger of same hand (Fig. 27).

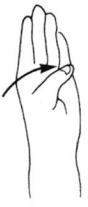 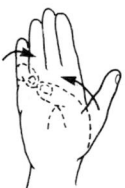

Fig. 26   Fig. 27

Hip

- *Flexion:* Move leg forward and up (ROM: 90-120) (Fig. 28).
- *Extension:* Move leg back beside other leg (ROM: 90-120) (Fig. 28).
- *Hyperextension:* Move leg behind body (ROM: 30-50) (Fig. 29).
- *Abduction:* Move leg laterally away from body (ROM: 30-50) (Fig. 30).
- *Adduction:* Move leg back toward medial position and beyond if possible (ROM: 30-50) (Fig. 30).
- *Internal rotation:* Turn foot and leg toward other leg (ROM: 90) (Fig. 31).
- *External rotation:* Turn foot and leg away from other leg (ROM: 90) (Fig. 31).
- *Circumduction:* Move leg in circle (ROM: 360) (Fig. 32).

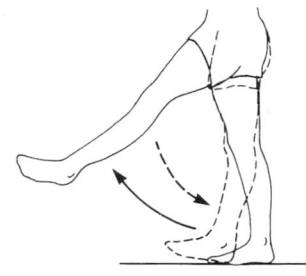
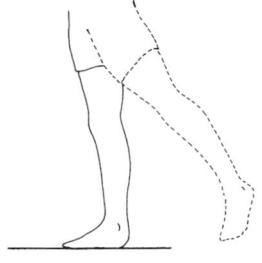

Fig. 28   Fig. 29

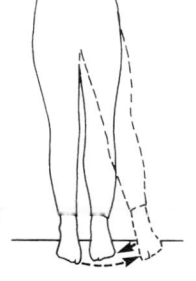
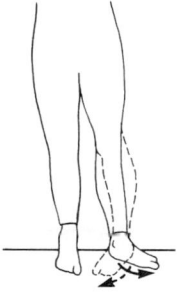
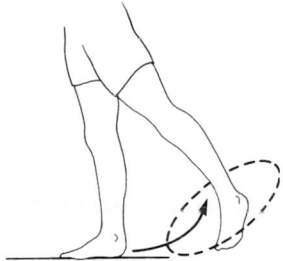

Fig. 30   Fig. 31   Fig. 32

Knee

- *Flexion:* Bring heel toward back of thigh (ROM: 120-130) (Fig. 33).
- *Extension:* Return leg to floor (ROM: 120-130) (Fig. 33).

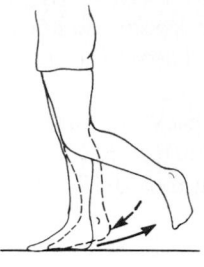

Fig. 33

Ankle

- *Dorsal flexion:* Move foot so toes are pointed upward (ROM: 20-30) (Fig. 34).
- *Plantar flexion:* Move foot so toes are pointed downward (ROM: 45-50) (Fig. 34).

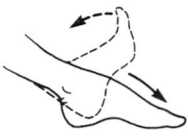

Fig. 34

Foot

- *Inversion:* Turn sole of foot medially (ROM: 10 or less) (Fig. 35).
- *Eversion:* Turn sole of foot laterally (ROM: 10 or less) (Fig. 35).
- *Flexion:* Curl toes downward (ROM: 30-60) (Fig. 36).
- *Extension:* Straighten toes (ROM: 30-60) (Fig. 36).
- *Abduction:* Spread toes apart (ROM: 15 or less) (Fig. 37).
- *Adduction:* Bring toes together (ROM: 15 or less) (Fig. 37).

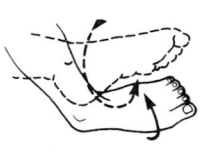
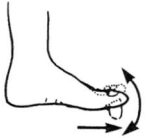
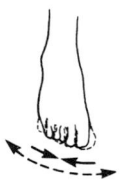

Fig. 35   Fig. 36   Fig. 37

Special Considerations

- It is essential to maintain joint flexibility. Contracted or immobile joints make protective positioning of a client difficult or impossible. It is hard to relieve pressure over bony prominences and to protect the client from pressure sores. Adequate skin care is difficult because it is hard to separate the skin folds adequately. If the client is in a curled or fetal position, chest expansion is restricted, and changes in abdominal pressure make elimination difficult.

- Contractures can begin shortly after onset of immobility. ROM exercises should be started as soon as possible. However, not all clients will require ROM exercises. Assess to determine which joints will get full ROM during client's normal activities and which will not and will require intervention.

- Some clients may need ROM exercises several times a day. Frequency depends on the individual client's medical diagnosis, present health condition, and willingness and ability to perform ROM exercises. Schedule exercises when it is convenient for the client. Bath time is a good time because bath water relaxes muscles, and joints are exposed so they are easy to manipulate and observe.

- When a person is immobile, the hip joint may become affected because full extension of the hip is difficult in all positions except relaxed standing. Partial flexion of the hip may occur. Elevation of the head, use of pillows under the knee, or elevation of the legs all increase flexion of the hip.

- Full extension of the knee while in bed seldom occurs without conscious effort. All positions, except prone, favor flexion. The dominant muscle of the lower leg, the hamstring muscle group, tends to draw the knee up into flexion. Other factors contributing to flexion of the knee include use of pillows under the knee, painful disabilities, and stationary positions.

- The ankle has a high risk for the development of flexion contractures (drop foot) because of gravity and the strength of the plantar flexion group. Plus, the weight of bedclothes contributes to the fatigue of the dorsal flexor muscles. Along with instituting ROM exercises of the ankle, a footboard or pillow may be useful in the prevention of footdrop. The client is instructed to place the feet against a pillow or footboard and to flex and extend the ankles against a pillow or footboard frequently throughout the day.

Walking with Crutches

Measurement

- Crutch measurement includes three areas: client's height, distance between crutch pad and axilla, and angle of elbow flexion. Use one of two methods: *Standing*—Position crutches with crutch tips at point 4 to 6 inches (14 to 15 cm) to side and 4 to 6 inches in front of client's feet and crutch pads 1½ to 2 inches (4 to 5 cm) below axilla. *Supine*—Crutch pad should be 3 to 4 finger widths under axilla with crutch tips positioned 6 inches (15 cm) lateral to client's heel.
- With either method elbows should be flexed 15 to 30 degrees. Elbow flexion is verified with goniometer.
- In addition to overall *length* of axillary crutch, *height* of handgrip is important. Both dimensions are adjustable on well-made crutch, and this is an important feature for a growing child. Handgrip should be adjusted so that client's elbow is *slightly flexed.* If handgrip is too low, radial nerve can be damaged even if overall crutch length is correct because extra length between handgrip and axillary bar can force bar up into axilla as client stretches down to reach handgrip. If handpiece is too high, client's elbow is sharply flexed and strength and stability of arms are decreased.

Teaching the Crutch Gait

Assist client in crutch walking by choosing appropriate gait.

To use crutches, client supports self with his or her hands and arms; therefore strength in arm and shoulder muscles, ability to balance body in upright position, and stamina are necessary. Type of gait client uses in crutch walking depends on amount of weight client is able to support with one or both legs.

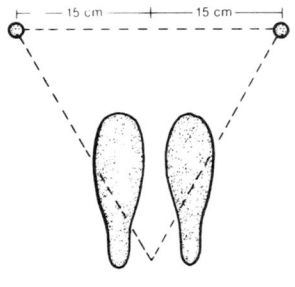

Fig. 38

Modified from Perry AG, Potter PA: *Clinical nursing skills and techniques,* ed 2, St Louis, 1990, Mosby; Potter PA, Perry AG: *Fundamentals of nursing,* ed 2, St Louis, 1989, Mosby.

A. The four-point gait is the most stable of crutch gaits because it provides at least three points of support at all times. Requires weight bearing on both legs. Often used when there is paralysis as in spastic children with cerebral palsy. May also be used for arthritic clients.

- Begin in tripod position (Fig. 38). Crutches are placed 6 inches (15 cm) in front and 6 inches to side of each foot. This improves client's balance by providing wider base of support. Posture should be erect head and neck, straight vertebrae, and extended hips and knees.
- Crutch and foot position are similar to arm and foot position during normal walking.
- Move right crutch forward 4 to 6 inches (Fig. 39).
- Move left foot forward to level of left crutch.
- Move left crutch forward 4 to 6 inches.
- Move right foot forward to level of right crutch.
- Repeat above sequence.

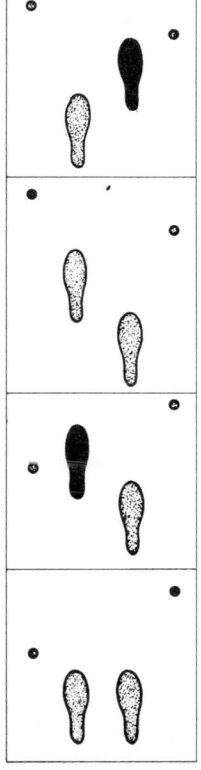

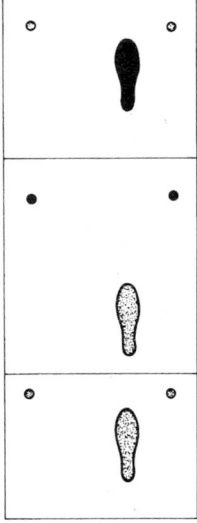

Fig. 39   Fig. 40

B. The three-point gait requires client to bear all weight on one foot. Weight is borne on uninvolved leg, then on both crutches. Affected leg does not touch ground during early phase of three-point gait. May be useful for client with broken leg or sprained ankle.

- Begin in tripod position. This improves client's balance by providing wide base of support.
- Advance both crutches and affected leg (Fig. 40).
- Move stronger leg forward.
- Repeat sequence.

C. The two-point gait requires at least partial weight bearing on each foot, and is faster than the four-point gait. Requires more balance because only two points support the body at one time.

- Begin in tripod position. This improves client's balance by providing wider base of support.
- Move left crutch and right foot forward (Fig. 41). (Crutch movements are similar to arm movement during normal walking.)
- Move right crutch and left foot forward.
- Repeat sequence.

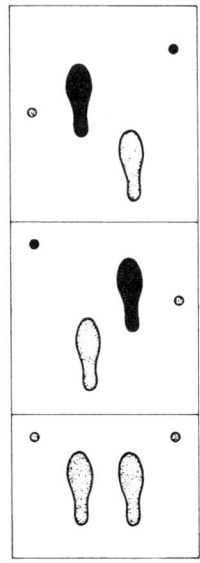

Fig. 41

Assist client in swing-to gait and swing-through gait. These are frequently used by clients whose lower extremities are paralyzed or who wear weight-supporting braces on their legs.

The swing-to gait is the easier of the two swinging gaits.

Swing-to gait:
• Move both crutches forward.
• Lift and swing legs to crutches letting crutches support body weight.
• Repeat steps 1 and 2.

Swing-through gait:
• Move both crutches forward. Initial placement of crutches is to increase the client's base of support so that when the body swings forward the client is moving the center of gravity toward the additional support provided by the crutches.
• Lift and swing legs through and beyond crutches.

Using Crutches while Walking on Stairs

A. Ascending stairs with crutches:

• Begin in tripod position.
• Transfer body weight to crutches. This prepares client to transfer weight to unaffected leg when ascending first stair.
• Advance unaffected leg to stair. The crutch adds support to affected leg. Client then shifts weight from crutches to unaffected leg.
• Align both crutches and unaffected leg on stairs to maintain balance and provide wide base of support.
• Repeat sequence until client reaches top of stairs.

B. Descending stairs with crutches:

• Begin in tripod position.
• Transfer body weight to unaffected leg. This prepares client to release support of body weight maintained by crutches.
• Move crutches to stair and instruct client to begin to transfer body weight to crutches and move affected leg forward. This maintains client's balance and base of support.
• Move unaffected leg to stair and align with crutches. This maintains balance and provides base of support.
• Repeat sequence until stairs are descended.

Sitting in a Chair when Using Crutches

As with crutch walking and crutch walking up and down stairs, the procedure for sitting in a chair involves phases and requires the client to transfer weight. First, the client gets positioned at the center front of the chair with the posterior aspect of the legs touching the chair. Second, the client holds both crutches in the hand opposite the affected leg. If both legs are affected, as with a paraplegic who wears weight-supporting braces, the crutches are held on the client's stronger side. With both crutches in one hand the client supports body weight on the unaffected leg and crutches. While still holding the crutches, the client grasps the arm of the chair with the remaining hand and lowers the body. To stand, the procedure is reversed, and the client when fully erect should assume the tripod position before walking.

Walker Use

Walkers are used by clients who are able to bear partial weight. Walkers need to be picked up, so clients need sufficient strength to be able to pick up walker. The four-wheeled model, which does not need to be picked up, is not as stable.

- Stand in center of walker and grasp handgrips on upper bars to balance self before attempting to walk.
- Take step forward into walker. This provides broad base of support between walker and client. Client then moves center of gravity toward the walker.
- Move walker 6 to 8 inches forward and take another step forward with either leg. If there is one-sided weakness, instruct the client after advancing walker to step forward with uninvolved leg, support self with the arms, and follow through with involved leg. If unable to bear weight on one leg, after advancing walker have the client swing on to it, supporting weight on hands.
- Repeat steps.

Modified from Perry AG, Potter PA: *Clinical nursing skills and techniques,* ed 2, St Louis, 1990, Mosby.

Transferring and Positioning
of Immobile Clients

The nurse will frequently encounter a semi-helpless, helpless, or immobilized client whose position must be changed or who must be moved up in bed. Proper use of body mechanics can enable the nurse (and a helper) to move, lift, or transfer such a client safely and at the same time avoid musculoskeletal injury.

Prepare the following equipment and supplies:
a. Pillows
b. Footboard
c. Trochanter roll
d. Sandbag
e. Hand rolls
f. Restraints (as appropriate)
g. Side rails

Raise level of bed to comfortable working height.
Remove all pillows and devices used in previous position.
Get extra help as needed.
Explain procedure to client.

Moving helpless client up in bed (one person):
a. Place client on back with head of bed flat. Stand on one side of bed.
b. Place pillow at head of bed.
c. Begin at client's feet. Face foot of bed at 45-degree angle. Place feet apart with foot nearest head of bed behind other foot (forward-backward stance). Flex knees and hips as needed to bring arms level with client's legs. Shift weight from front to back leg and slide client's legs diagonally toward head of bed.
d. Move parallel to client's hips. Flex knees and hips as needed to bring arms level with client's hips.
e. Slide client's hips diagonally toward head of bed.
f. Move parallel to client's head and shoulders. Flex knees and hips as needed to bring arms level with client's body.
g. Slide arm closest to head of bed under client's neck, with hand reaching under and supporting client's shoulder.
h. Place other arm under client's chest.
i. Slide client's trunk, shoulders, head, and neck diagonally toward head of bed.

Modified from Perry AG, Potter PA: *Clinical nursing skills and techniques,* ed 2, St Louis, 1990, Mosby.

j. Repeat procedure, switching sides until client reaches desired height in bed.

k. Center client in middle of bed, moving body in same three sections.

Assisting client to move up in bed (one person or two):

a. Place client on back.

b. Place pillow at head of bed.

c. Face head of bed.

- Each person should have one arm under client's shoulders and one arm under client's thighs.

- Alternate position: position one person at client's upper body. Person's arm nearest head of bed should be under client's head and opposite shoulder; other arm should be under client's closest arm and shoulder. Position other person at client's lower torso. This person's arms should be under client's lower back and torso.

d. Place feet apart with foot nearest head of bed behind other foot (forward-backward stance).

e. Ask client to flex knees with feet flat on bed.

f. Instruct client to flex neck, tilting chin toward chest.

g. Instruct client to assist moving by pushing with feet on bed surface.

h. Flex knees and hips, bringing forearms closer to level of bed.

i. Instruct client to push with heels and elevate trunk while breathing out, thus moving toward head of bed on count of 3.

j. On count of 3, rock and shift weight from front to back leg. At the same time, client pushes with heels and elevates trunk.

Positioning client in lateral (side-lying) position:

- Position client to side of bed.

- Turn client onto side:

    To turn helpless client onto side, flex knee that will not be next to mattress. Place one hand on client's hip and one hand on shoulder.

    Roll client onto side.

- Place pillow under client's head and neck.

- Bring shoulder blade forward.

- Position both arms in slightly flexed position. Upper arm is supported by pillow level with shoulder, other arm by mattress.

- Place tuck-back pillow behind client's back. (Make by folding pillow lengthwise. Smooth area is slightly tucked under client's back.)

- Place pillow under semiflexed upper leg level at hip from groin to foot.

- Place sandbag parallel to plantar surface of dependent foot.

Transferring client from bed to chair:

a. Assist client to sitting position on side of bed. Have chair in position at 45-degree angle to bed.

b. Apply transfer belt and transfer aids, if needed.

c. Ensure that client has stable, nonskid shoes. Weight-bearing, or strong leg forward, weak foot back.

d. Spread feet apart.

e. Flex hips and knees, aligning knees with client's.

f. Grasp transfer belt from underneath, if used, or reach through client's axilla and place hands on client's scapulae.

g. Rock client up to standing position on count of 3 while straightening hips and legs, keeping knees slightly flexed. Client may be instructed to use hands to push up if applicable.

h. Maintain stability of client's weak or paralyzed leg with knee.

i. Pivot on foot farther from chair.

j. Instruct client to use arm rests on chair for support and ease into chair.

k. Flex hips and knees while lowering client into chair.

l. Assess client for proper alignment for sitting position. Provide support for paralyzed extremities. Lap board or sling will support flaccid arm. Stabilize leg with bath blanket or pillow.

m. Praise client progress, effort, performance.

◊ Intravenous Care

Intravenous Therapy

1. Observe for signs and symptoms indicating fluid or electrolyte imbalances:
   a. Sunken eyes.
   b. Periorbital edema.
   c. Greater than 2% increase or decrease in body weight.
   d. Dry mucous membranes.
   e. Flattened or distended neck veins.
   f. Change from baseline vital signs.
   g. Irregular pulse rhythm.
   h. Auscultation of rales or rhonchi in lungs.
   i. Poor skin turgor.
   j. Increased or decreased bowel sounds.
   k. Decreased urine output.
   l. Behavioral changes.
   m. Confusion.
2. Review client's medical record for physician's order, stating type and amount of IV fluid and rate of fluid administration.
3. Assemble necessary equipment for initiating IV line:
   a. Correct solution.
   b. Proper needle for venipuncture (Fig. 42).

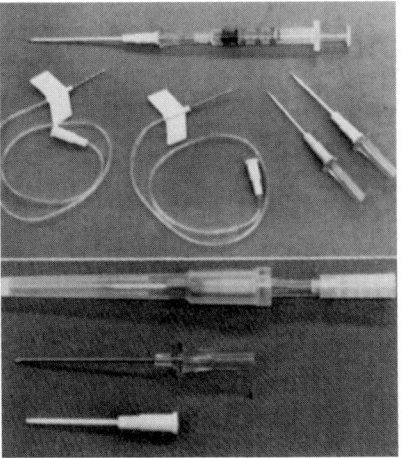

Fig. 42

Modified from Perry AG, Potter PA: *Clinical nursing skills and techniques,* ed 2, St Louis, 1990, Mosby.

   c. Infusion set (infants and children require a 60 gtt/ml drip and often a volume control device).

   d. IV tubing.

   e. Alcohol and povidone-iodine cleansing swabs.

   f. Disposable gloves.

   g. Tourniquet.

   h. Arm board.

   i. Gauze and povidone-iodine ointment or transparent dressing and povidone-iodine solution.

   j. Tape, cut and ready to use.

   k. Towel to place under client's hand.

   l. IV pole; coat rack or bed post.

4. Identify accessible vein for placement of IV needle or catheter (Fig. 43, *A-C*).

   a. Avoid bony prominences.

   b. Use most distal portion of vein first.

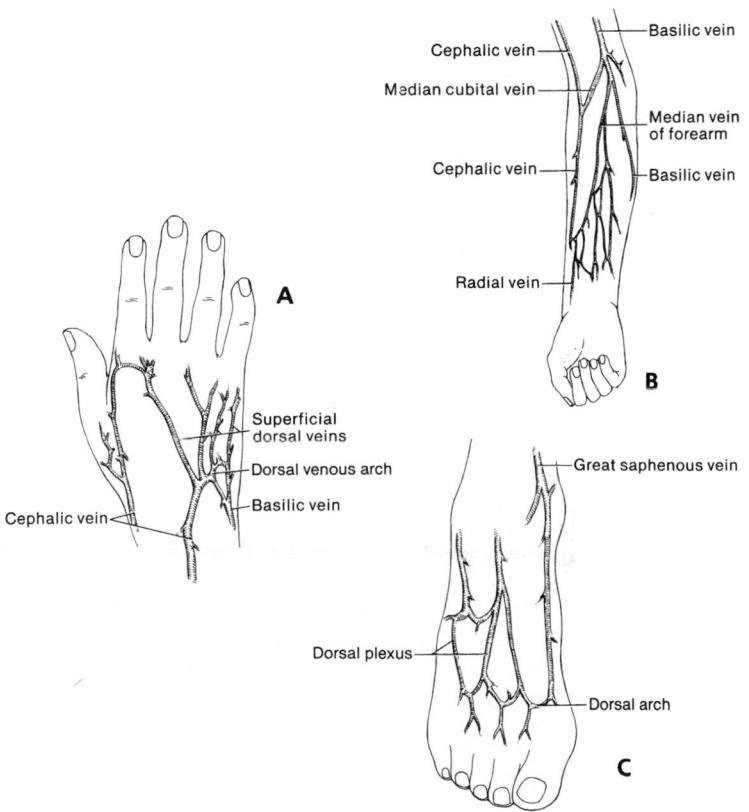

Fig. 43

    c. Avoid placing IV over client's wrist.

    d. Avoid placing IV in client's dominant hand.

Prepare client and family by explaining procedure, its purpose, and what is expected of client.

5. Wash hands.
6. Organize equipment on clutter-free bedside stand or over-bed table, if available in home.
7. Open sterile packages using aseptic technique.
8. Check solution, using "five rights" of drug administration. Make sure prescribed additives, such as potassium and vitamins, have been added. Check solution for color, clarity, and expiration date. *Note:* When using bottled IV solution, remove metal cap and metal and rubber disks beneath cap. For plastic IV solution bags, remove plastic sheath over IV tubing port.
9. Open infusion set, maintaining sterility of both ends.
10. Place roller clamp about 2 to 4 cm (1 to 2 in) below drip chamber.
11. Move roller clamp to "off" position.
12. Insert infusion set into fluid bag or bottle.

    a. Remove protective cover from IV bag without touching opening (Fig. 44, *A*).

    b. Remove protector cap from tubing insertion spike, not touching spike, and insert spike into opening of IV bag (Fig. 44, *B*). Or insert spike into black rubber stopper of IV bottle. Cleanse rubber stopper with antiseptic.

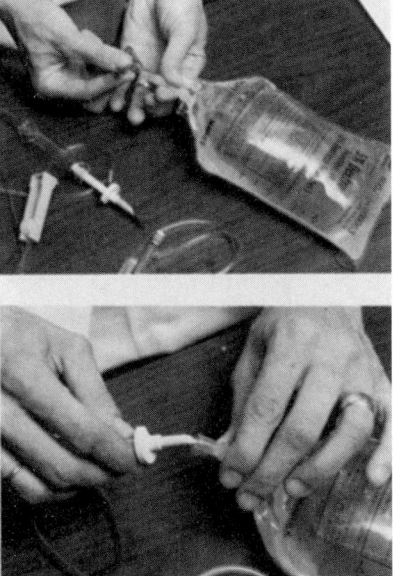

Fig. 44

13. Fill infusion tubing.
    a. Compress drip chamber and release.
    b. Remove needle protector and release roller clamp to allow fluid to travel from drip chamber through tubing to needle adapter. Return roller clamp to off position after tube is filled.
    c. Be certain tubing is clear of air and air bubbles.
    d. Replace needle protector.
14. Select appropriate IV needle or angiocatheter.
15. Select distal site of vein to be used.
16. If large amount of body hair is present at needle insertion site, shave it off.
17. If possible, place extremity in dependent position.
18. Place tourniquet 10 to 12 cm (5 to 6 in) above insertion site. Tourniquet should obstruct venous, not arterial, flow. Check presence of distal pulse.
19. Apply disposable gloves.
20. Select well-dilated vein. Client may have to make fist if vein in hand or arm is selected.
    Note: Be sure needle adapter end of infusion set is nearby and on sterile gauze or towel.
21. Cleanse insertion site with povidone-iodine solution, followed by alcohol.
22. Perform venipuncture. *Butterfly needle:* needle at 30-degree angle with bevel up about 1 cm (½ in) distal to actual site of venipuncture (Fig. 45). *Angiocatheter:* inserted bevel up at 30-degree angle distal to actual site of venipuncture.
23. Look for blood return through tubing of butterfly needle or angiocatheter, indicating that needle has entered vein. Advance catheter into vein until hub rests at venipuncture site. Remove stylet from angiocatheter, leaving catheter in place. Small, flexible catheter remains to permit entry of IV fluids.

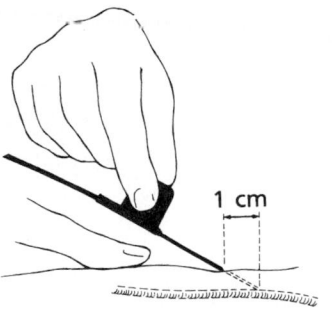

Fig. 45

24. Connect needle adapter of infusion set to hub of angiocatheter or needle. To maintain sterility, do not touch point of entry of needle adapter or hub of angiocatheter.
25. Stabilizing catheter with one hand, release tourniquet. Release roller clamp to begin infusion at a rate to maintain patency of IV line.
26. If gauze dressing is used, place povidone-iodine ointment at venipuncture site. If transparent dressing is used, place povidone-iodine solution at site.
27. Secure IV catheter or needle.
    a. Place narrow piece (½ in) of tape under catheter and cross tape over catheter.
    b. Place second piece of narrow tape directly across catheter.
    c. Place third piece of narrow tape under IV insertion needle adapter and cross tape over infusion tubing. Place 2 × 2 gauze pad over catheter and secure with 1 in piece of tape or place transparent dressing over IV site in direction of hair growth (Fig. 46).
    d. Secure infusion tubing to dressing with piece of 1 in tape.
28. Write date and time of placement of IV line on dressing.
29. Adjust flow rate to correct drops per minute.
30. Remove gloves. Discard supplies and wash hands.
31. Teach caregiver to observe client every hour to determine response to therapy.
    a. Correct amount of solution infused as prescribed.
    b. Proper flow rate gtt/minutes.
    c. Patency of IV catheter or needle.
    d. Absence of infiltration, phlebitis, or inflammation.

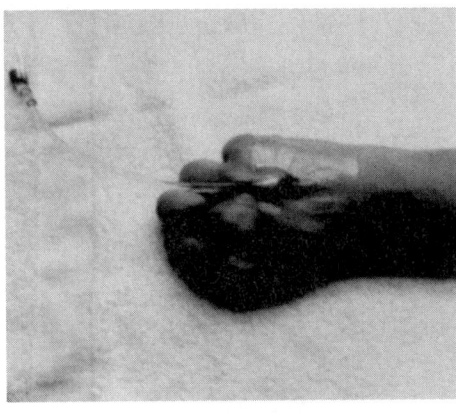

Fig. 46

Special Considerations

- Women of childbearing age may note fluctuation in weight of 2 to 5 lb between ovulation cycle and onset of menstruation. This does not indicate fluid imbalance but rather normal physiological response to fluctuating hormone levels.
- Most IV infusions in pediatric clients require a 21- or 23-gauge butterfly needle. When child is critically ill or long-term IV access is anticipated, surgical cutdown may be used to access larger vein.
- Assessment for potential venipuncture sites should consider conditions, cautions, and contraindications that exclude certain sites. Because very young and elderly clients have fragile veins, the caregiver should avoid sites that are easily moved or bumped. It is often difficult to insert IV lines in clients who have had numerous venipunctures because their veins may be sclerosed with scar tissue. Obese clients present problems for venipuncture because of difficulty in locating superficial veins. IVs should not be introduced into lower extremities unless specifically ordered by physician. Lower extremities are more likely to develop thrombophlebitis.
- Avoid using extremities with circulatory or neurological impairments.
- Venipuncture is contraindicated in site with signs of infection, infiltration, or thrombosis. Infected site is red, tender, swollen, and possibly warm to touch. Exudate may be present. Infected site is not used because of danger of introducing bacteria from skin surface into bloodstream.
- When it is anticipated that blood or blood components are going to be administered, a large-gauge (19 or 18) needle should be used for infusion of more viscous solution.
- Critically ill clients at all stages of life require more frequent assessment to monitor status of therapy.
- When infiltration occurs, infusion must be discontinued and, if necessary, reinserted into another extremity. Nursing measures to reduce discomfort caused by infiltration are elevation of extremity, which promotes venous drainage and helps decrease edema, and wrapping extremity in warm towel for 20 minutes every 4 hours, which increases circulation and reduces pain and edema.
- When phlebitis is present, IV line must be discontinued and new line inserted in another vein. Warm, moist heat on site of phlebitis can offer some relief.
- Phlebitis is potentially dangerous because blood clots (thrombophlebitis) can occur and in some cases result in emboli.

- When solution has less than 100 ml remaining, the caregiver should have new solution at client's bedside and slow flow rate. This reduces risk of solution emptying before it can be replaced.
- Assess client and family/primary caregiver's willingness to participate in client's care, including procurement of supplies and ability to handle emergency situations.
- Assess home environment for possible safety hazards, cleanliness, adequate storage for supplies, electrical wiring, and availability of running water.
- Coordinate client teaching and develop plan of care to be followed by client and primary caregiver.

Home Care Teaching for IV Therapy

Home care teaching includes all procedures that the client will need to care for the IV at home, such as the following:

1. Work area: away from family living area, preferably not a bathroom, and no drafts
2. Work surface: sturdy with a washable surface (clean with 70% isopropyl alcohol before and after each procedure)
3. Hand washing
4. Dressing changes
5. Injection cap changes (if applicable)
6. Flushing and heparin/saline use (as applicable)
7. Signs and symptoms of complications (when to call the MD)

Those procedures that the client must perform should be demonstrated to the nurse to ensure proper understanding.

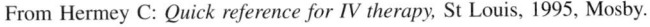

From Hermey C: *Quick reference for IV therapy,* St Louis, 1995, Mosby.

Collecting Blood
Specimens by Venipuncture

The three primary methods of obtaining blood specimens are venipuncture, skin puncture, and arterial stick.

Venipuncture, the most common method, involves inserting a hollow-bore needle into the lumen of a large vein to obtain a specimen. The nurse may use a needle and syringe or a special Vacutainer that allows the drawing of multiple blood samples. Because veins are major sources of blood for laboratory testing and routes for IV fluid or blood replacement, maintaining their integrity is essential. The nurse should be skilled in venipuncture to avoid unnecessary injury to veins.

Skin puncture is the least traumatic method of obtaining a blood specimen. A sterile lancet or needle is used to puncture a vascular area on a finger, toe, or heel. A drop of blood is placed on a test slide or collected within a thin glass capillary tube for laboratory analysis.

The most traumatic form of obtaining blood specimens is arterial stick. A small-gauge needle is inserted directly into the lumen of an artery to collect a specimen. Of all methods for obtaining blood specimens, arterial stick poses the greatest risks.

1. Determine understanding of purpose of procedure and method to be used.
2. Determine if special conditions need to be met before specimen collection (i.e., client to the NPO, specific time for collection after medication or meal).
3. Assess client for possible risk for venipuncture: anticoagulant therapy, low platelet count, bleeding disorders (history of hemophilia or ecchymosis).
4. Determine ability to cooperate with procedure.
5. Assess client for contraindicated sites for venipuncture: presence of IV fluids, hematoma at potential site, history of mastectomy, hemodialysis recipient.
6. Review physician's orders for type of tests.
7. a. Obtain appropriate specimen under required conditions (according to agency laboratory policy).
   b. Minimize discomfort at venipuncture site.
   c. Minimize trauma at needle insertion site.
   d. Prevent infection at venipuncture site.
   e. Minimize client's anxiety.

Modified from Perry AG, Potter PA: *Clinical nursing skills and techniques,* ed 2, St Louis, 1990, Mosby.

8. Prepare equipment and supplies:
   a. Alcohol or antiseptic swab.
   b. Disposable gloves.
   c. Small pillow or folded towel.
   d. Sterile gauze pads (2 × 2).
   e. Rubber tourniquet.
   f. Band-Aid or adhesive tape.
   g. *Syringe method:*
      - Sterile needles (20 to 21 gauge for adults, 23 to 25 gauge for children).
      - Sterile syringe of appropriate size.
   h. *Vacutainer method:*
      - Vacutainer tube with needle holder.
      - Sterile, double-ended needles (20 to 21 gauge for adults, 23 to 25 gauge for children). (Some nurses prefer to use butterfly or scalp vein needles.)
   i. Appropriate blood tubes.
   j. Completed identification labels according to agency policy.
   k. Completed laboratory requisition (date, time, type of test).
9. Explain procedure to client: describe purpose of tests; explain how sensation of tourniquet, alcohol swab, needle stick feel.
10. Wash hands.
11. Bring equipment to bedside.
12. Assist client to supine or semi-Fowler's position with arms extended to form straight line from shoulders to wrists. Place small pillow or towel under upper arm.
13. If client is a child, ask parent to restrain child so venipuncture site is immobilized.
14. Apply disposable gloves.

15. Apply tourniquet 5 to 15 cm (2 to 6 in) above venipuncture site selected (antecubital fossa site is most often used). Encircle extremity and pull one end of tourniquet tightly over other, looping one end under other. Apply tourniquet so it can be removed by pulling end with single motion.
16. Palpate distal pulse (e.g., radial) below tourniquet. If pulse not palpable, reapply tourniquet more loosely.
17. Keep tourniquet on no longer than 1 to 2 minutes.
18. Ask client to open and close fist several times, finally leaving fist clenched.
19. Quickly inspect extremity for best venipuncture site, looking for straight, prominent vein without swelling or hematoma.
20. Palpate selected vein with index finger. Note if vein is firm and rebounds when palpated or if vein feels rigid and cordlike and rolls when palpated.

21. Select venipuncture site. (If tourniquet on arm is too long, remove, and assess other extremity or wait 60 seconds before reapplying.)
22. Obtain blood sample:
    a. *Syringe method:*
       - Have syringe with appropriate needle securely attached.
       - Cleanse venipuncture site with alcohol swab, moving in circular motion from site for approximately 5 cm (2 in). Allow to dry.
       - Remove needle cover and inform client "stick" lasting only few seconds will be felt.
       - Place thumb or forefinger of nondominant hand 2.5 cm (1 in) above or below site and pull skin taut.
       - Hold syringe and needle at 15- to 30-degree angle from client's arm with bevel up.
       - Slowly insert needle into vein.
       - Hold syringe securely and pull back gently on plunger.
       - Look for blood return.
       - Obtain desired amount of blood, keeping needle stabilized.
       - After specimen is obtained, release tourniquet.
       - Apply 2×2 gauze pad or antiseptic swab over puncture site without applying pressure and quickly but carefully withdraw needle from vein.
    b. *Vacutainer method:*
       - Attach double-ended needle to Vacutainer tube.
       - Have proper blood specimen tube resting inside Vacutainer but do not puncture rubber stopper.
       - Cleanse venipuncture site with alcohol swab, moving in circular motion out from site for approximately 5 cm (2 in).
       - Remove needle cover and inform client that "stick" lasting only few seconds will be felt.
       - Place thumb or forefinger of nondominant hand 2.5 cm (1 in) above or below site and pull skin taut. Stretch skin down until vein is stabilized.
       - Hold Vacutainer at 15- to 30-degree angle from arm with bevel up.
       - Slowly insert needle into vein.
       - Grasp Vacutainer securely and advance specimen tube into needle of holder (do not advance needle in vein).
       - Note flow of blood into tube (should be fairly rapid).
       - After specimen tube is filled, grasp Vacutainer firmly and remove tube. Insert additional specimen tubes as needed.
       - After last tube is filled, release tourniquet.

- Apply 2×2 gauze pad over puncture site without applying pressure and quickly but carefully withdraw needle from vein.
23. Immediately apply pressure over venipuncture site with gauze or antiseptic pad for 2 to 3 minutes or until bleeding stops. *Option:* apply pressure over site and tape gauze dressing securely.
24. For blood obtained by syringe, transfer specimen to tubes. Insert needle through stopper of blood tube and allow vacuum to fill tube. Do not force blood into tube.

    or

    Remove needle from syringe and stopper to each test tube. Gently inject required amount of blood into each tube. Reapply stopper.
25. Take blood tubes containing additives and gently rotate back and forth 8 to 10 times.
26. Inspect puncture site for bleeding and apply adhesive tape with gauze.
27. Check tubes for any sign of external contamination with blood. Decontaminate with 70% alcohol if necessary.
28. Remove disposable gloves after specimen obtained and any spillage cleaned.
29. Assist client to comfortable position.
30. Securely attach properly completed identification label to each tube and affix proper requisition.
31. Dispose of needles, syringe, soiled equipment in proper container. Do not cap needles.
32. Wash hands after procedure.
33. Send or take specimens immediately to laboratory.
34. Reinspect venipuncture site.
35. Determine if client remains anxious or fearful.
36. Check laboratory report for test results.
37. If hematoma develops, obtain order from physician to apply cold compress. After bleeding subsides, order for hot compress can be obtained.
38. Inform clients who are to receive further venipunctures about reasons for tests.

Special Considerations

- Check policy regarding designated container for disposal of contaminated needles and syringes.
- If gloves become contaminated with blood, replace with clean pair after proper disposal of contaminated ones. Touch nothing and do not handle supplies with contaminated gloves.

- Infants and young children need to be restrained, as do restless, confused, or combative clients. Check policy on need for physician's order if restraint is necessary. Parent may hold child to facilitate cooperation and decrease anxiety.

- Samples taken from vein near IV infusion may be diluted or contain concentrations of IV fluids. Postmastectomy client may have reduced lymphatic drainage in arm on operative side increasing risk of infection from needle sticks. Arteriovenous shunt should never be used to obtain specimens because of risks of clotting and bleeding. Hematoma indicates existing injury to vessel's wall.

- If drawing sample for blood alcohol level, use only antiseptic swab to ensure accurate test results.

- Clients receiving anticoagulants require pressure over site for at least 5 minutes.

- If child needs to be restrained during procedure, let parents choose if they want to assist. Person restraining client should speak in calm, reassuring tone. By leaning across child, nurse maintains body and eye contact, which can help reduce fear.

- If client has large distended veins, tourniquet may not be needed.

- Clients undergoing frequent venipunctures may have preferred or undesirable site. Most commonly used vein is median cubital in antecubital fossa. In children, use veins on dorsal aspect of foot or scalp veins. Avoid vessels that pulsate; this indicates artery.

- If vein cannot be palpated or viewed easily, remove tourniquet and apply warm, wet compress over extremity for 10 to 20 minutes. Heat causes local vasodilation.

- With experience nurse will feel "pop" as needle enters vein. If plunger pulled back too quickly, pressure may cause vein to collapse.

- Instruct client to briefly apply pressure to venipuncture site. Clients with bleeding disorders or on anticoagulant therapy should apply pressure for at least 5 minutes.

- Instruct client to notify nurse, agency, or physician if persistent or recurrent bleeding or expanding hematoma occurs at venipuncture site.

Vascular Access Devices

Clients with chronic diseases often need long-term IV therapy, which requires safe, repeated access to the venous system for administration of drugs, fluids, nutrition, and blood products. Frequent venipuncture and multiple IV lines pose problems and risks, including infection, pain, and bruising. Clients with chronic diseases are generally more susceptible to infection and bleeding. Clients receiving multiple doses of chemotherapeutic drugs experience vein sclerosis or hardening. Eventually, no suitable peripheral veins remain for drug administration.

The need for safe and convenient long-term IV therapy has led to the development of VADs, which are catheters, cannulas, or infusion ports designed for long-term, repeated access to the venous or arterial systems. The nurse must be able to maintain the integrity of central venous catheters and implanted infusion ports and educate clients about the care of catheters for home use.

Home health nurses frequently administer parenteral nutrition and chemotherapy in the home using VADs. The trend in the care of oncology clients is expanded home health services. VADs allow clients to go home earlier and to receive continued care rather than remain in acute-care settings for several weeks.

Nurses play a role in identifying clients who may benefit from VADs. For example, a client with severe nutritional deficiencies may need long-term parenteral nutrition. The nurse may be the first to recognize the client's intolerance to oral or enteral feedings.

The types of VADs and their therapeutic uses vary according to the diagnosis. Nurses must have the necessary knowledge, skill, and judgment to maintain and troubleshoot VADs. Client education is also important. Clients and families learn to change dressings around catheters and to recognize signs of complications such as infection, bleeding, or leakage at insertion sites.

To manage long-term IV therapy effectively the nurse must know the types of VADs, including central venous catheters, external catheters, and implanted infusion ports.

Central venous catheters are inserted by the physician into a large vein, typically the superior vena cava that leads to the right atrium of the heart (Fig. 47). The large vessel lumen minimizes the risks of vessel irritation, inflammation, or sclerosis that commonly occur when smaller peripheral veins are used.

Atrial catheters are surgically inserted with the client in the operating room under general or local anesthesia. First a tunnel is made through subcutaneous tissue, usually between the clavicle and

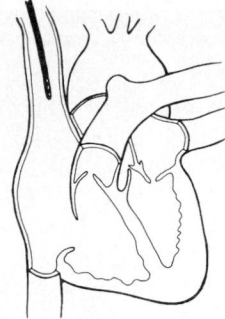

Fig. 47

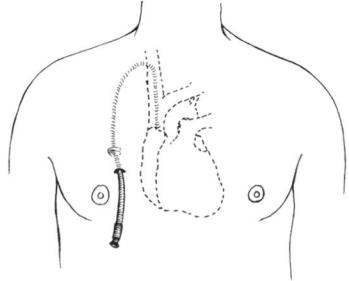

Fig. 48

nipple. The tunnel allows the catheter to remain in place longer because it creates space between the end of the catheter and the actual vein. The risk of infection is less. Then the catheter tip is inserted through the cephalic, internal, or external jugular vein, or a similar large vein, and is threaded into the right atrium (Fig. 48). These catheters have single or double lumens; i.e., one or two hollow tubes extend within the inside of the catheter and allow for administration of more than one type of infusion simultaneously.

A second type of external catheter is the small-gauge central venous catheter, which is inserted directly through the skin and into the subclavian vein of the neck or the basilic vein in the antecubital fossa of the arm. The catheter is threaded into the right atrium but can only be used a short time. Intermittent or continuous intravenous infusions can be given.

The third type of VAD is the implanted infusion port, which consists of a self-sealing injection port housed in a plastic or metal case (Fig. 49) and connected to a silicone venous catheter. The port is also now available with a double-lumen catheter. The physician implants the infusion port under sterile conditions in an operating

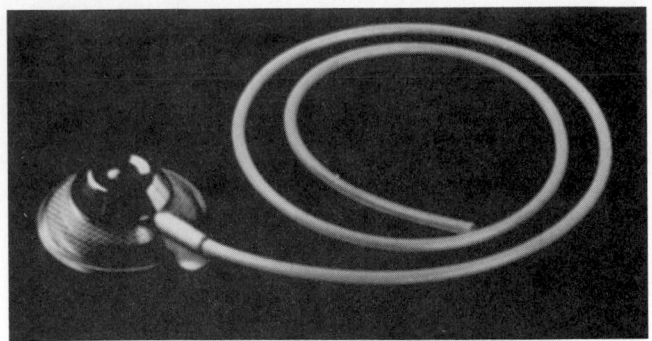

Fig. 49

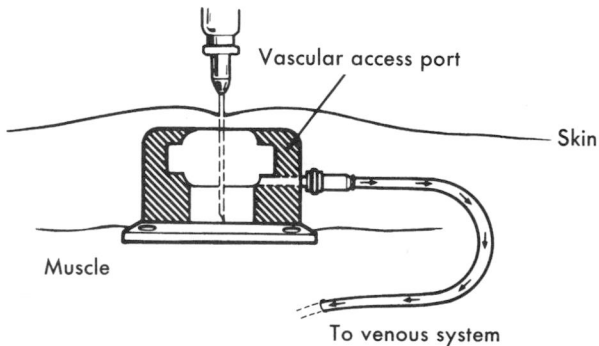

Fig. 50

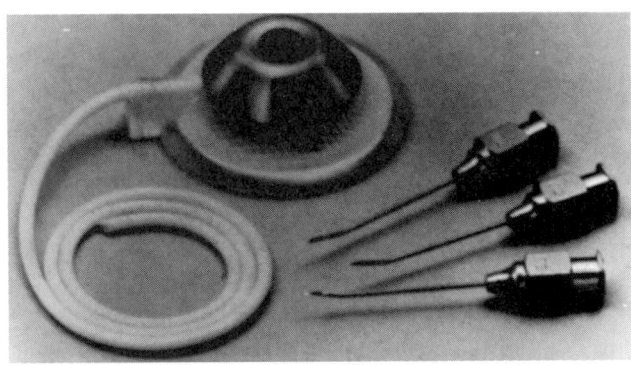

Fig. 51

room with the client under local anesthesia. The infusion port usually rests in a subcutaneous pocket in the infraclavicular fossa, and the catheter is inserted into a large vein and threaded into the right atrium (Fig. 50). The port can be easily palpated to determine placement. Specially designed Huber needles (straight or with 90-degree angles) are inserted through the skin to enter the port (Fig. 51). Implanted infusion ports are used for administration of injections and for continuous infusions of all types: medications, chemotherapy, parenteral nutrition, and blood products. The nurse or client heparinizes the port every 4 weeks when not in use to maintain its patency.

Care of VADs is simple as long as nurses and clients are aware of the purpose and function of the devices and the two most common complications, infection and clotting. In the home, most clients learn to use clean technique for dressing changes and catheter care. Within 2 to 3 weeks an adhesive bandage is sufficient to cover catheter insertion sites. Clients can learn to initiate infusions, heparinize devices, and discontinue infusions.

Accessing the Porta-Cath for Flushing with Heparinized Saline, Administration of Medication, or Drawing Blood

A. Supplies
B. Site preparation
C. Points to remember
D. Heparin flush to maintain system patency
E. Procedure for bolus injection
F. Procedure for continuous infusion
G. Procedure for drawing blood

Supplies

1. Sterile gloves
2. (3) Povidone swabs
3. (4) Alcohol swabs
4. Sterile Huber point (a noncore needle); straight for bolus injection, 90-degree angle for continuous infusion
5. IV extension tubing with Luer-Lok fittings, flow value, and inline filter for continuous infusion
6. Sterile normal saline
7. Heparinized saline (100 U heparin/ml)

Modified from Porta-Cath Pharmacies, Deltec, Inc; Visiting Nurse And Home Care, Inc, 1991, Waterbury, Conn.

8. For continuous infusion: an occlusive dressing (Tegaderm) 2 × 2, tape, and betadine ointment
9. 10-ml syringes
10. 20-ml syringe if drawing blood

Site Preparation

1. Wash hands.
2. Assess IVAD site for warmth, edema, skin excoriation, drainage, distended veins.
3. Locate the portal by palpation.
4. Cleanse the site with (3) povidone-iodine swabsticks followed by (3) alcohol swabsticks. Start at the center of site and clean outward in a circular motion (for 2- to 4-in diameter).
5. Let the alcohol dry.

Points to Remember

1. *Always* access system under aseptic conditions.
2. *Always* use a Huber point noncore needle to access.
3. *Always* insert needle *perpendicular* to the portal septum.
4. *Always* make sure the needle is inside the portal chamber and *against the needle stop* (the back of port) before starting the injection or infusion.
5. *Never* tilt or rock the needle once the port has been entered.
6. *Never* leave an open line while the needle is in the portal chamber because this could cause an air emboli to develop.
7. *Always* flush the system with normal saline *before and after each drug* infusion to check for flow and provide a buffer between drugs.
8. *Never* use a syringe smaller than 10 ml to avoid excess pressure.
9. *Always* continue injecting fluid slowly into the system while opening or closing the clamp of any extension tube.
10. *Always* stop injection or infusion if unusual resistance develops and report this to physician.
11. *Always* maintain *positive* pressure while withdrawing needle to prevent reflux.
12. *Always* leave vascular systems filled with heparinized saline and intraperitoneal systems filled with normal saline.

Procedure for Heparinized Saline Flush to Maintain Patency

1. Prepare site as described.
2. Attach a Huber 22-gauge Porta-Cath needle to a 10-ml syringe filled with 5 ml of heparinized saline for injection (100 U/ml).
3. Locate the portal septum by palpation.

4. Insert the needle perpendicular to the septum. Push firmly through the skin to the bottom of the chamber.
5. Flush the system with 3 to 5 ml of heparinized saline.
6. Press down on the portal with two fingers and maintain positive pressure as the needle is withdrawn.

Procedure for Bolus Injection

1. Prepare site as described.
2. Connect an extension tube to a straight Huber point needle on one side and a 10-ml syringe filled with 5 ml of normal saline at the other end.
3. Prime the tubing with normal saline and *close the clamp.*
4. Prepare heparinized saline (100 U heparin/ml) 3 to 5 ml in a 10-ml syringe.
5. Prepare medication to be administered.
6. With gloved hand locate the portal septum by palpation.
7. Push the *Huber* needle firmly (the port's septum requires pressure to access) until it hits the bottom of the portal chamber (which is metal).
8. As you open the extension tubing clamp, flush the system with the normal saline.
9. *Close the clamp* and remove the syringe from the extension tube.
10. Attach the syringe with the medication to be administered.
11. As you start the injection, release the flow clamp.
12. As you complete the injection, close the flow clamp and remove the syringe. If more than one drug is administered, follow each injection with a normal saline flush.
13. After removing the drug administration syringe, connect your heparinized (100 U/ml) normal saline to the extension tube.
14. Open the clamp and flush the system with 3 to 5 ml of the heparinized normal saline leaving a "heparin lock." The clamp is closed while maintaining positive injection pressure.
15. To avoid reflux when removing the Huber needle from the port, maintain positive injection pressure while simultaneously withdrawing the needle and pressing down on the portal with two fingers to stabilize it.
16. Cleanse the site with an alcohol swab.

Procedure for Continuous Infusion

1. Prepare the site as described.
2. Prepare normal saline flush (5 ml in a 10-ml syringe) and 3 to 5 ml of heparinized saline (100 U of heparin/ml) in a 10-ml syringe.
3. Connect an extension tube to a sterile *90-degree Huber point needle* and with a 10-ml syringe filled with about 5 ml of normal saline.

4. Prime the tubing with the normal saline and clamp.

5. Locate portal septum by palpation with gloved hand. Push needle firmly through skin and portal septum until it hits the bottom of portal chamber.

6. Apply an occlusive dressing. First put a folded 2 × 2 gauze pad under the bend of the needle, betadine ointment at entry site. Cover with a sterile dressing and tape all connections.

7. As you open the clamp, flush the system with the normal saline (3 to 5 ml) and confirm that fluid flows through the system.

8. Close the clamp and remove the syringe from the extension tube.

9. Connect previously primed IV infusion to the extension tube.

10. Open the flow clamp and start infusion. *If* a pump is to be used, turn it on just before opening the clamp.

11. When the infusion is finished, close the clamp. If a pump was used, turn it off *after* closing the clamp.

12. If more than one drug is administered, follow each infusion with a normal saline flush and clamp. This provides a buffer between different drugs.

13. Cleanse the IV or pump tubing connection with alcohol, and disconnect from the extension tube.

14. Attach a 10-ml syringe filled with 5 ml of heparinized (100 U/ml) saline to the extension tube.

15. Open the clamp and flush the system with 3 to 5 ml of heparinized saline leaving a "heparin lock."

16. Slowly close the clamp while maintaining positive injection pressure.

17. To remove the Huber needle, stabilize the port with thumb and index finger, and while maintaining positive pressure withdraw the needle.

Procedure for Drawing Blood

1. Prepare site as described.

2. Prepare normal saline flush (5 ml in 10-ml syringe) and heparinized saline (100 U heparin/ml) 5 ml in a 10-ml syringe, plus 20 ml normal saline flush.

3. Connect straight Huber needle to IV extension tubing and 5 ml of normal saline in a 10-ml syringe.

4. Prime the tubing with normal saline and clamp.

5. Locate the portal septum by palpation with gloved hand.

6. Push the straight Huber needle firmly through the skin and portal septum until it hits the bottom of the portal chamber.

7. As the clamp is released, flush the port with 3 ml of normal saline to confirm that fluid flows through the system.

8. As soon as you complete the flush, withdraw at least 3 ml of

blood, then clamp the extension tubing and discard the syringe. Attach a new 10-ml syringe.

9. As you unclamp, withdraw the desired volume of blood, then clamp.

10. *Immediately* after withdrawing the blood sample, clamp the extension tubing, attach the heparinized saline 100 U/ml flush and as you unclamp, flush the system with 3 ml heparinized saline to avoid clots forming inside the catheter. Clamp and attach 20 ml normal saline flush.

11. As you unclamp, flush the system with 20 ml of normal saline. Then clamp, and attach 5 ml of heparinized saline (100 U/ml).

12. As you unclamp, flush the system with 5 ml of heparinized (100 U/ml) saline, leaving a "heparin lock," maintaining positive pressure as the extension tube is clamped.

13. Remove the Huber needle maintaining positive pressure.

Documentation Guidelines for IVAD

Baseline

Type of IVAD location
Date of insertion

Flowsheet Parameters
Site inspection/palpation

Redness
Edema
Warmth
Distended veins
Skin excoriation
Tenderness
Movement of port

Temp
Routine heparinization

Frequency
Heparin flush strength/amount

Date for changing

Needle
Dressing
Luer-Lok cap
Tubing

Modified from Visiting Nurse and Home Care, Inc, 1991, Waterbury, Conn.

Medication administration
Amount/time (rate, if continuous)
Side effects
Heparin flush (amount)
Laboratory test results

Obtaining blood sample
Amount
Heparin flush strength/amount
Saline flush 20 ml
Tests ordered
Lab sent to

Additional findings
Client's response to procedure
Difficulties encountered
Unusual circumstances

Assessment of client status
Care given
Instructions

Criteria for Admission of Client
Utilizing Portable Infusion Pumps

1. Client or family must have had complete instructions in the hospital regarding use of portable infusion pump. Written instructions should accompany client home.
2. Agency personnel must have had prior instruction regarding use of the pump as well as demonstration in the hospital with the client.
3. Family must be willing, available, and reliable in their participation in client care and use of infusable pump.
4. Clients must be followed on a regular basis at least every 2 weeks by a physician initially and when condition stabilizes, at least once a month.
5. Blood values must be done at least every 2 weeks by a physician and when condition stabilizes, at least once a month.

Modified from Visiting Nurse and Home Care, Inc, 1991, Waterbury, Conn.

Portable Infusion Pump Procedure

Portable infusion pumps deliver intermittent drugs or fluids over a period of time. The solution is delivered subcutaneously. The pump is battery operated. A physician regulates the settings on the pump. These settings indicate flow rate of the solution. The pump is designed to hold any standard brand syringe. A physician's order must be obtained for the nurse to use the pump as well as to draw up and inject the prescribed solution. An order is also necessary to instruct the client and/or responsible individuals in the use of the pump.

Equipment

Infusable pump with dials preset by physician
Medication or solution
Deseret needle (27 gauge)
Nonallergic tape
Alcohol wipes
Gauze as needed

Procedure	Point of emphasis
1. Check order for amount and type of solution.	
2. Draw up solution into syringe to specified amount.	Use sterile technique.
3. Attach Deseret needle (27 gauge) to the syringe.	
4. Flush tubing of Deseret needle with the solution.	
5. Attach needle and tubing to the pump.	
6. Select site for injection and cleanse with alcohol (sites are abdomen, thighs, or arms).	Instruct client or responsible individual to rotate sites each time injection necessary.
7. Inject needle into the skin at a 45-degree angle.	
8. Secure needle in place with tape and gauze.	A pillow may be made of gauze to place under needle to position needle.
9. Turn on pump.	
10. When solution is finished, remove needle and wipe skin with alcohol.	Store equipment in clean area.

Modified from Visiting Nurse and Home Care, Inc, 1991, Waterbury, Conn.

Hickman Broviac Catheter: Site Care

Purpose
To prevent infection.
To monitor for signs and symptoms of infection.

Equipment
Sterile gloves
Alcohol swabs (3)
Povidone-iodine swabs (3)
Betadine ointment
Sterile applicator
Transparent dressing (e.g., Opsite or Tegaderm), or if ordered, sterile
    2×2 gauze
Silk tape—1 or 2 in—optional for framing.

Procedure
1. Wash hands thoroughly.
2. Remove old dressing. Check dressing for drainage and discard.
3. Check exit site for signs of infection.
4. Put on sterile gloves.
5. Cleanse site with alcohol swab, starting near catheter and working outward $1\frac{1}{2}$ in. Repeat ×2. Let alcohol dry. Then, with third alcohol swab, cleanse catheter from exit site for 2 in.
6. Cleanse site with povidone-iodine swab in same manner—allow to dry. Then, cleanse from exit site for 2 in with third betadine swab.
7. Apply betadine ointment over exit site using a sterile applicator.
8. Cover exit site with a transparent dressing (e.g., Opsite or Tegaderm) and frame with tape.
9. If catheter is long enough, loop it, and tape it to the client's chest. This helps prevent accidental dislodgement. Optional: as a comfort measure, put 2×2 gauze under cap end of catheter before taping to chest.
10. Record dressing change and site characteristics in client's record.
11. Frequency of site care:
    If transparent dressing, usually 2 to 3 ×/wk.
    If gauze dressing, usually daily.

Modified from Visiting Nurse and Home Care, Inc, 1991, Waterbury, Conn.

Hickman Broviac Catheter: Irrigation

The Hickman Broviac indwelling catheter is commonly used for total parenteral nutrition or the administration of chemotherapeutic agents. It provides ready access to the client's circulation. The catheter is inserted in the operating room. A subcutaneous tunnel is formed exiting at the area between the sternum and the nipple. The catheter is pulled through the tunnel, inserted into the cephalic vein, and positioned in the superior vena cava at the entrance to the right atrium.

Purpose

To maintain patency of catheter by flushing and filling the catheter with heparin solution when the catheter is not in use or after infusion. If the client is receiving frequent intermittent infusions (e.g., antibiotics q4h) and the amount of heparin may surpass therapeutic range and affect bleeding times, normal saline may be used for flushing.

Equipment

Heparin lock flush 100 U per ml
5-ml syringe with needle
Alcohol swabs

Procedure

1. Obtain written orders from physician.
2. Wash hands.
3. Assemble equipment.
4. Check physician's orders and label on medication bottle.
5. Draw 3 ml of heparin lock flush 100 USP per ml.
6. Clamp catheter over thickened portion of catheter; use cannula ("bulldog") clamp—*never Kelly clamp.*
7. Clean catheter plug at connection with alcohol wipe.
8. Insert needle into catheter plug.
9. Release clamp as you start to inject to maintain positive pressure.
10. Clamp catheter as last ½ ml of solution is injected and leave clamped as needle is removed. Apply pressure on syringe plunger as you remove it from catheter plug. (If catheter is unclamped before the needle is removed there may be a backup of blood into the catheter.)

Modified from Visiting Nurse and Home Care, Inc, 1991, Waterbury, Conn.

11. Secure catheter to dressing so that it is not "kinked." (Clamp may be left on catheter between flushes or removed, depending on physician's orders.)
12. Record in client's record.

Hickman Broviac Catheter: Plug Change

Purpose
To prevent infection.
To prevent leakage.

Equipment
Sterile gloves
Alcohol swabs
Plastic hemostat or plastic tipped hemostat
Sterile catheter plug

Procedure
1. Wash hands thoroughly.
2. Close clamp on Hickman Broviac over thickened portion of catheter.
3. Put on gloves
4. Swab old plug and junction with alcohol.
5. Loosen old plug slightly.
6. Pick up sterile plug.
7. Remove old plug and insert new plug—securely.
8. Swab junction again with alcohol swab.
9. Unclamp hemostat.

Modified from Visiting Nurse And Home Care, Inc, 1991, Waterbury, Conn.

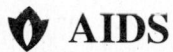 **AIDS**

Administration of Pentamidine Aerosol Therapy

Since 1989 aerosolized pentamidine isethionate has been one of the methods recommended by the Centers for Disease Control to prevent AIDS-related *Pneumocystis carinii* pneumonia (PCP). Based on clinical trials, the current recommendation for aerosol therapy is 300 mg of pentamidine isethionate, administered once every 4 weeks via the Respirgard II jet nebulizer.

I. **Preadministration assessment** (to be performed before the first treatment)

A. Has the client ever received pentamidine isethionate either systemically or via aerosol? If yes, have any adverse events occurred?

B. Review the pulmonary system, noting:
   1. Past history of respiratory infections
   2. Past history of asthma, bronchitis, emphysema
   3. Current history of AIDS-related pulmonary malignancy or opportunistic infection
   4. Has the client been evaluated for pulmonary TB?
       a. Chest x-ray?
       b. Sputa for AFB?
   5. If the client has been diagnosed as having pulmonary TB, has sputum been examined for evaluation of treatment response?
   6. History of smoking including tobacco, marijuana, crack/cocaine

C. Review of metabolic system, including diabetes or hypoglycemia. This is a frequently encountered side effect of systemic pentamidine therapy, which is rarely seen in persons receiving aerosolized pentamidine; however, it has been reported.

D. Female clients:
   1. Are they currently or do they plan on becoming pregnant?
   2. Are they breast-feeding?

Modified from Ungvarski P: Nursing care of the client with infection due to *Pneumocystis carinii.* In Flaskerud J, Ungvarski P, editors: *HIV-AIDS: a guide to nursing care,* ed 2, appendix II, Philadelphia, 1992, WB Saunders; *Managing early HIV infection: quick reference guide,* USDHHS, AHCPR, Pub #94-0573, 1994, Rockville, Md.

II. **Equipment needed**
   A. Pentamidine isethionate, 300 mg
   B. One 10-ml vial of sterile water USP, for injection (preservative-free; do not use bacteriostatic sterile water)
   C. One 10-ml syringe with an 18-gauge needle
   D. Respirgard II nebulizer system
   E. Handheld micronebulizer
   F. Unit dose bronchodilator prescribed by client's physician
   G. Gas source (can use compressed air or oxygen, or a freestanding air compressor):
      1. If using compressed air or oxygen, a flow meter is required to adjust gas flow rate.
      2. If using a freestanding air compressor, select one with 40 to 50 pounds per square inch (PSI), a variable-pressure regulating knob, and a PSI gauge. In addition, a nipple adaptor and an in-line bacterial filter are needed to filter air going to the client's lungs.
   H. A cup of liquid (selected by client, either hot or cold) to be sipped during procedure to moisten upper airway
   I. Protective wear for the person administering the treatment

III. **Pretreatment teaching**
   A. Explain the procedure.
   B. Give breathing instructions:
      1. Breathe only through the mouth so that any exhaled drug or microorganisms will be trapped by the nebulizer's exhalation filter. Some clients may benefit from nose clips to prevent nasal breathing.
      2. Breathe at a normal rate, but take a deep breath at least once every minute by exhaling all the air from the lungs and then inhaling deeply to fill them. If possible, hold this breath for a few seconds before exhaling.
   C. When the client takes a break during the treatment, turn *off* the gas supply before removing the mouthpiece, to prevent environmental contamination and facial exposure to the drug. Encourage client to take deep breaths at the beginning of the break. Periodic breathing from residual volume may provide a more equal distribution of the aerosol to the lungs.
   D. Give positioning instructions
      1. Aerosol distribution in the lungs is more uniform when administered to clients lying in the supine position.
   E. Remind client to report any problems during the treatment.

IV. **Preparing the medication**
   A. Wash hands thoroughly.
   B. Reconstitute medication by injecting 6 ml of sterile water, USP, into the medication vial.

C. Shake well, until all particles are dissolved.

D. Withdraw all of the solution into the syringe.

V. **Preparing the nebulizer**

A. Assemble the nebulizer according to the packaged instructions.

B. Once assembled, inject the pentamidine solution into the nebulizer reservoir.

C. Attach the connecting tubing to the selected gas source:

1. For in-wall or compressed oxygen or air, set the flow rate between 5 and 9 L per min.

2. For a freestanding compressor, attach the nipple adaptor and in-line bacterial filter first (before attaching the connecting tubing); adjust the pressure setting to 22 to 25 PSI.

VI. **Administer the treatment**

A. Give mouth care to the client before the treatment.

B. Position the client in the supine position.

C. Take blood pressure, pulse, respirations, and auscultate breath sounds before treatment; record on client's record.

D. Before starting treatment, remind client to take rest periods. Be sure to turn off the gas source before removing mouthpiece.

E. Have client insert mouthpiece and then turn on gas source.

F. Auscultate breath sounds during procedure to detect rhonchi (wheezes) that may indicate ensuing bronchoconstriction. If wheezing is detected, turn off the gas source and administrate the bronchodilator ordered by the physician. Allow the client to rest briefly. If respiratory symptoms are not relieved, discontinue therapy and notify the physician.

G. If the client demonstrates symptoms of dyspnea, chest pain, or fever, discontinue the therapy and notify the physician.

H. Continue the therapy until the nebulizer's reservoir is dry (about 30 to 45 min).

I. Assess the client's response to treatment: take blood pressure, pulse, respirations, and auscultate breath sounds. Record findings on client's record.

J. Do not reuse the Respirgard II. The possibility of occluded jet orifices, sticking one-way valves, and the potential for bacterial growth do not justify reusing the system.

VII. **Adverse experiences**

A. Fatigue—can be minimized by scheduling therapy in the evening rather than at the beginning of the day.

B. Cough—can be minimized by having the client sip liquids during treatment. Antitussive agents may be of benefit.

C. Shortness of breath—can be minimized by taking rest periods during treatment.

D. Residual metallic taste—related to the drug. Encourage client to perform mouth care after as well as before the treatment. Hard candies (e.g., licorice, butterscotch flavors) or breath mints may help.

E. Decreased appetite—client may need nutritional supplements.

F. Dizziness or lightheadedness—often associated with deep, rapid breathing during the treatment. Encourage client to breathe normally and take rest periods.

G. Wheezing—may indicate bronchospasm and need for bronchodilator therapy.

H. Fever or rash—may indicate drug reaction. Stop treatment and notify physician.

References

Baskin M, Abd A, Ilowite J: Regional deposition of aerosolized pentamidine: effects of body position and breathing pattern, *Ann Intern Med* 113:677-683, 1990.

Centers for Disease Control: Guidelines for prophylaxis against *Pneumocystis carinii* pneumonia for persons with human immunodeficiency virus, *MMWR Morb Mortal Wkly Rep* 38(suppl 5):1-9, 1989.

Lindley D, Schleupner C: Aerosolized pentamidine and conjunctivitis, *Ann Intern Med* 109:988, 1988.

Lymphomed: *Nebu Pent* (pentamidine isethionate) (product monograph). Rosemont, Ill, 1989, Lymphomed.

Sarti G: Aerosolized pentamidine in HIV: promising new treatment for Pneumocystis carinii pneumonia, *Postgrad Med* 86(2):54-56, 59-60, 63, 1990.

Smith C: Nursing management of aerosolized pentamidine administration, *AIDS Patient Care* 4(1):13-17, 1990.

Guidelines—Infection Control for Home Health Care of Persons with AIDS and Other Infectious Diseases

The infection control guidelines for persons with acquired immune deficiency syndrome (AIDS) and their caregivers below are based on Centers for Disease Control (CDC) recommendations and epidemiological data. The guidelines have provided the basis for the infection control policy and procedures at the AIDS Home Care and Hospice Program in San Francisco.

Hand Washing

Hand washing is the single most important way to prevent the spread of an infectious organism. Soap and water should be used at all times. Hand washing should be done before and after all aspects of client care, including preparation and serving of meals to clients in their homes. If running water is not available, gloves should be worn. Hand washing is advised after removing and disposing of gloves.

Gloves

Gloves serve to block the transmission of any infectious agent to a potential host. The caregiver should wear gloves in the following situations:

- When caring for open skin lesions or wounds
- When handling secretions or excretions, such as emesis, urine, stool, blood, or wound secretions
- When handling soiled diapers, incontinence pads, linens, or clothing
- When providing oral care, if contact with oral lesions or blood is likely
- When providing perineal care to the person who is incontinent, or to a woman who is menstruating or who has postpartum bleeding

Gloves *are not required* when bathing AIDS clients without skin lesions, when assisting AIDS clients with transfers or ambulation, when feeding AIDS clients, or when talking with or counseling an AIDS client.

Protective Smocks

Protective smocks are not required for routine caregiving, but aprons or gowns may be used if soiling of the caregiver or his or her clothing is likely.

From Hughes A, Martin J, Franks P: *AIDS home care and hospice manual,* VNA of San Francisco, 1987, AIDS Home Care and Hospice Program.

Handling of Needles and Other Sharp Instruments

Needles, scalpels, and other sharp instruments must be handled with particular caution because the virus is capable of being transmitted through blood contact. *Needles should not be recapped* or resheathed after use but disposed of intact in a puncture-resistant container. These containers may be available through supply companies. Household metal tins or heavy plastic bottles may be substituted. To prevent injury, the container should be discarded and replaced when it is three-fourths filled.

Disposal of Supplies

Soiled disposable supplies used in the care of the person with AIDS (gloves, diapers, incontinence pads, toilet paper, dressing supplies, respiratory therapy tubing, or nebulizers) may be placed in a heavy-duty plastic bag that can be securely fastened at the top. If a heavy-duty plastic bag is not available, double bagging should be done. Removal of these plastic bags, as well as the sharps containers, should be in conformity with local solid waste disposal regulations used by the community. Usually this is the regular trash disposal system. The local public health department should be aware of these regulations and be able to assist in their interpretation and implementation.

Environmental Safety

Environmental safety is maintained by usual household cleaning methods. Standard household detergents are appropriate to maintain a safe environment for the person with AIDS and other members of his or her household.

For floor or counter surfaces soiled by secretions or excretions, removal of surface debris and cleansing with hot soapy water, followed by disinfecting with a 10% bleach solution (1 part bleach: 9 parts water) is adequate. The bleach solution also can be used to disinfect the toilet, tub, and shower after routine cleaning.

Bedpans and commodes should be cleaned regularly with household detergents and hot water. Soiled linens or clothing may be laundered in the household or laundromat washing machine. One cup of bleach along with the regular detergent should be added to water prior to placing clothes in the washer. (This procedure will help prevent discoloring of clothes.)

Items that are shared with other clients, such as toilets, showers, or bedpans, do not require different handling or cleansing. The cleaning procedures described earlier are sufficient: removing surface debris; cleaning with hot soapy water; and disinfecting with a 10%

bleach solution. This procedure should be done between clients if a client is incontinent, has diarrhea, or has open genital lesions.

The dishes of the person with AIDS can be cleaned with those of other household members using hot soapy water. Utensils do not need to be isolated.

Weekly cleaning of the interior surface of the refrigerator, as well as the bathroom fixtures (toilet, shower, and bathtub), will help to control the growth of molds or fungi. Routine household cleaning agents can be used.

Pets

Pets may pose a particular threat to the person with AIDS. Organisms sometimes present in the excrement of cats, birds, and fish may cause serious illness because the immune system of the person is compromised. As a result, for clients who wish to keep pets, someone other than the person with AIDS should be responsible for cleaning the bird cage, cat litter box, or fish tank.

Pregnant Caregivers and AIDS

Women who are pregnant or who may be pregnant should be excused from providing direct care to a person with AIDS. The rationale for this policy is that persons with AIDS are prone to two viruses— cytomegalovirus and herpesvirus—that have been known to cause serious birth defects and spontaneous abortions (miscarriages). Although the infection control guidelines discussed earlier would prevent caregivers from acquiring these infections if followed, the serious, harmful effects to the fetus of these viruses require particular caution. Further support for this position is found in the restriction of pregnant women from other potential occupational exposures, such as radiation therapy, that pose a threat to the fetus.

Durable Medical Equipment and AIDS

The management and cleaning of durable medical equipment (DME) is an issue of particular concern for home health care providers caring for persons with AIDS. The CDC has issued no specific guidelines for the provision or cleaning of DME used in the home of a person with AIDS. However, the CDC has recommended the use of a 10% bleach solution wipe down of *soiled* DME that cannot be sterilized by ethyl oxide or autoclaved. Most DME used at home for clients with AIDS (hospital beds, commodes, walkers, wheelchairs) cannot be autoclaved or sterilized.

San Francisco vendors who were surveyed reported that before DME is returned to the supplier, the DME is expected first to be cleaned by usual cleaning methods (using household detergents with hot water following the removal of any surface debris). The DME is then labeled "AIDS." The supplier disinfects it with a 10% bleach solution. After disinfection, the DME is returned to the inventory for general circulation—*its use is not restricted to AIDS clients.*

Dealing with Loss of Appetite, Nausea, and Vomiting in AIDS

Loss of appetite and nausea and vomiting are common symptoms of HIV infection, opportunistic infections, and treatment. There are a variety of ways to relieve nausea and vomiting and help increase appetite.

Loss of Appetite

Loss of appetite can be a serious problem; it can lead to malnutrition and severe weight loss. When your body is trying to fight infection, it needs nutrition. It needs enough protein and calories to function at its best, to give you energy, and to help reduce the effects of the disease and its treatment.

Eating enough of the right kinds of foods can be difficult when you don't feel like eating at all. Here are some tips to help you increase your appetite:

- Take a walk before mealtime. Mild exercise can stimulate your appetite.
- Avoid drinking liquids before a meal, because they can fill you up. If you want to drink, drink juices or milk—something nutritious.
- Eat with family or friends if possible. If eating is a social event, it will seem less of a chore.
- Eat a variety of foods. Spice up your food with herbs, spices, and sauces. Use butter, bacon bits, croutons, wine sauces, and marinades to provide taste-pleasing meals.
- Don't fill up on salads or "diet" foods. Eat vegetables and fruits along with meats, poultry, and fish to make sure you get enough calories and nutrition.
- Eat smaller meals more often, especially if you fill up before you've eaten all your meal.

If you still are not getting enough calories or protein, your health care provider may recommend dietary supplements that can be added to milk, soup, or pudding.

Nausea and Vomiting

Nausea and vomiting are common side effects of many treatments and infections. Doctors frequently prescribe an *antiemetic* to combat this. The antiemetic usually is given a few hours before the treatment and then every 3 or 4 hours after the treatment for a day or two. It may take some experimenting with dosage and timing to come up with the best schedule for you.

The following are other remedies and preventive measures you can try to help prevent or alleviate nausea and vomiting:

• Eat soda crackers and suck on sour candy balls throughout the day to relieve queasiness.
• Choose cold or room-temperature foods instead of hot ones; hot and warm foods seem to cause nausea.
• Avoid salty, fatty, and sweet foods or any food with strong odors—opt instead for bland, creamy foods, such as cottage cheese, toast, and mashed potatoes.
• Stay away from nauseating odors, sights, and sounds. Get as much fresh air as possible. A leisurely walk can help alleviate nausea.
• Don't eat right before your treatment. Eat lightly for a few hours after your treatment.
• Try relaxation therapy, self-hypnosis, or imagery to alleviate nausea-inducing tension.
• Distract yourself with a book, TV, or activity.
• Sleep during episodes of nausea if possible.

If vomiting does occur, eat or drink nothing until your stomach has settled, usually a few hours after the last vomiting episode. Then begin sipping clear liquids or sucking on ice cubes. If you tolerate the liquids, you may begin eating bland foods a few hours after you started the liquids.

Safety Tips for the Caregivers of Persons with Confusion or Impaired Judgment Associated with AIDS

The mental status of a person with HIV infection may change suddenly, leading the person to exhibit symptoms ranging from confusion and forgetfulness to severe dementia and psychosis.

The person who has confusion or impaired judgment may be unable to remember where dangers lie or to judge what is dangerous (steps, stoves, medications). Fatigue and inability to make the body do what one wants also can lead to injury. Therefore it is important that this person live in an environment that has been made as safe as possible. The following are some safety guidelines to use in your home:

- Keep clutter out of the hallway and off stairs or anywhere the person is likely to walk. Remove small rugs that could cause tripping.
- Remove breakables and dangerous objects (matches, knives, guns).
- Keep medications in a locked cabinet or drawer.
- Limit access to potentially dangerous areas (bathrooms, basement) by locking doors if the person tends to wander. Have the person wear an identification bracelet in case he or she wanders outside.
- Dress the person appropriately for the season.
- Put name labels in clothing. Make sure clothing is not too baggy and that shoes fit well and have nonskid soles.
- Keep the person's bed low. If he or she falls out, you may want to place the mattress on the floor or install side rails.
- Make sure rooms are well lit, especially in the evening. Night-lights can help prevent falls.
- Have someone stay with the person who is severely confused or agitated or place the person in a day care center.
- Encourage rest periods if the person tires easily.
- Keep exit doors locked. Consider some type of exit alarm, such as a bell attached to the door.
- Consider a mat alarm under a bedside rug to alert others of the person getting up during the night.

It is also helpful to do the following:

- Have the person rest frequently. Don't let the person get fatigued.
- Avoid crowded places, such as shopping malls and stadiums.
- Have someone with the person when he or she goes outdoors.
- Keep meal times quiet and calm.
- Limit the number of visitors.
- Have the person do one activity at a time.
- Keep activities simple—this will minimize fatigue.
- Plan activities ahead of time.
- Ensure that medications are taken as prescribed.
- Keep a calendar of activities visible on the wall. Cross off days as they pass.
- Maintain a photo album with labeled pictures of family members, friends, home, and so on.
- Include the person in family activities and conversations.
- Remember to treat the person with respect and maintain his or her privacy.
- Discuss all medication use with the health care provider.

Some things to avoid during periods of confusion include the following:

- Alcohol
- Contact sports
- Horseback riding
- Swimming
- Hunting
- Power tools or sharp implements
- Driving
- Riding recreational vehicles, such as bicycles, skateboards, motorcycles, or snowmobiles
- Cooking without supervision

Use of Antiretroviral Drugs

No drug cures infection with the human immunodeficiency virus (HIV). However, a number of drugs have been shown to reduce the rate at which HIV multiplies within the body. Each of these drugs seems to be reasonably effective for certain time periods. However, after some time passes, the drug seems to lose some or all of its ability to prevent multiplication of the virus. When this occurs, you may be switched to another antiretroviral drug or you may be given a second drug to take with the first drug. The length of time it takes for a drug to lose its potency varies with each person. For some this takes only a few months, whereas others obtain benefit from the same antiretroviral drug for years.

Because it is not clear why some people do well for only a short time and others do well for a long time, your response to the drugs will be watched closely. Your doctor will schedule you to return for examination and blood testing on a regular basis. It is important that you keep your medical appointments so that your doctor can determine if your drug therapy is working. If it is not, your physician will want to change drugs or add another drug to the one you are taking.

Antiretroviral drugs are powerful and may cause physical reactions, called side effects, even while they are doing their job of preventing HIV from multiplying. Some of the side effects are temporary and go away after a few weeks. Other side effects will continue as long as you take the drugs. Most of these side effects can be described as being uncomfortable or inconvenient but not harmful. Other side effects, however, may be permanently damaging or even life-threatening. Therefore, it is important that you learn what to expect when you take these drugs. You are the best judge of how you feel and what is happening to your body. The physicians and nurses caring for you need your assistance in watching for potentially harmful side effects. Therefore, the following guide has been prepared to help you understand and report your symptoms.

If You Are Taking AZT (Zidovudine)—Possible Side Effects: What You Should Do

Nausea or vomiting: usually disappears within 4 to 6 weeks of starting the drug. Report these symptoms to your health care provider if they last longer than this, cause you to lose weight, or return after being absent.

Headache: usually disappears within 4 to 6 weeks of starting the drug. Report this symptom to your health care provider if it persists past 6 weeks, does not respond to usual pain-relieving remedies, or returns after being absent.

Fatigue: usually disappears within 4 to 6 weeks. You can cope with it by reducing the amount you expect to accomplish and by getting plenty of rest. Report this symptom to your health care provider if fatigue persists past 6 weeks, returns after being absent, or interferes with your ability to live your life.

Muscle pain, severe upper abdominal pain, shortness of breath, unusual bleeding or bruising, sore throat, fever, injury that will not heal: these may indicate more serious reactions; report any of these symptoms to your health care provider.

If You Are Taking ddI (didanosine)—Possible Side Effects: What You Should Do

Diarrhea: a fairly common side effect; discuss remedies with your health care provider at the next visit. Report this symptom sooner if the diarrhea is severe, lasts for several days, or causes you to lose weight.

Upper abdominal pain, persistent nausea and vomiting; pain, tingling, or numbness in your hands or feet; convulsions; shortness of breath; mental confusion; unusual bleeding or bruising: report these symptoms to your health care provider as soon as possible.

If You Are Taking ddC (zalcitabine)—Possible Side Effects: What You Should Do

Canker sores in mouth; rashes and itching skin: see your dentist; avoid using soaps or powders that may further dry or irritate the skin; use lotions to moisturize the skin. Report these symptoms to your health care provider if they persist.

Upper abdominal pain; persistent nausea and vomiting; pain, tingling, or numbness in your hands or feet; convulsions; shortness of breath; mental confusion; unusual bleeding or bruising: report these symptoms to your health care provider as soon as possible.

Other Reactions While Taking Antiretrovirals

All three of these drugs may cause side effects that are not listed here in some people, because individuals respond differently to different drugs. In addition, unusual symptoms may be related to other infections and not to the drugs that you are taking. Symptoms that are disabling or that interfere with your ability to live a reasonably normal life should be reported to your health care provider as soon as possible. Also, symptoms that involve pain, weakness, unusual weight loss, or bleeding should be reported soon. Problems that are merely annoying can usually wait until the next scheduled visit.

Diagnosis of Infection in HIV-Exposed Infants

Age	Test	If test is positive	If test is negative
1 month	HIV culture or PCR[1]	Repeat test to confirm diagnosis of infection	Repeat test at age 3 to 6 months
3 to 6 months	HIV culture or PCR[1]	Repeat test to confirm diagnosis of infection	Test with ELISA at age 15 months
15 months	ELISA	Repeat test at age 18 months	Repeat test at age 18 months
18 months or older	ELISA	Child is infected[2]	Child is not infected[3]

[1]If HIV culture and PCR are unavailable, p24 antigen testing may be used after 1 month of age.
[2]Serological diagnosis of HIV infection requires two sets of confirmed HIV serologic assays (ELISA/Western blot) performed at least 1 month apart after 15 months of age.
[3]Confirmation of seronegativity requires two sets of negative ELISAs after 15 months of age in a child with normal clinical and immunoglobulin evalation.
NOTE: This chart presents recommendations only for the items reviewed by the HIV panel.

HIV-Associated Conditions
in Pediatric HIV Infection

Failure to thrive
Generalized lymphadenopathy
Hepatomegaly
Splenomegaly
Persistent oral candidiasis
Parotitis
Recurrent or chronic diarrhea
Encephalopathy
Lymphoid interstitial pneumonitis (LIP)
Hepatitis
Cardiomyopathy
Nephropathy
Recurrent bacterial infections
Opportunistic infections (recurrent viral infections [herpes simplex, herpes zoster], fungal, parasitic)
Malignancies (lymphoma)

From *Managing early HIV infection: quick reference guide,* USDHHS, AHCPR, Pub. #94-0573, 1994, Rockville, Md.

Testing and Preventive Therapy
for Tuberculosis Infection

The reemergence of tuberculosis (TB) as a major public health concern is especially important for HIV-infected individuals because the immunosuppression caused by the virus permits *Mycobacterium tuberculosis* infection to progress at an accelerated pace, and they are more likely to develop active TB. TB merits special consideration in the treatment of HIV-infected clients because it is readily communicable to others, management is different for HIV-infected clients than for non–HIV-infected clients, and, unlike many other opportunistic infections, it is preventable and may be curable if treated promptly.

Screening

- The medical history for all HIV-infected individuals should include the following steps: (a) assessment of previous TB infection or disease, past treatment or preventive therapy, and history of exposure to *M. tuberculosis;* (b) assessment of the risk

---

From *Managing early HIV infection: quick reference guide,* USDHHS, AHCPR, Pub. #94-0573, 1994, Rockville, Md.

for *M. tuberculosis* infection, including predisposing social conditions (e.g., household contacts, country of origin, homelessness, history of incarceration, residence in a congregate living situation); and (c) suggestive symptoms (e.g., cough, hemoptysis, fever, night sweats, weight loss). During the physical examination, the provider should seek indications of active disease (e.g., abnormal pulmonary signs, documented weight loss).

- The medical history for all HIV-infected individuals should also include an assessment of health and social conditions that may affect an individual's ability to complete a course of therapy, specifically, repeated failure to keep medical appointments, alcoholism, mental illness, and substance use.

- All HIV-infected individuals, including those who have received BCG vaccination, should be screened, using purified protein derivative (PPD) for infection with *M. tuberculosis* during their initial evaluation.

- All HIV-infected individuals should be screened for anergy using two control antigens in addition to PPD during their initial evaluation.

- All HIV-infected individuals who are PPD-positive or anergic should receive a chest x-ray and clinical evaluation, and those who have symptoms suggestive of TB should receive a chest x-ray, regardless of their PPD or anergy status.

- PPD and anergy testing should be repeated annually in persons who are neither PPD-positive nor anergic on initial evaluation. Persons who reside in areas where TB prevalence is high should be tested every 6 months.

- All PPD-negative or anergic HIV-infected individuals who have recently been exposed to persons with suspected or confirmed TB should be immediately tested with PPD and anergy antigens. Repeat testing should be performed in 3 months.

- PPD testing should be performed by the Mantoux method, using an intradermal injection of 0.1 ml 5 TU PPD (intermediate strength).

- Reactions should be assessed by a trained observer between 48 and 72 hours after injection. Reactions of 5 mm or greater induration should be considered positive in persons with HIV infection, regardless of prior BCG vaccination.

- Two of the following three antigens can be used for anergy testing: candida, mumps, or tetanus toxoid. Any degree of induration observed in response to intradermal injection of these antigens constitutes a positive reaction and indicates that the individual is not anergic.

- Chest x-rays should be obtained to exclude the presence of active pulmonary TB in all HIV-infected individuals who are PPD-positive, anergic, or have symptoms suggestive of TB.
- If the chest x-ray reveals any abnormality, multiple sputum smears and cultures should be performed.
- If a sputum smear is positive, the client should be started on anti-TB therapy immediately, pending culture results. Acid-fast bacillus (AFB) isolation should be initiated promptly if the client is coughing. If the sputum smears are negative and if there is no other etiology for the abnormal chest x-ray, bronchoscopy should be performed and empiric anti-TB therapy should be initiated, pending the results of the mycobacterial culture. AFB isolation should be maintained until the diagnosis is confirmed by smear or culture.
- In many of these clinical situations, diagnostic evaluation and management will need to be individualized. Consultation with an infectious disease or pulmonary specialist may be necessary.

Preventive Therapy

- Preventive therapy for TB should proceed according to the following protocol: (1) isoniazid (INH) preventive therapy should be initiated and continued for 12 months in all HIV-infected individuals who have a positive PPD test but do not have active disease, regardless of their age; (2) preventive therapy should be strongly considered for anergic clients who are known contacts of clients with TB and for anergic clients belonging to groups in which the prevalence of TB infection is 10% or higher. Such individuals include injection drug users, prisoners, homeless persons, persons living in congregate housing, migrant laborers, and persons born in countries where rates of TB are high.
- Clinicians should consider factors specific to their geographic areas, including the incidence and prevalence of TB infection, when considering the decision to start preventive therapy.
- In persons with HIV who are exposed to drug-resistant strains of *M. tuberculosis,* an alternative preventive therapy should be considered. Consultation should be sought with a pulmonary or infectious disease specialist.
- The presence of AFB on sputum smear should prompt immediate empiric anti-TB therapy tailored to community drug-susceptibility patterns, pending final determination of drug-susceptibility testing.

◊ Special Training

Bowel and Bladder Training

Bowel and bladder training refers to a program to assist in controlling urinary and bowel elimination. Urinary or bowel incontinence may be a result of decreased cerebral function, such as lack of awareness, medications, lack of control over sphincter muscle, trauma, surgical procedures, and medical disorders. The training program focuses on stool evacuation and bladder emptying at set times that are as close to the usual elimination patterns as possible.

Interventions
Bowel elimination

1. Assess bowel patterns for usual habits, stool characteristics, and frequency of incontinence.
2. Establish time for daily defecation, preferably 30 minutes to 1 hour after meal.
3. Inform client of need for 2 to 3 L of fluids per day if permitted.
4. Encourage bowel movement at regular times by offering warm fluids, abdominal massage, and digital stimulation of anal area; allow 1 hour for defecation.
5. Administer enema at regular times to empty bowel until next scheduled defecation; suppositories may also be used.
6. Tell client to avoid foods that produce gas and foods that might produce diarrhea and stool incontinence.
7. Encourage a routine time each day for bowel elimination; provide bathroom facilities, bedpan, or commode at that time.
8. Revise training program if it is not successful; report failure to achieve goals.

Bladder elimination

1. Assess urinary patterns for usual habits, characteristics, and frequency of incontinence.
2. Establish schedule for micturition; allow specific amounts of fluid during and between meals.
3. Restrict fluid intake after 9 PM or after retiring.
4. Schedule voiding every 2 hours during the day and every 4 hours during the night; extend periods of time between voidings when continence is established.

From Jaffe M, Skidmore-Roth L: *Home health nursing care plans,* ed 2, St Louis, 1995, Mosby.

5. Tell client to avoid drinks containing caffeine and diuretics.
6. Monitor intake and output ratio.
7. Palpate for bladder distention that may cause incontinence.
8. Advise client to strengthen perineal muscles with Kegel exercises, tensing muscles by pressing buttocks together and holding for 3 to 5 minutes and repeat 10 times per hour; answer a call to void immediately.
9. Catheterize if program is unsuccessful; revise training program.

Fecal Impaction

When an impaction is present, the fecal mass may be too large or hard to be passed voluntarily. Suppositories and enemas may be ordered to promote evacuation of stool. However, if the enema fails to promote defecation, the nurse must use the fingers to break up and remove the fecal mass. This procedure can be uncomfortable and embarrassing for the client. Excessive rectal manipulation may cause irritation to the mucosa, bleeding, and stimulation of the vagus nerve, which can cause a reflex slowing of the heart rate.

1. Assemble supplies needed before beginning procedure:
   a. Disposable gloves
   b. Water-soluble lubricant
   c. Waterproof absorbent pad
   d. Bedpan
   e. Bedpan cover
   f. Bath blanket or cotton blanket
   g. Face cloth, towel, basin
2. Explain procedure to client. Indicate that manipulation of rectum can cause discomfort.
3. Wash hands.
4. Obtain assistance to help change client's position, if necessary. Assist client to left side-lying position with knees flexed.
5. Provide for privacy: close door to room, drape bath blanket over client so client is minimally exposed.
6. Drape client's trunk and lower extremities with bath blanket.
7. Place waterproof pad under buttocks.
8. Place bedpan next to client.
9. Don disposable gloves.
10. Lubricate glove's index finger with lubricating jelly.
11. Insert index finger into rectum and advance finger slowly along rectal wall toward umbilicus.

Modified from Perry AG, Potter PA: *Clinical nursing skills and techniques,* ed 2, St Louis, 1990, Mosby.

12. Gently loosen fecal mass by massaging around it. Work finger into hardened mass.
13. Work stool downward toward end of rectum. Remove small sections of feces.
14. Periodically assess heart rate and look for signs of fatigue. Stop procedure if heart rate drops or rhythm changes.
15. Continue to clear rectum of feces and allow client to rest at intervals.
16. After disimpaction, provide washcloth and towel to wash buttocks and anal area.
17. Remove bedpan and dispose of feces. Remove gloves by turning inside out and discarding in proper receptacle.
18. Assist client to toilet or clean bedpan.
19. Wash hands. (Procedure may be followed by enema or cathartic.)
20. Perform rectal examination for stool.
21. Reassess vital signs and compare to baseline values.
22. Assess bowel sounds.
23. Abdomen is soft and nontender.

Expected Outcomes

1. Impacted stool is successfully removed.
2. Client is able to subsequently evacuate stool voluntarily.
3. Vital signs remain normal.

Special Considerations

- Some allow only physician to perform this procedure. Check policy manuals.
- Physician may order oil-retention enema several hours before this procedure to soften stool for easier extraction.
- Physician may order analgesic to be administered before procedure.
- Physician may order procedure to be followed by administration of cleansing enema or cathartics.
- If constipation and subsequent impaction is diet related, teach client about high-fiber nutritional products to increase bulk.
- If necessary, teach ancillary caregivers about the effects of immobility, hydration, nutrition on normal bowel elimination.

Ostomy Care

Equipment

1. Ostomy appliance
2. Protective cover
3. Plastic bag or Chux
4. Soap and warm water, basin, washcloth, and towels
5. Disposable nonsterile gloves

Procedure

1. Explain the procedure to the client/caregiver.
2. Assemble the equipment at a convenient work area.
3. Place the client in a comfortable position with the abdominal area exposed.
4. Place a plastic bag or Chux under the client if he or she is bed-bound.
5. Remove the appliance and discard it.
6. Cleanse peristomal area with soap and water. Use a spiral pattern at the stoma site, and work outward. Rinse, and pat dry.
7. Examine the stoma for integrity versus any signs of necrosis or infection. Report any abnormal findings to the physician.
8. Position the appliance to fit well around the stoma. (The appliance will depend on the type of stoma.)
9. Provide client comfort measures.
10. Clean and replace the equipment. Discard disposable items in a plastic trash bag, and secure.

Nursing Considerations

Consider referral to the enterostomal therapist to establish stoma and peristomal care regimen.

Documentation Guidelines

Document the following on the visit report:

- The procedure and client toleration
- Color, shape, and size of stoma
- Type of stoma
- Condition of the surrounding skin
- Function, character, and amount of drainage

From Rice R: *Handbook of home health nursing procedures,* St Louis, 1994, Mosby.

- Any client/caregiver instructions and compliance with the proce dure, including the client's reaction to and ability to perform ostomy care
- Other pertinent findings

Update the client care plan.

Contraindications to Colostomy Irrigation

- Ascending colostomies
- Temporary colostomies
- Disease in remaining colon (diverticulosis, inflammatory disease)
- Infant or child
- Physical limitations (arthritis, paralysis)
- Mental limitations (confusion, dementia, retardation)
- Inadequate sanitary facilities
- Stomal abnormalities (prolapse, hernia)

From Potter A, Perry A: *Fundamentals of nursing: concepts, process, and practice,* ed 3, St Louis, 1993, Mosby.

Pouching an Enterostomy

Assessment

1. Observe pouch for leakage and length of time in place; observe stoma for color and healing; observe abdominal incision (if present) for relationship to stoma for proper placement of pouch. Observe drainage from stoma and keep a record of intake and output. Ask client about skin tenderness.
2. Assess abdomen for best type of pouch to use:
   a. Contour
   b. Presence of scars, incisions
   c. Location of stoma
3. After pouch removal, assess skin around stoma, noting scars, folds, skin breakdown, and peristomal suture line if present.
4. Auscultate for bowel sounds.
5. Determine client's emotional response and knowledge and understanding of ostomy.

From Potter A, Perry A: *Fundamentals of nursing: concepts, process, and practice,* ed 3, St Louis, 1993, Mosby.

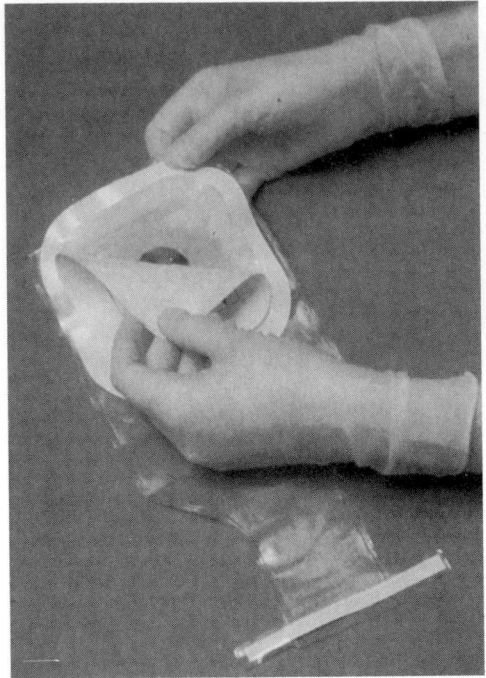

Fig. 52

Implementation

1. Position client supine or standing and drape.
2. Prepare pouch by removing backing from barrier and adhesive. If using cut-to-fit pouch, cut opening $\frac{1}{16}$ to $\frac{1}{8}$ inch larger than stoma before removing backing (Fig. 52). With ileostomy, apply thin circle of barrier paste around opening in pouch; allow to dry.
3. Wash hands and don gloves.
4. Place towel or disposable waterproof barrier under the client.
5. Remove used pouch gently by pushing the skin away from the barrier.
6. Cleanse peristomal skin gently with warm tap water using gauze pads or clean washcloth; do not scrub the skin; dry completely by patting the skin with gauze or towel or use cool setting on handheld blow dryer. Measure the stoma (see 5 above).
7. Apply the pouch:
   a. If there are creases next to stoma, use barrier paste to fill in; let dry 1 to 2 minutes.
   b. Hold pouch by barrier, center over stoma, and press down gently on barrier; bottom of pouch should point toward client's knees.

c. Use skin sealant wipes on skin directly under adhesive; allow to dry. Press the adhesive smoothly against the skin, starting from the bottom and working up and around the sides.

d. Maintain gentle finger pressure around the barrier for 1 to 2 minutes.

e. If using a two-piece pouch, apply flange (barrier with adhesive) as in steps 10a through c. Then snap on pouch and maintain finger pressure.

8. Fold bottom of the pouch up once and apply clamp (or follow instructions for closure).

9. Properly dispose of old pouch and soiled equipment.

10. Remove gloves and wash hands.

11. Change pouch every 3 to 7 days unless leaking; pouch can remain in place for tub bath or shower; after bath, pat adhesive dry or use handheld dryer set on cool.

Evaluation

1. Note appearance of stoma around skin and existing incision (if present) while pouch is removed and skin is cleansed. Reinspect condition of skin barrier and adhesive.

2. Ask if client feels discomfort around stoma.

3. Observe client's nonverbal behaviors as pouch is applied. Ask if client has any questions about pouching.

4. Auscultate bowel sounds and observe characteristics of stool.

Expected outcomes are based on goals of care:

- Client denies discomfort.
- Stoma is functioning with moderate amount of liquid or soft stool and flatus in pouch. (Flatus is noted by bulging of pouch in absence of drainage.)
- Client observes stoma and steps of procedure carefully.
- Ostomy is moist and reddish-pink. Skin is intact and free of irritation; sutures are intact.
- Client asks questions about procedure and may attempt to assist with pouch change.

Unexpected outcomes that may occur include:

- Skin around stoma is irritated, has burning sensation. Mucosal layer of stoma separates from skin.
- Necrotic stoma is manifested by purple or black color, dry instead of moist texture, failure to bleed when washed gently, tissue sloughs.
- Client complains of irritation and burning around stoma.
- Client refuses to view stoma or participate in care.

PART SIX
TEACHING TOOLS

◆ Anticipatory Guidance

Preventing Respiratory Infections

Respiratory infections can be a serious complication for anyone with a chronic lung disease. Unfortunately, people with chronic lung diseases are more susceptible to respiratory infections; even an ordinary cold that causes only sniffles in someone else can turn into pneumonia. Because of this, clients must make every effort to prevent infection. The client must also learn the early danger signs and the importance of seeing a doctor at once when any symptoms appear. Some specific guidelines for clients follow.

Preventing Infection

Follow your doctor's orders. Take your medications exactly as ordered. Perform chest physiotherapy as directed. If oxygen therapy is prescribed, take it as ordered.

Take care of yourself every day. Drink at least six glasses of water daily (unless your doctor tells you differently). Eat a nutritious, well-balanced diet. Sleep 7 or 8 hours every night. Take several short rests during the day. Learn to conserve your energy and avoid getting too tired.

Stay away from people who have colds and flu, if at all possible. If this can't be avoided, wear a disposable mask (available at medical supply companies and many grocery stores) when around people with colds or flu.

Avoid air pollution, including tobacco smoke, wood or oil smoke, car exhaust, and industrial pollution.

Take special precautions with your personal hygiene. Wash your hands before taking your medication or handling your oxygen equipment. Wash your hands after handling soiled tissues and

From *Mosby's patient teaching guides,* St Louis, 1995, Mosby.

before and after using the bathroom. Always rinse your oral inhaler after each use.

Ask your doctor about flu vaccines.

Detecting Infections

Symptoms of respiratory infections can appear suddenly and worsen quickly. When an infection develops, it's important to start treatment right away. Your doctor may decide to prescribe antibiotics or other drugs to get the infection under control before it becomes serious. (**Don't try to treat yourself.** Over-the-counter cold remedies may worsen the problem, so don't use them unless your doctor tells you it's okay.) Call your doctor immediately if any of these signs occur:

Fever

Increased coughing, wheezing, or trouble breathing

Mucus changes in any of these ways: the mucus is thicker; the amount is either more or less than usual; it has a foul odor; or the color is green, yellow, brown, pink, or red

Stuffy nose, sneezing, or sore throat

Increased fatigue or weakness

Weight gain or loss of more than 5 pounds within a week

Swollen ankles or feet

Confusion, memory loss, or persistent drowsiness

Infection Control

Infection occurs as a result of transmission of an infectious agent to a susceptible host. Home health nurses must keep in mind that an infected individual will not necessarily show signs or symptoms of the infection but may nonetheless be capable of infecting others. Below are common signs and symptoms of infection.

Signs and Symptoms of Infection
Inflammatory response

- Redness
- Heat
- Swelling
- Pain

Other possible signs and symptoms

- Sore throat, cough
- Sputum production, change in color or amount of sputum
- Elevated temperature

From *Mosby's home health nursing pocket consultant,* St Louis, 1995, Mosby.

- Tachycardia, tachypnea
- Rash, dermatitis of the skin
- Loose stool, diarrhea
- Nausea, vomiting
- Weight loss (inappropriate)
- Green or yellow exudates or drainage from the wound bed
- Burning or painful urination

Understanding mechanisms of transmission provides insight into the management of communicable diseases. The following procedures will reduce the transmission of communicable disease:

- The infectious agent is eradicated by a method of disinfection/ sterilization.
- The infectious agent is prevented from entering the host (actual or potential).
- Prevalence of the infectious agent is reduced by enhancing host response by means of antibiotic administration or immunizations.
- The infectious agent's reservoir is neutralized.

These procedures, along with a philosophy that all clients should be treated as though they have an infectious disease, form the basis for infection control guidelines recommended by the Centers for Disease Control (CDC).

Universal Precautions

Universal precautions are those actions taken to prevent transmission of microorganisms from one person to another. They include care of hands, care of inanimate objects or articles used, and use of barriers and techniques to protect against transmission to client or caregiver.

Since a health history and physical assessment cannot reliably identify all clients who have a communicable disease, the CDC and Occupational Safety and Health Administration (OSHA) recommend that universal blood and body fluid precautions be followed with all clients. All health care workers should wear gloves when touching mucous membrane or nonintact skin of all clients (e.g., wound care, suctioning care). Masks, goggles, and gowns should be worn if aerosolization or splashes are likely to occur.

Provision of care

- Routine precautions should be taken when there is any possibility of exposure to blood or body fluids of any client (wound care, suctioning, any care involving body orifices or injections). Aprons or gowns are required for procedures involving extensive contact with blood or body fluids. Gloves are required when handling items soiled with blood or body fluids (soiled linens, dressings, catheter/enema equipment).

- Immediately after contact with blood or body fluids all contaminated skin surfaces should be washed completely. Hands should be washed with soap and water immediately after gloves are removed. Wearing gloves does not eliminate the necessity for hand washing after each client contact. Do not reuse disposable gloves. Gloves should be changed between contact with clients to prevent cross-contamination. General utility gloves should not be worn if they are peeling, cracked, or discolored, as this is evidence of deterioration.
- All health care workers who perform or assist in invasive procedures must use extraordinary care to prevent injuries caused by needles, glucose monitoring lancets, and other sharp instruments or devices. After use, disposable syringes, needles, and other sharp items should be placed in a puncture-resistant container for disposal. To prevent needlestick injuries, needles should not be recapped, purposely bent or broken, removed from disposable syringes, or otherwise bent by hand.
- Although saliva has not been implicated in HIV transmission, mouthpieces or other ventilation devices should be available for employees to minimize the risk involved in emergency mouth-to-mouth resuscitation.
- Health care workers who have exudative lesions, weeping dermatitis, or breaks in the skin should wear gloves when doing any procedural treatment for the client or family.

Disinfection (at the home health agency)

- Wash all equipment thoroughly with soap and water, rinse, and dry.
- Always read the label of the disinfectant and follow directions. After washing equipment with soap and water, disinfect, rinse, and dry. According to OSHA, after initial cleanup one of the following disinfectants should be used for cleaning equipment exposed to blood or body substances:
  - Chemical germicides that are approved for use as hospital disinfectants and are tuberculocidal when used at recommended dilutions
  - Products registered by the Environmental Protection Agency (EPA) as being effective against HIV with an accepted "HIV (AIDS Virus)" label
  - A solution of 5.25% sodium hypochlorite (household bleach) diluted between 1:10 and 1:100 with water; mix a fresh supply of bleach every day for effective disinfection
- *Remember:* Disinfectants are designed for inanimate objects and are

damaging to the skin. Wear gloves to protect the hands and goggles if there is a possibility of splashes to the eye. Disinfectants should be used in a well-ventilated room. If possible, totally submerge contaminated articles in the disinfecting solution for the required period of time.

- Since most durable medical equipment (DME) used in the home cannot be autoclaved, disinfection is recommended. Submerge or wipe down DME with soap and water and disinfect. Remember, bleach is caustic to metal.

Disposal techniques for waste: environmental considerations

- Sharps: Injection needles with syringes, glucometer lancets, vacutainer needles, etc., should be contained in a puncture-resistant container marked with the biohazard symbol and sealed to prevent leakage.
- Blood, body fluids, and secretions generated by clients in their own homes may be disposed of via the sanitary sewer.
- All antineoplastic chemotherapeutic wastes are considered a hazardous waste by most health departments and must be neutralized by dilution. Review regulations with local health departments and the EPA.

Special Precautions in Home Care

These guidelines are based on practical adaptations of universal/body substance isolation (BSI) precautions for home health nurses and may be individualized to meet specific client needs.

Provision of care for clients with communicable diseases

- Explain all procedures and their rationale to clients. Respect clients' rights to privacy and confidentiality.
- Wash hands with soap and water before and after client care and during care if soiled.
- Wear gloves on both hands whenever there is any possibility of contact with blood or body substances (oral or body secretions, feces, urine, vomitus, tissues, wound or other drainage). Change gloves between procedures as appropriate.
- Wear a mask if clients are coughing productively or when suctioning. Masks may be worn if the client has active TB, influenza, mumps, measles, chickenpox, or pertussis.
- Routinely wipe down the bell/diaphragm of the stethoscope with an alcohol prep-pad between clients.
- Do not recap used syringes/needles; place them in a puncture-resistant container for storage.

- Wipe down blood specimen tubes with a 10% bleach solution, if possible; otherwise, use an alcohol prep-pad. Label tube "blood precautions" and store in a sealed plastic bag for laboratory delivery.
- Do not replace any contaminated equipment in the nursing bag until it has been disinfected.

Guidelines for Preventing and Controlling Nosocomial Infections

Control of External Environment (Exogenous Sources of Infection)
Health care providers
1. In good health—do not care for clients when ill
2. Keep immunizations current
3. Practice effective hand washing between each client
   If skin dry, rough, or broken, seek appropriate attention
   If active herpes simplex infection of hand (herpetic whitlow), do not give direct client care until lesion healed
4. Wear gloves when contact with any body substance is anticipated

Housekeeping and sanitation
1. Bed linens not shaken in air or thrown on floor
2. Proper disposal of wastes—solid and liquid
3. Proper cleaning and sterilization of contaminated articles
4. Proper ventilation for adequate air exchanges
   Modern hospitals—clients' room air is under negative pressure
   Negative pressure keeps air from clients' rooms from moving into hallways
5. Proper mopping and damp dusting to remove dust and other environmental reservoirs of infection

Control of Internal Environment (Endogenous Sources of Infection)
1. Preventive measures aimed at increasing client's defense mechanisms and thus reducing risk of infection
   Teach client about good nutrition
   Teach client about personal hygiene, especially hand washing

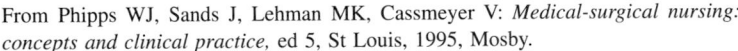
From Phipps WJ, Sands J, Lehman MK, Cassmeyer V: *Medical-surgical nursing: concepts and clinical practice,* ed 5, St Louis, 1995, Mosby.

2. Be aware that normal flora of client can be disrupted when client
   is receiving antibiotics or chemotherapy and colonization may
   occur
   >Give antibiotics on time as scheduled
   >Teach client about appropriate use of antibiotics and dangers
   >of taking them when not prescribed by physician

Notes

Insulin Adjustment During Jet Travel across Multiple Time Zones

Daily insulin regimen	Day of departure	First morning at destination	10 hours after morning dose	Second day at destination
Eastbound				
Single-dose schedule	Usual dose	2/3 usual dose	Remaining 1/3 AM dose if blood sugar over 240	Usual dose
Two-dose schedule	Usual morning and evening doses	2/3 usual morning dose	Usual evening dose plus remaining 1/3 of AM dose if blood sugar over 240	Usual two doses

Daily insulin regimen	Day of departure	18 hours after departure	First day at destination	
Westbound				
Single-dose schedule	Usual dose	1/3 usual dose followed by snack if blood sugar over 240	Usual dose	
Two-dose schedule	Usual morning and evening doses	1/3 usual AM dose followed by snack if blood sugar over 240	Usual two doses	

Reprinted with permission from Edward A. Benson, MD (Virginia Mason Clinic—Seattle, Wash).

A Guide for the Nurse to Assist Clients in Taking Medications at Home

The following categories have been identified as areas in which clients may need support in taking medications at home. Strategies are to be used by the nurse.

Problem category	Strategy
Understanding schedule and route	Provide adequate oral explanation.
	Give simple written instructions.
	Suggest using a daily tear-off calendar for once-a-day medication, tearing off page when medication is taken.
	Use larger calendar for multiple medications, placing a check mark in the dated square after taking each medication.
	Put each medication in a transparent envelope and attach to dated squares. Write name of medicine, time, and dose to be taken on that day.
	Obtain a commercial drug caddy for client for multiple medication needs for a day or week (or use an egg carton).
	Seek or write simple pamphlets and booklets in appropriate language, i.e., English, Spanish. Take into account age, sight, and memory changes of ill clients.
	Use simple audio-visual aids for teaching. Take into home to teach; i.e., questions to ask about medication, medication effects, and proper medication taking.
Opening the bottle	Request pharmacists to place medications in screw- or flip-top container rather than "child-proof" container.
Reading the label	Ask pharmacist to place medications in over-sized bottle and prepare label with large print.
	Ask pharmacist to write directions in simple terms and appropriate language, i.e., English, Spanish, etc.
	Devise a color code for multiple medications and include the color key to be kept with medications.
	For visually impaired, seek braille labels for clients.

Modified from Ebersole P, Hess P: *Toward healthy aging,* ed 3, St Louis, 1990, Mosby.

Continued.

A Guide for the Nurse to Assist Clients in Taking Medications at Home—cont'd

Problem category	Strategy
Taking too much or too little	Adjust medication schedule to life pattern and habits of client.
	Ask physician to give medication dosages which can be taken at morning and bedtime (2× daily).
	Ask physician to give multiple medications, all of which can be taken at the same times each day.
	Check with physician and pharmacist about compatibility of these multiple drugs and potential drug interactions.
	Monitor effects of medication and ask physician to discontinue medicine as soon as possible if client not compliant.
Difficulty swallowing medications	Ask if medication comes in liquid form and change from tablets/capsules.
	Teach client to put *tablet* on *back* of tongue and take with liquid.
	Teach client to put *capsule* on *front* of tongue and take with liquid.
	Teach client to *avoid* crushing coated, plastic metric, and layered tablets.

◊ Therapeutic Interventions

Breathing Exercises to Relieve Dyspnea

The feeling of not being able to get enough air into your lungs is frightening. Shortness of breath or difficulty breathing—called dyspnea—is a problem for people with chronic lung diseases. However, there are several things clients can do to help themselves breathe more easily. Some suggested client guidelines follow.

Avoiding Trouble

Breathing pollutants can aggravate dyspnea. Avoid heavy traffic and smog as much as possible. Don't use aerosol sprays. Stay away from products that produce fumes, such as paint, kerosene, and cleaning agents.

Cold weather can trigger dyspnea. If you must go outside when it's cold, cover your mouth with a scarf or mask.

Very dry air increases dyspnea and thickens the mucus in your lungs. A portable room humidifier is helpful, especially in the winter.

Physical exertion brings on dyspnea. Learn to conserve your energy by resting frequently, alternating light and heavy tasks, and minimizing movement. Instead of standing, sit. Instead of pushing or lifting objects, pull. Be creative in managing tasks—for example, a cart or child's wagon can be used to haul groceries, and wheels can be installed on furniture that is frequently moved.

Breathing Exercises

There are two simple exercises that can help you breathe more easily. You can do pursed lip breathing anywhere. With abdominal breathing, you will need to lie down. Practice them daily so when you are having problems with dyspnea, you will immediately know what to do.

Pursed lip breathing

Pursed lip breathing will help get rid of the stale air trapped inside the lungs. It will slow down your breathing so it is more efficient. (Breathing fast only makes the dyspnea worse.)

1. Breathe in slowly through your nose. Hold your breath for three seconds (count to yourself by saying one 100, two 100, three 100). Be sure to breathe through your nose to avoid gulping air.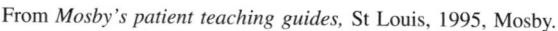
2. Purse your lips as if you were going to whistle or give someone a kiss.

From *Mosby's patient teaching guides*, St Louis, 1995, Mosby.

3. Breathe out slowly through your pursed lips for 6 seconds (count one 100, two 100, three 100, four 100, five 100, six 100.) The sound you make breathing out will be like a soft whistle.

Abdominal breathing

Abdominal breathing will also slow down your breathing to make it more effective. It also helps relax your entire body and is a wonderful technique to use before you go to sleep.

1. Lie on your back in a comfortable position with a pillow under your head. Place another pillow under your knees to help relax your abdomen.

2. Rest one hand on your abdomen just below your rib cage. Rest the other hand on your chest.

3. Slowly breathe in and out through your nose using your abdominal muscles. The hand resting on your abdomen will rise when you breathe in, and it will fall when you breathe out. The hand and the chest should be almost still.

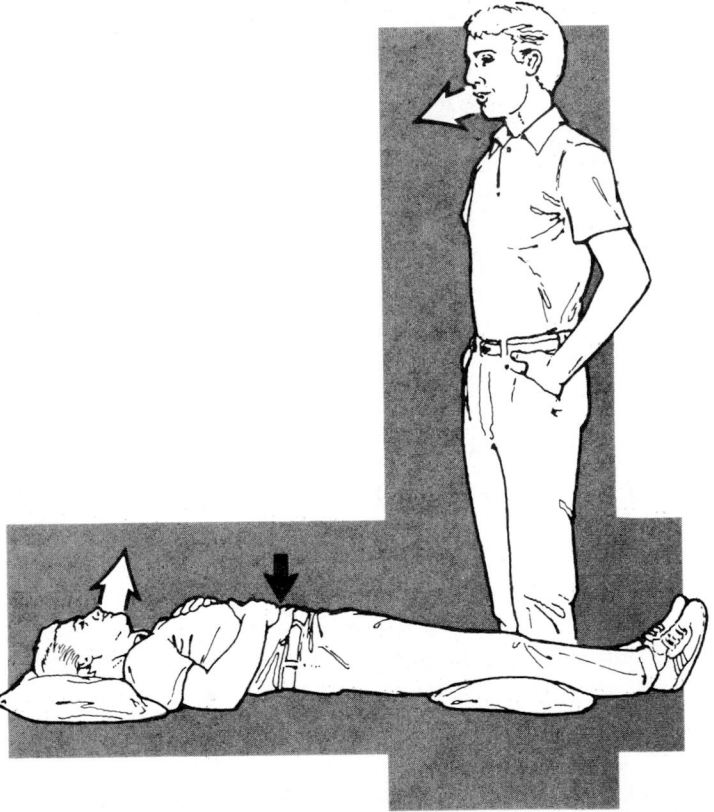

Aerosol Therapy (Nebulizer)

Client Teaching Information

Take your treatment for _____ minutes or until medication is gone.

Do not overuse. If you feel you need the treatment more often than ordered, be sure to call your doctor.

Instruct clients to follow these simple steps

1. Sit up straight in a chair that will give back support.
2. Make sure the equipment is clean, dry, and located at table height.
3. Put the medication in as directed.
4. Turn the machine on and check for a mist at the mouthpiece.
5. Put your lips around the mouthpiece to form a seal.
   Inhale through your mouth only. If this is hard for you to do, you may need a nose clip.
   Hold your breath for two seconds.
   Exhale slowly and completely through your mouth.
6. Never hold in a cough during the treatment. Stop and cough. Turn the machine off or tip the nebulizer cup sideways until you are ready to start again. Then continue your treatment.
7. Drink water or rinse your mouth during the treatment if your mouth becomes dry.
8. Notify your doctor if you have any discomfort during or after the treatment.
9. Do not allow anyone else to use the machine.
10. Do not use your machine if you have any doubts that it is not working properly. If you are in the hospital when this happens, notify your nurse or therapist. If you are at home, call your supplier.
11. Rinse out your medication containers and mouthpiece after each use.
12. Keep the machine covered with a clean towel when not in use.
13. Rinse your mouth before and after each treatment for cleanliness and comfort.

Cleaning your equipment

All equipment that you use to breathe in medication must be cleaned every day. If germs (bacteria) are not cleaned from your equipment, they may cause an infection. An infection would make extra work for your heart and lungs and make it harder for you to breathe.

Modified from *Living with lung disease,* American Lung Association of Connecticut, 1989.

Your supplier is responsible for providing you with written instructions concerning the appropriate method for cleaning your equipment.

Metered Dose Inhaler

Client Information

A metered dose inhaler (MDI) is a handheld pressurized device that delivers a premeasured amount of medication to your lungs.

1. Assemble the MDI for use according to package directions.
2. Shake the MDI.
3. Open mouth wide.
4. Place MDI about 1 inch in front of your lips. Do not close lips around mouthpiece.
5. Exhale fully.
6. Press your MDI once as you begin to inhale slowly and deeply.
7. Hold your breath for 5 to 10 seconds if possible at the peak of your deep breath.
8. Exhale slowly through pursed lips.
9. Repeat steps 5 through 7 for each puff as ordered by your doctor. Wait 2 to 5 minutes between puffs if using a fast-acting bronchodilator.
10. If you use both a bronchodilator and other medication MDIs, always use the bronchodilator first. It is most effective to allow 15 minutes between two medications.
11. Rinse your mouth out with water after using steroid sprays.
12. To check the amount of medicine left in your MDI, place the canister in water.

Do not overuse your MDI. Use only as ordered by your doctor.

Instructor Information

The medication brochure may not reflect current information regarding appropriate instructions for use. It is important to review these concepts carefully with the client for most effective results.

Some clients have difficulty coordinating their breathing with pressing the MDI. Various types of spacers allow the aerosolized particles to collect in a chamber. The client then inhales from the chamber. Assemble and use as instructed on package insert. If clients will be using a spacer, alter the instructions for use (especially step 4) to correspond with the package insert.

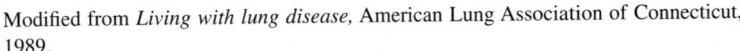

Modified from *Living with lung disease,* American Lung Association of Connecticut, 1989.

Note: Some medications (e.g., ipratropium bromide) are better administered by using closed mouth technique or a spacer. Some of the atropine-containing MDIs may cause pupillary dilation if sprayed in the eyes, which can be disabling.

If possible, watch clients do this entire procedure. If they are not properly performing the procedure, they may not be receiving their proper medication dosage.

If clients are using a fast-acting bronchodilator (e.g., metaproterenol, albuterol) instruct them to wait 2 to 5 minutes between puffs to allow the medication time to open the bronchi so the next puff can go deeper into the lungs.

There are also inexpensive arthritic aids available for people who have difficulty compressing the MDI.

Metered Dose Bronchodilator Inhalation Technique

It is important that the client be instructed in the correct use of a metered dose nebulizer before it is needed to relieve an asthma attack. The prescriber will indicate whether the closed-mouth or the open-mouth technique is to be used. If it is optional, encourage the client to use the open-mouth technique for better inhalation of the drug. If used incorrectly, the dose may be dispersed into the air or even swallowed. Since only 10% of an inhaled dose reaches the lungs under the best of conditions, the ability to use the metered dose nebulizer appropriately is essential for the client.

A placebo nebulizer should be used for demonstration. This will enable the client to repeat the demonstration a number of times until the nebulizer can be easily and correctly used.

The Closed-Mouth Technique

1. Shake the container for 2 to 5 seconds.
2. Hold the nebulizer with the drug container upside down.
3. Place the mouthpiece in the mouth, closing lips tightly around it.
4. Exhale steadily and completely through nose.
5. Inhale slowly and deeply, and at the same time press the container down on the mouthpiece.
6. Hold breath for as long as possible before exhaling and remove mouthpiece from your mouth.
7. Wait 15 seconds.
8. Repeat steps 1 through 6 above.
9. If no relief is achieved after 5 minutes and condition worsens, contact physician.

From McKenry L, Salerno E: *Mosby's pharmacology in nursing,* ed 19, St Louis, 1995, Mosby.

The Open-Mouth Technique

1. Shake the container for 2 to 5 seconds.
2. Hold the nebulizer with the drug container upside down.
3. Hold the mouthpiece two finger widths (about 1½ inches) in front of widely opened mouth. Hold container upright.
4. Exhale deeply, then inhale slowly through mouth and at the same time press down firmly on the container. Continue to breathe deeply.
5. Hold breath for a few seconds, then exhale slowly. Wait approximately 15 seconds, and then repeat steps 3 through 5 for second inhalation.

   (Keep eyes closed—temporary blurring of vision may occur if the aerosol is sprayed into the eyes.)

Metered Dose Inhaler

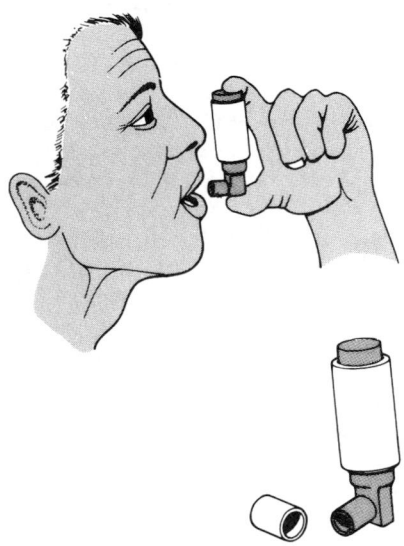

Advise client that rinsing the mouth after using the nebulizer prevents systemic absorption and minimizes dryness of the mouth. The mouthpiece should be rinsed at least once daily to avoid clogging. Stress the importance of keeping the equipment clean to prevent infection. If using a refillable nebulizer, do not place more than a day's supply of drug in nebulizer. Change solution daily.

Clients with asthma benefit greatly from the use of sympathomimetic inhalers; however, they should be discouraged from using over-the-counter inhalers because of the nonselective beta-agonist drug effect of the epinephrine base. The nurse needs to recognize the possibility of misuse and the consequences of abuse in order to successfully help the client with inhalant drug therapy.

How to Use Eyedrops or Ointment

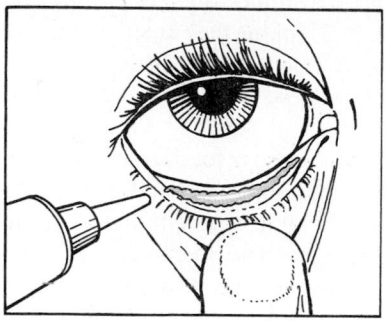

Administering ophthalmic ointments.

From Clayton BD, Stock YN: *Basic pharmacology for nurses,* ed 9, St Louis, 1989, Mosby.

To Instill Eyedrops

Wash your hands and put on gloves if necessary.

Gently cleanse exudate from the eye, if necessary.

Ask the client to tilt the head toward the side of the affected eye.

Gently pull the lower eyelid down and ask the client to look up.

Instill the correct number of drops in the sac formed by the lower eyelid.

Take care not to touch the dropper to the eye or eyelashes.

Gently apply pressure for 30 seconds to 1 minute over the inner canthus next to the nose to prevent absorption through the tear duct and premature drainage of the medication away from the eye.

Ask the client to gently close the eye, which distributes the solution. Warn against squeezing the eye tightly, which will force out the medication.

Wipe away any excess medication.

If both eyes are to be medicated, do the second instillation quickly before the client begins to blink and tear as a reaction to the burning sensation occurring in the first eye medicated.

To Instill Eye Ointment

The procedure is the same except the ointment is expressed directly onto the exposed conjunctival sac from inner to outer canthus with a small individual tube and closed eye; gently massage to distribute the medication.

From McKenry L, Salerno E: *Mosby's pharmacology in nursing,* ed 19, St Louis, 1995, Mosby.

Eyedrops and Look-alikes

Containers that are facsimiles are the culprits behind many oph-thalmic emergencies. Thinking they are instilling eyedrops, adults and children have instead dropped in superglue, contact lens cleaners, ear drops, and perfumes. These products are often sold in bottles that are similar in shape, size, and color. The elderly, who may have poor eyesight, are particularly at risk for mistaking one product for another.

In most cases, the injured eye responds to copious flushing to dilute and wash out the offending agent, followed by topical antibiotics, lubricants or cycloplegics, and patching, if needed. If the client has instilled glue in the eye and has no significant pain, irrigation and a sterile eyepatch soaked in tap water and left overnight are sufficient. The solvents to dissolve the glue are too toxic for the eye, so if the conservative approach does not work, the client may need to be referred to an ophthalmologist, who may cut the eyelids apart to prevent corneal abrasion.

Advise all clients to keep their eyedrops in one particular place away from other chemicals. Recommend that they check the labels on the container while still wearing their glasses or contact lenses to ensure they have the right medicine before administering their eyedrops.

The client should be asked to look up so that the cornea reflex is diminished, and the dropper should be introduced from the side. The lower lid is gently retracted, and the drops are instilled into the conjunctival sac. Drops should not be placed directly onto the cornea. After the drops are instilled, the lid is gently released.

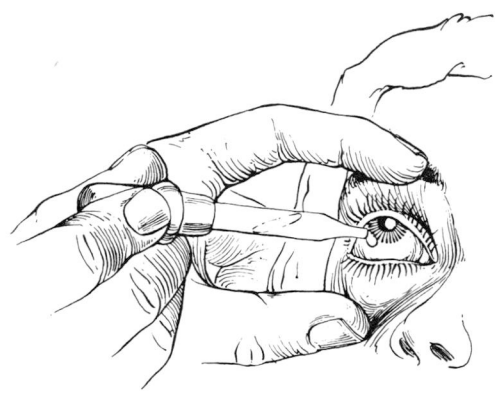

Instillation of drops onto the conjunctiva of the lower lid of the eye.

From McKenry L, Salerno E: *Mosby's pharmacology in nursing,* ed 19, St Louis, 1995, Mosby.

Instructions for Use of
Ear Wash and Drops

You have been given a prescription that you should have filled at your own drugstore. You will also need a 2- or 3-ounce ear syringe, which you can buy at a drugstore if you do not have one. Someone else should wash your ear for you; you cannot do it as well yourself. The instructions below should be followed carefully:

1. Wash hands before and after this procedure.
2. Fill the ear syringe with the solution.
3. The solution must be at body temperature. If the solution is too warm or too cool, you will feel dizzy. Warm the solution by placing the syringe in a pan of hot water. Do *not* warm the solution on the stove.
4. Lie down with the ear to be washed facing up and pull up and out on the external ear. Place the tip of the ear syringe into the ear canal. Do not be afraid to push it down into the ear. However, you should get a return flow. If you do not, you have it in too far. Pull the syringe out slightly.
5. Pump the warmed solution from the syringe back and forth into the ear by squeezing and releasing the bulb of the syringe. Do this vigorously and repeatedly. The ear wash must be forced back and forth, in and out of the ear canal.
6. Lean over and let the solution run out of the ear.
7. Pull the ear up, back, and out to straighten the ear canal.
8. Put three to five warmed drops into the ear.
9. If the solution burns too much at first, you may dilute the solution. Mix 2 ounces of water with 2 ounces of the solution. Later, decrease the amount of water used with each irrigation.
10. Use the solution and drops twice a day for 2 weeks and then until the ear stops running or becomes dry. If you are not sure that the ear is dry, check it by putting a cotton swab down into the ear canal. If the cotton swab comes out dry, stop using the solution and drops. If the cotton swab is wet or there is an odor, continue using the solution and drops for 4 days.
11. Do not use the solution and drops as long as the ear remains dry and is not running, and as long as there is no odor. Should the ear start to run after being dry for a period of time, start using the ear solution and drops until the ear is dry again.
12. **Do not get any water in your ears.** You should not go swimming until you are told you may do so. Whenever there is a chance of

getting water in your ears, such as when you shower or wash your hair, use cotton in the ear. First, place a dry piece of cotton in the ear and then a second piece that has been saturated with petroleum jelly.

13. If you have any questions, call your doctor.

Administration of Eardrops

The infant or child is positioned on the unaffected ear. The nurse pulls the pinna down and back to administer eardrops to infants and children under 3 years of age.

When administering eardrops to children older than 3 years and adults, the nurse gently pulls the pinna up and back. The nurse should stabilize his or her hand on the client's head for safety and instill the prescribed number of drops. The drops are directed toward the ear canal to avoid hitting the tympanic membrane, which can cause pain. The client should remain in the position for 5 to 10 minutes. Otic drops should be warmed before they are instilled, to prevent nausea or vertigo.

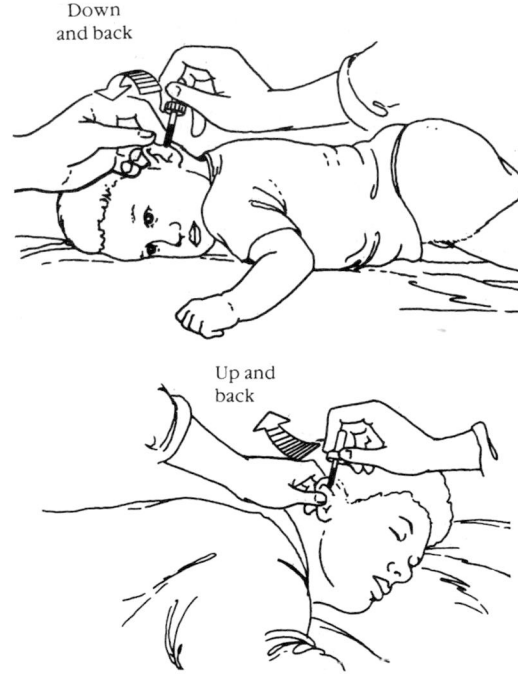

Down and back

Up and back

From Myers J: *Quick medication administration reference,* ed 2, St Louis, 1995, Mosby.

Administering a Rectal Suppository

Position client on side and drape. Unwrap suppository and remove from package. Apply water-soluble lubricant. Gently insert suppository about an inch past the internal sphincter.

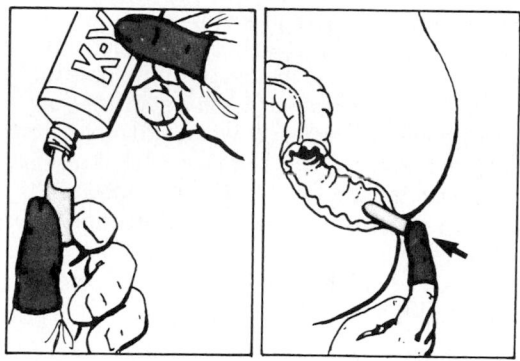

Administration of Vaginal Medication

Gently insert the vaginal applicator as far as possible into the vagina and push plunger to deposit the medication.

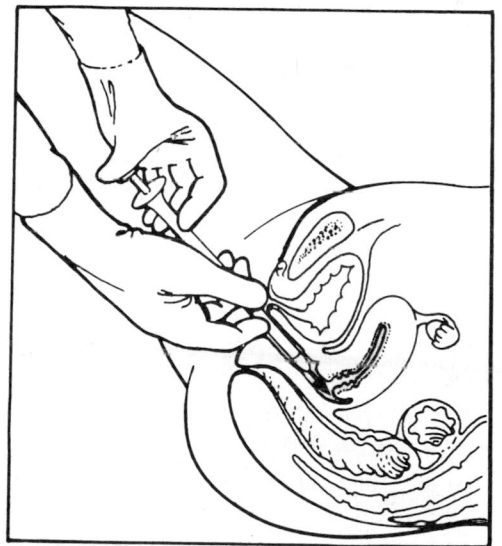

From Myers J: *Quick medication administration reference,* ed 2, St Louis, 1995, Mosby.

Using Oxygen at Home Teaching Guide

Your doctor has prescribed extra oxygen at a flow rate of _____ liters per minute for _____ hours every day. The medical supply company will show you how to set the flow rate and how to care for the equipment. Keep the supplier's phone number handy so that you can call if the system doesn't work properly.

You will be using a liquid oxygen unit, an oxygen tank, or an oxygen concentrator. You will breathe the oxygen through either a mask or a nasal cannulae (two short prongs that fit just inside your nostrils). The system will also have a humidifier to warm and moisturize the oxygen.

It's a good idea to also have a small portable oxygen tank for an emergency backup system in case of power failure.

Here are some general guidelines and safety tips for using oxygen equipment.

General Guidelines

Always keep your oxygen flow rate where your doctor prescribes.

Sometimes it's hard to tell whether oxygen is flowing through the tubes. If you have doubts, check to be sure that the system is turned on and there are no kinks in the tubing. If you still aren't sure, place the nasal cannulae in a glass of water with the prongs up and watch for bubbles. (Always shake the water off before inserting the cannulae into your nostrils.) If no bubbles appear, oxygen is not flowing through the tubes and you need to call your supplier.

Each time before using your oxygen, check the humidifier bottle. If it's near the fill line, empty the bottle and refill it with sterile or bottled water.

Even with the humidifier, oxygen can dry the inside of your nose. A water-soluble lubricant (such as K-Y Jelly) helps ease dryness and cracking. Don't use petroleum-based products such as Vaseline because this will make the dryness worse.

To avoid running out of oxygen, reorder your new supply when the register reads $1/4$ full—2 or 3 days before you need a new tank.

Safety First

Oxygen is highly combustible. By following these rules, you can be confident that your oxygen system is not posing a serious fire hazard:

- Keep your oxygen unit away from open flames and heat. This includes smoking—don't smoke and don't allow others to smoke around you. If you have a gas stove, gas space heater, or kerosene heater or lamp, stay out of the room while it's on.

- To prevent leakage, always keep your oxygen system upright, and make sure the system is turned off when not in use. Don't place carpets, bed clothes, or furniture over the tubing, since this may cause a leak.
- Keep an all-purpose fire extinguisher close by.
- If a fire should occur, turn off the oxygen and leave the house at once.
- Notify your local fire department that you have oxygen in the house. In most areas, the fire department offers free safety inspections, which can help make your home even safer for using oxygen.

Call your doctor immediately if:

- Your breathing is difficult, irregular, shallow, or slow.
- You become restless or anxious.
- You are tired, drowsy, or have trouble waking up.
- You have a persistent headache.
- Your speech becomes slurred, you can't concentrate, or you feel confused.
- Your fingernails or lips are bluish.

These symptoms may arise when you are not getting enough oxygen or when you are getting too much oxygen. Only your doctor can determine how much oxygen you need. Therefore, you must never change the flow rate without instructions from your doctor.

Chest Physiotherapy

In some lung conditions, such as chronic bronchitis, emphysema, and cystic fibrosis, thick mucus collects in the lungs. This makes breathing more difficult and increases the chance of getting pneumonia or other infections. To help loosen the mucus and move it out of the lungs, your doctor has suggested that you perform chest physiotherapy. This consists of postural drainage, chest percussion, and coughing.

You should do chest physiotherapy twice a day (unless your doctor tells you otherwise)—once when you first get up in the morning and once in the evening before you go to bed. Whenever you have more mucus than usual, you should do chest physiotherapy more often.

Remember that drinking a lot of fluids (at least 2 quarts daily) will also help thin the mucus.

You can do the postural drainage and coughing by yourself. Someone will need to help you with chest percussion.

Postural Drainage

1. Place pillows on the floor beside the bed and a box of tissues close by.
2. Lie on the bed with your trunk over the side, head and arms resting on the pillows. You will lie on your stomach and on each side. Stay in each position 10 to 20 minutes.

Chest Percussion

Here's where a friend or family member will have to help you. You will stay in the postural drainage position for percussion.

1. The helper should make a cup with his or her hands. This is done by keeping fingers together, flexing the fingers, and tucking the thumb tightly against the index finger.
2. The helper firmly pats your back rhythmically, alternating the cupped hands, for 3 to 5 minutes. When done correctly, this will make a sound like a galloping horse. (With just a little practice, this technique is easy to master.)

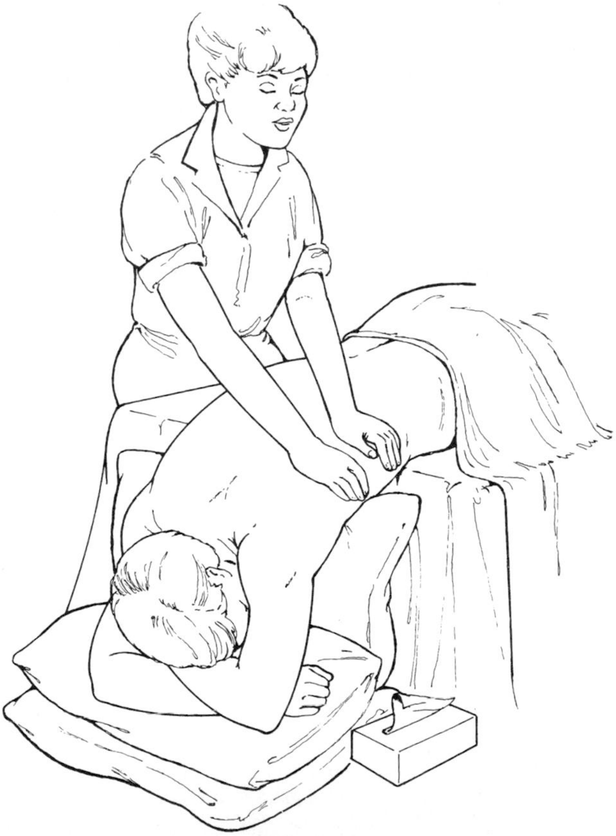

Coughing

Stay in the postural drainage position.

1. Take a slow, deep breath through your nose. Hold your breath for 3 seconds. (Counting one 100, two 100, three 100 will help you hold your breath long enough.)
2. Open your mouth slightly, coughing three times as you breathe out. A good cough that helps bring up mucus sounds hollow, deep, and low. (A high-pitched cough is not effective.)
3. Take a slow, deep breath through your nose and breathe normally for a few minutes. Then repeat the coughing procedure several more times.
4. Be sure you spit the mucus into a tissue. (Do not swallow it, since this can cause nausea.)

Guidelines for Women with Lymphedema

Lymphedema

Swelling of the arm may occur in women who have had a mastectomy and removal of lymph glands under the arm and after other operations or radiation therapy that involves these glands.

Precautions to Observe

- Care for simple cuts, scratches, or burns by careful washing and covering them with a protective dressing. Be sure to change plastic Band-Aids or bandages often to avoid infection.
- Wear loose-fitting gloves and avoid wearing anything that will constrict the hand or arm, such as tight sleeves or jewelry.
- Let technicians, nurses, and doctors know of the surgery and the need for care in taking blood pressure and giving vaccinations and injections on the operated side.
- Manicure nails carefully. Avoid cutting or tearing cuticles. Cuticles can be kept soft with a lanolin-based cream.
- Protect fingers from punctures by sharp objects such as needles and pins.
- Protect hand and arm when gardening by wearing gloves. This avoids punctures from thorns of roses or other plants or tools.

Modified from *Reach to recovery: an ounce of prevention: suggestions for hand and arm care,* Pamphlet No 4605-PS, Z-86.

- Protect arm and chest from overexposure to the sun, particularly if the client has received radiation therapy. Apply a sunscreen liberally to exposed areas.
- Think through a task before starting it to see if there are precautions that should be taken to protect hands and arms.

Swelling (Lymphedema)

Swelling does not mean a recurrence of cancer, but it is a side effect that occurs in some women following surgery or radiation. Swelling can occur immediately after surgery (may be only temporary), or months, or even years later. If the hand and arm swell, contact physician. The physician may refer the client to a specialist in physical medicine or to the physical therapy department of a hospital.

Corrective Measures to Use for Swelling

The physician may prescribe antibiotics if there is evidence of infection or the physician may recommend treatment with a compression unit. A compression unit with a lymphedema sleeve is a sleevelike apparatus into which the affected arm is placed while the sleeve inflates and forces the fluids back into the lymph system to attempt to reduce the swelling. The physician will prescribe the length of time to leave the affected arm in the compression unit and the correct pressure setting. The sleeve will help control the swelling with regular use, but the technique is usually not curative. Some physicians advise clients to use the unit once or twice a day, or suggest treatments at the hospital as an outpatient. Ask the physician to write a prescription detailing the need, and check with the insurance company to see if payment or partial payment will be made for treatments or for the purchase of a portable unit. Some units are portable and can be used at home. The unit should be taken to the physiatrist (doctor of physical medicine) or physical therapy department at a hospital for setting and instruction.

Guidelines for Care of Client with Chronic Renal Failure

Do's	Don'ts
1. If blood needs to be drawn, use the nonvascular access limb.	1. No blood pressure or venipuncture in vascular access limb.
2. Use of glucose meter for determining blood glucose levels is more accurate.	2. Do not check urine samples of a diabetic client for glucose; diminished renal function renders the procedure useless.
3. Use concentrated glucose (sugar, candy bar, soft drinks) to treat hypoglycemia in a diabetic renal client.	3. Do not give orange juice to a hypoglycemic diabetic renal client; the potassium could be lethal.
4. Encourage use of various spices such as onion powder, garlic powder, Mrs. Dash, and so on to spice up food without adding salt.	4. Permit no salt substitute; they substitute potassium chloride for sodium chloride.
5. Always do a multipositional blood pressure assessment (lying to sitting to standing).	5. Never accept a lying (supine) hypertensive blood pressure reading without following up with a sitting/standing assessment.
6. Assess vascular access function by listening for bruit or feeling for thrill as evidence the access is patent.	6. Never occlude the vascular access with constrictive clothing, B/P cuff; remind client not to carry heavy objects on the arm.
7. Do encourage the client to assume as much responsibility for self-care as possible.	7. Do not encourage dependency and complacency because these contribute to decreased quality and quantity of life.
8. Do encourage the client to follow the prescribed regimen of diet, medications, and dialysis (if applicable).	8. Remind client that noncompliance can be very uncomfortable and lead to death in a renal client.

Modified from Martinson I, Widmer J, editors: *Home health care nursing,* Philadelphia, 1989, Saunders.

Pharmacological Issues

In working with individuals in the home and community, the nurse often finds that medications present major issues for clients. To properly comply with taking medications, clients want to understand the importance of the medicine to their overall care and how they will be affected. The following information will give the nurse cues to medication interactions with other drugs, foods, and physiological responses of clients to certain pharmacological agents. The use of proper agents is emphasized.

Summary of Essential Equivalents

Household	Apothecary	Metric
Volume		
1 tsp = 4 to 5 ml	1 fl dr = 4 ml or 1 tsp	5 ml = 1 tsp
3 tsp = 1 tbsp	4 drams = ½ oz	15 ml = 1 tbsp
1 tbsp = ½ oz or 15 ml	8 drams = 2 tbsp (1 oz)	30 ml = 2 tbsp
	16 minims = 1 ml	1 ml = 16 minims†
2 tbsp = 1 oz or 30 ml	1 pt* = 16 oz or 480 ml	500 ml = 0.5 L or 1 pt
	1 qt* = 32 oz or 960 ml	
Teacup = 6 oz		1000 ml = 1 L or 1 qt
Glass or cup = 8 oz		
Weight		
	$\frac{1}{60}$ grain = 1 mg	
	1 grain = 60 mg or 0.060 g	
	15 grains = 1 g or 1000 mg	
	2.2 lbs = 1 kg	
	1 mg = 1000 µg	

Reprinted from Hegsted L, Hayek W: *Essential drug dosage calculations,* Table 5-1. Copyright © 1983 by Robert J Brady Company. Reprinted by permission of Appleton & Lange.

*The pint is considered to be 500 ml and the quart is considered to be 1000 ml when used in medication orders.

†Sixteen minims is used as the equivalent rather than 15 because the equipment for dispensing medications is calibrated in 16 minims per ml.

Polypharmacy Risk Factors

More than six medicines
Multiple prescribers
Multiple pharmacies
Lack of defined indications for drugs
Duplicate medications (same class)
Multiple minor complaints
Confusion or dementia
Apparent improvement on discontinuation of drug(s)
History of drug allergy or toxicity

Oral Medication Assessment

Observation	Assessment
Old prescriptions	Lack of recent physician assessment, possible inappropriate drug use
Duplicate prescriptions	Possibility of overdosage
Others' medications	Possibility of inappropriate drug use
Inappropriate storage	Possibility of lack of drug effect
Outdated medications	Possibility of lack of drug effect
"Stockpiling" (inappropriate quantities)	Possibility of overdosage or outdated medication

From Martinson I, Widmen J, editors: *Home health care nursing,* Philadelphia, 1989, Saunders.

Calculating Pediatric Dosage

Clark's Rule

Because this formula is based on weight alone, it is often considered an imprecise calculation for children.

$$\frac{\text{Average adult dose} \times \text{Weight of child in pounds}}{150} = \text{Estimated safe dose}$$

Example: How much acetaminophen (Tylenol) should a 1-year-old child weighing 21 pounds receive if the average adult dose is 10 grains?
   Answer:

$$\frac{10 \text{ (grains)} \times 21 \text{ (weight in pounds)}}{150} = \text{gr } 1\tfrac{2}{5}$$

From McKenry L, Salerno E: *Mosby's pharmacology in nursing,* ed 19, St Louis, 1995, Mosby; Wong D: *Whaley and Wong's nursing care of infants and children,* ed 5, St Louis, 1995, Mosby.

$$\frac{\text{BSA of child}}{\text{BSA of adult}} \times \text{Adult dose} = \text{Estimated child's dose}$$

$$\text{BSA of child (m}^2) \times \text{Dose/m}^2 = \text{Estimated child's dose}$$

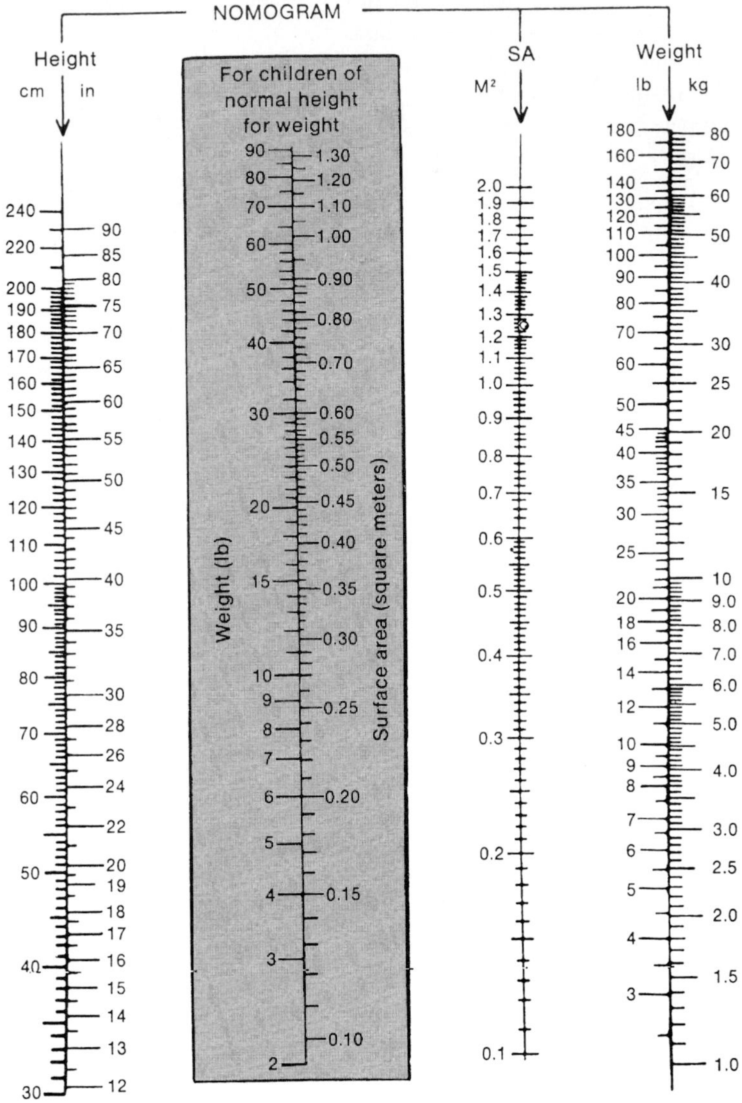

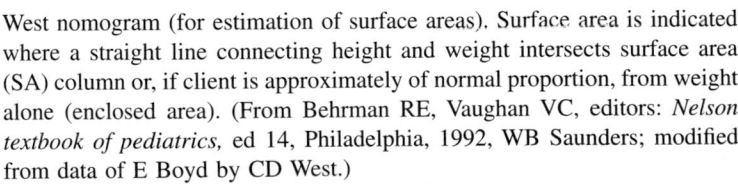

West nomogram (for estimation of surface areas). Surface area is indicated where a straight line connecting height and weight intersects surface area (SA) column or, if client is approximately of normal proportion, from weight alone (enclosed area). (From Behrman RE, Vaughan VC, editors: *Nelson textbook of pediatrics,* ed 14, Philadelphia, 1992, WB Saunders; modified from data of E Boyd by CD West.)

Calculation of IV Rates

A. *Flow rate*

(must know amount of solution ordered and amount of time of infusion)

EXAMPLE: infuse D5NS, 1000 ml, over 8 hours using a macro drip set (15 gtt/ml)

1. Calculate amount of solution per hour:

$$\frac{1000 \text{ ml}}{8 \text{ hr}} = 125 \text{ ml/hr}$$

2. Calculate gtt/min:

$$\frac{\text{gtt/ml of tubing}}{60 \text{ min/hr}} \times \frac{\text{Amount of fluid}}{1}$$

$$\frac{15}{60} \times \frac{125}{1} = \frac{1875}{60} = 31 \text{ gtt/min}$$

B. *Flow rate in mg*

(must know amount of solution, amount of drug, gtt factor/ml, and amount of drug to be administered)

EXAMPLE: lidocaine drip, 2 g, in D5W, 500 ml, to infuse at 2 mg/min

1. Calculate amount of drug/ml in mg:

$$2 \text{ g} = 2000 \text{ mg}$$

$$\frac{2000 \text{ mg}}{500 \text{ ml}} = 4 \text{ mg/ml}$$

2. Calculate number of gtt for 1 mg:

$$\frac{4 \text{ mg}}{1 \text{ ml}} = \frac{4 \text{ mg}}{60 \text{ gtt}} = \frac{1 \text{ mg}}{15 \text{ gtt}}$$

3. Calculate number of desired mg:

$$\frac{1 \text{ mg}}{15 \text{ gtt}} = \frac{2 \text{ mg}}{X}$$

$$X = 30 \text{ ml}$$

C. *µg/kg/min*

(to determine number of µg/kg/min when drip factor is known, must know client weight, amount of drug, amount of solution, gtt factor/ml, and gtt being administered)

EXAMPLE: client weighing 154 lb is receiving dopamine, 400 mg, in D5W, 500 ml, at 30 gtt/min

1. Convert pounds to kg:

$$\frac{154}{2.2} = 70 \text{ kg}$$

2. Calculate number of mg in 1 ml of solution:

$$\frac{400 \text{ mg}}{500 \text{ ml}} = 0.8 \text{ mg/ml}$$

From Hermey C: *Quick reference for IV therapy,* St Louis, 1995, Mosby.

Continued.

3. Convert mg to μg:
$$0.8 \text{ mg} \times 1000 = 800 \text{ μg}$$

4. Divide μg by weight to obtain μg/kg/ml:
$$\frac{800 \text{ μg}}{70 \text{ kg}} = 11.4 \text{ μg/kg/ml}$$

5. Find μg/kg/gtt:
$$\frac{11.4 \text{ μg/kg}}{60 \text{ gtt}} = \frac{X}{1 \text{ gtt}}$$
$$X = 0.19 \text{ μg/kg/gtt}$$

6. Multiply current drip rate by number calculated to obtain μg/kg/min:
$$0.19 \times 30 = 5.70 \text{ μg/kg/min}$$

D. *gtt/min*
(to determine number of gtt/min when μg/kg/min is ordered, must know client weight, amount of drug, amount of solution, gtt factor/ml, and dosage to be administered)
EXAMPLE: client weighs 154 lb; MD orders 5 μg/kg/min of dopamine, 400 mg, in D5W, 500 ml
1. Convert lb to kg:
$$\frac{154}{2.2} = 70 \text{ kg}$$

2. Calculate number of mg in 1 ml of solution:
$$\frac{400 \text{ mg}}{500 \text{ ml}} = 0.8 \text{ mg/ml}$$

3. Convert mg to μg:
$$0.8 \times 1000 = 800 \text{ μg}$$

4. Divide μg by weight to obtain μg/kg/ml:
$$\frac{800 \text{ μg}}{70 \text{ kg}} = 11.4 \text{ μg/kg/ml}$$

5. Calculate rate needed to administer ordered dose of drug:
$$\frac{11.4 \text{ μg/kg/ml}}{60} = \frac{5 \text{ μg/kg/min}}{X}$$
$$X = 26 \text{ gtt/min}$$

E. *Pediatric dosage*
$$\frac{\text{BSA of child}}{\text{BSA of adult}} \times \text{Adult dosage} = \text{Pediatric dosage}$$

New Classification of Tuberculin Skin Test Reactors

The Centers for Disease Control (CDC) has received a number of inquiries about the new classification of tuberculin skin test reactors contained in the recently distributed tuberculin skin test videotape. (The videotape is available in the Health Services Film Library, 404-566-4290.) The videotape reflects changes contained in the revision of "Diagnostic Standards and Classification of Tuberculosis," which will be published as joint American Thoracic Society/Centers for Disease Control (ATS/CDC) statements in the *American Review of Respiratory Diseases*. To avoid sending a videotape that would soon be out of date, the CDC decided to incorporate the new classification criteria into the skin test videotape that was released last summer, in advance of the "official" ATS/CDC recommendations.

As shown in the videotape, reactions to the intracutaneous Mantoux test (with 5TU tuberculin PPD) should now be interpreted as follows:

- A reaction of *5 millimeters or more of induration* is classified as positive in the following groups:
  1. Persons who have had close recent contact with tuberculosis
  2. Persons who have chest radiographs consistent with tuberculosis
  3. Immunosuppressed persons
- A reaction of *10 millimeters or more of induration* is classified as positive in persons who do not meet the above criteria but who have other risk factors for tuberculosis. This includes:
  1. Foreign-born persons from high prevalence countries in Asia, Africa, and Latin America
  2. Intravenous drug users
  3. Homeless individuals
  4. Residents of nursing homes
  5. Residents of correctional institutions
  6. Persons with the following factors that increase the risk of tuberculosis: silicosis; diabetes mellitus; immunosuppressive therapy; some hematological and reticuloendothelial disease; and clinical situations associated with substantial rapid weight loss or undernutrition.
- A reaction of *15 millimeters or more of induration* is classified as positive in all other persons.

For each of the above categories, reactions below the cut-point are considered negative.

From Centers for Disease Control, Atlanta, March, 1990.

Biological Agents for Diagnostic Tests for Tuberculosis

Biological product	Purpose, preparation, and storage	Alerts
Biological diagnostic tests Tuberculin, old; tine test	Multiple-puncture, disposable test device for the detection of tuberculin reactivity; especially useful in mass screening; initial test should be done at or before rubeola immunization, thereafter annually or biannually or as indicated by individual risk of exposure (repeated testing may increase the size of reaction but will not sensitize to tuberculin). Apply the disk with its four coated prongs quickly and firmly to the volar surface of the forearm so that puncture sites and disk impression are seen. Reaction read 48 to 72 hr (criteria for positive reaction—extent of induration or vesiculation as per enclosed ruler in package—2 mm or greater). Store unrefrigerated below 30°C (86°F).	Precautions: test with caution those with active tuberculosis (possible activation of quiescent lesions); hypersensitivity to acacia gum; immunosuppression or recent vaccination with live virus vaccines may suppress reactivity; doubtful or positive reaction—further test using Mantoux, chest roentgenogram, sputum culture Side effects: local vesicles, ulceration, or necrosis in highly sensitive persons; pain or pruritus may be relieved by cold packs
Tuberculin purified protein derivatives—PPD test (Mantoux) (Aplitest, multipuncture)	Solution obtained from human strain of *Mycobacterium tuberculosis* for more conclusive results than the tine test. Given intradermally 0.1 ml strength either 1 US unit (for those who are highly sensitized), 5 US units, or 250 US units (for those failing to react), which should never be used as initial dose. Given	Contraindications: never inject a 250 US unit/ 0.1 ml dose as initial test Precautions: immunosuppression or concurrent or recent immunization with certain virus vaccines or recent viral infection (may cause suppressed reactivity). Those over 55 years of age may need second testing

	intracutaneously. Positive reaction when read 48 to 72 hr later: an induration 10 mm or more; 5 to 9 mm is "doubtful" reaction except in case of known exposure. Positive reaction only indicates previous exposure to tuberculosis, not necessarily active disease; further testing for diagnosis is thus required. Store at 2° to 8°C.	Side effects: see package insert for details
Allergenic extracts	Several hundred individual purified fluid allergens for diagnosis and hyposensitization for specific allergies pollens, poison ivy/oak, foods, dusts, skin contactants, insects, fungi, yeasts, autogenous bacteria, based on intracutaneous skin test responses. Treatment is periodic subcutaneous injection of gradually increasing potency of dilutions of specific allergen(s); schedule and dosages are highly individualized.	Contraindications: severe anaphylaxis Precautions: severe anaphylaxis (reduce dose); keep on hand epinephrine, antihistamines, oxygen, etc. Side effects (grass allergens most reactive of all): local—edema, redness, pain (reduce dose); systemic—urticaria, sneezing, dyspnea (give epinephrine, antihistamines, steroids; reduce dose)

From McKenry L, Salerno E: *Mosby's pharmacology in nursing*, ed 19, St Louis, 1995, Mosby.

Common Tests for Screening Selected Conditions

Preparation	Condition monitored or detected	Procedure
Acetone tests (Acetest, Chemstrip K, Ketostix)	Tests of urine or blood for ketones, in diabetes mellitus	Tablets, papers, or strips
Albumin (Albustix)	Protein detection in urine	Strips
Bacteria in urine tests (Microstix-Nitrite; Microstix-3 Strips, Uricult)	Tests for nitrite to detect bacteria in urine	Strips
Bilirubin test (Ictotest)	Tests for bilirubin in urine	Tablets
Blood urea nitrogen test (Azostix)	Tests for urea nitrogen in blood	Strips
C-reactive protein (LAtest-CRP)	Serum test for acute inflammation	Kit

From McKenry L, Salerno E: *Mosby's pharmacology in nursing*, ed 19, St Louis, 1995, Mosby.

Food-Drug Interactions

Drug category/medication	Foods to avoid	Rationale
Antacids		
Calcium carbonate (Tums)	Avoid large amounts of dairy products. If used as a calcium supplement, avoid concurrent administration of bran and whole grain breads or cereals.	Milk or cream may increase acid secretion. Reduces absorption of calcium.
Antibiotics		
Erythromycin, penicillins*	Meals, acidic fruit juices, citrus fruits, or acidic beverages, such as cola drinks	The antibiotics are acid labile (reduced absorption). Take medication 1 hour before meals or apart from acidic foods or 2 hours after meals.
Tetracyclines	Calcium-containing foods: milk, ice cream, yogurt, cheeses, and others	Calcium may complex with tetracycline, resulting in reduced absorption of the antibiotic. Most tetracyclines, with the exception of doxycycline and minocycline, should be administered 1 hour before or 2 hours after meals.

From McKenry L, Salerno E: *Mosby's pharmacology in nursing,* ed 19, St Louis, 1995, Mosby.
*Erythromycin base (E-Mycin, Ey-Tab, E-Mycin Eryc) or stearates (Erypar, Erythrocin Stearate, Ethril, Wyamycin S) are best absorbed in the fasting state. Erythromycin ethylsuccinate (E.E.S.), estolate (Ilosone), and enteric-coated erythromycin may be given before or with meals. Penicillin, such as penicillin G, ampicillin, cloxacillin, cyclacillin, dicloxacillin, nafcillin, and oxacillin may have decreased absorption if given with food or acidic-type products.

Continued.

Food-Drug Interactions—cont'd

Drug category/medication	Foods to avoid	Rationale
Anticoagulants Warfarin (Coumadin), Dicumarol, heparin	Beef liver and green leafy vegetables contain vitamin K (spinach, cabbage, brussels sprouts)	Vitamin K can counteract therapeutic action of anticoagulants. A normal, balanced diet will not interfere with this medication. Fad or extreme diets with foods high in vitamin K can affect anticoagulant activity.
Laxative Mineral oil (Agoral plain, mineral oil)	Take 2 hours apart from food. Do not administer at bedtime.	May decrease absorption of vitamins A, D, E, and K. Also reduces absorption of calcium. Aspiration of mineral oil may induce lipid pneumonitis.
MAO inhibitors Isocarboxazid (Marplan), phenelzine (Nardil), tranylcypromine (Parnate)	Foods with high tyramine content, such as aged cheese (brie, cheddar, processed American, camembert, and others), aged meat, sour cream, yogurt, pickled herring, chicken liver, canned figs, raisins, bananas, avocados, soy sauce, yeast extract, meat tenderizers, alcoholic beverages such as beer and wine (chianti, sherry, or hearty red wines), sausages, chocolate, anchovies	Concurrent use may result in severe headache, nosebleed, chest pain, eyes sensitive to light, or severe hypertension which may result in a hypertensive crisis.

Drug Interactions with Antibiotics

Drug	Possible effect and management
Anticoagulants, oral coumarin or indanedione, heparin or thrombolytic agents	Increased risk of bleeding when given with high doses of parenteral carbenicillin or ticarcillin, as these drugs inhibit platelet aggregation. Monitor closely for signs of bleeding. Concurrent use of these penicillins with thrombolytic agents also increases the risk for severe bleeding; thus concurrent drug administration is not recommended.
Antiinflammatory nonsteroidal analgesics, platelet aggregation inhibitors (such as salicylates, dextran, dipyridamole, valproic acid), and sulfinpyrazone	With high doses of carbenicillin or ticarcillin (parenteral dosage forms), an increased risk for bleeding or hemorrhage exists. These drugs inhibit platelet function and large doses of salicylates may induce hypoprothrombinemia and also gastrointestinal ulcers (from NSAIDs, salicylates, or sulfinpyrazone), all adding to the potential risk of hemorrhage.
Captopril, potassium-sparing diuretics, enalapril, lisinopril, potassium-containing drugs, or potassium supplements	If given concurrently with parenteral penicillin G potassium, serum potassium levels may increase, causing hyperkalemia. Monitor closely; dosage adjustments may be necessary.
Cholestyramine or colestipol	May decrease absorption of oral penicillin G if given concurrently. Advise clients to take antibiotic first and other medications 3 hours later.
Estrogen-containing contraceptives	When used concurrently with ampicillin, bacampicillin, or penicillin V, the effectiveness of the oral contraceptives may be decreased because of increase in estrogen metabolism or reduction in enterohepatic circulation of estrogens. Advise clients to use an alternate method of contraception while taking these antibiotics.

From McKenry L, Salerno E: *Mosby's pharmacology in nursing,* ed 19, St Louis, 1995, Mosby.

Continued.

Drug Interactions with Antibiotics—cont'd

Drug	Possible effect and management
Probenecid	Decreases renal tubular secretion of penicillins, resulting in elevated serum levels and an increase in half-life. It may also increase toxicity. Several combinations of penicillin and probenecid are marketed to take advantage of this effect.

Selected Types of Laxatives

- **Saline laxatives**—retain and increase water content of feces by virtue of osmotic qualities
- **Stimulant laxatives**—increase peristalsis in the colon by irritating intramural sensory nerve plexi endings in the mucosa
- **Bulk laxatives**—absorb water and increase the volume, bulk, and moisture of nonabsorbable intestinal contents, thereby distending the bowel and initiating reflex bowel activity
- **Intestinal lubricants**—mechanically lubricate feces to facilitate defecation
- **Emollients, or fecal softening agents**—act as dispersing wetting agents, facilitating nature of water and fatty substances within the fecal mass; when a homogeneous mixture is produced, the feces become soft
- **Hyperosmotic agents**—increase the introluminal osmotic pressure in the bowel; because they are not absorbed, they draw water into the intestine, resulting in an increased volume that stimulates peristalisis

From McKenry L, Salerno E: *Mosby's pharmacology in nursing,* ed 19, St Louis, 1995, Mosby.

Laxatives: Over-the-Counter and Prescription Varieties

	No prescription required				Prescription required	
	Irritant contact stimulant type	Osmotic saline type	Stool softener surfactant or wetting agent type	High-fiber and bulk-forming type	Lubricant	Lactulose syrup/ PEG 3350*
Disadvantages with repeated frequent (long-term) administration	Watery stools, griping	Watery stools, cramps	Unreliable results, may contribute to liver toxicity	Obstruction of narrowed lumen, some difficulty in chewing and swallowing	Anal leakage, lipid pneumonia	Early, transient flatulence and cramps; nausea reported
Increases rate of transit in small bowel	Yes	Yes	Yes	Yes	Unknown	Possibly
Causes net secretion of water and electrolytes in small bowel	Yes	Yes	Yes	Yes	No	No
Inhibits absorption in small bowel	Yes	Yes	Yes	Yes	Yes	Not reported
Increases mucosal permeability in small bowel	Yes	Not studied	Yes	Not reported	Not reported	No

Continued.

From McKenry L, Salerno E: *Mosby's pharmacology in nursing,* ed 19, St Louis, 1995, Mosby.
*PEG 3350, polyethylene glycol electrolyte solution.

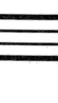

Laxatives: Over-the-Counter and Prescription Varieties—cont'd

	No prescription required					Prescription required
	Irritant contact stimulant type	Osmotic saline type	Stool softener surfactant or wetting agent type	High-fiber and bulk-forming type	Lubricant	Lactulose syrup/ PEG 3350*
Causes mucosal damage in small bowel	Yes	Not studied	Yes	Not reported	Not reported	No
Acts only in colon (not small bowel)	No	No	No	No	Yes	Yes
Indicated for long-term treatment	No	No	No	Probably	No	Yes—lactulose No—PEG
Examples of type	Anthraquinone, bisacodyl, phenolphthalein, castor oil, danthron	Magnesium salts, MOM, sodium salts, glycerin	DSS, DCS Poloxamer 188	Methylcellulose, karaya gum, sodium CMC, malt soup extract, psylium seed, agar, plantago bran (unprocessed), polycarbophil	Mineral oil	Chronulac (lactulose) CoLyte GoLYTELY (PEG 3350)

Physical or chemical property responsible for action	Mucosal surface irritation to stimulate or increase intestinal motor function or activity	Hyperosmolar ingredients trap water in intestinal lumen; hypertonicity of colon increases liquid in colon; hyperosmotic or saline	Changes surface tension of fecal mass, provides increased penetration of colonic water; penetrates and softens fecal mass by wetting agents	Absorbs water surface, increases soft fecal mass, adds bulk and moisture to feces causing distention and elimination	Coats over fecal mass, passes with ease, lubricates gastrointestinal tract and softens feces	Colon-specific increase in stool water content and stool softening by increase in osmotic pressure (hyperosmotic) and colon acidification

Laxatives and Suppositories

Laxatives

Category examples*	Actions/uses	Nursing considerations
Bulk forming		
Powders Unprocessed bran Fiberall (sugar free) Metamucil Hydrocil Instant Modane Bulk	Stimulate intestinal motility and bulks stool by absorbing water; usually begin to act in 12 to 24 hr but delay of 3 days is not unusual	Dose should be taken with at least 8 oz of fluid; interferes with absorption of digitalis, nitrofurantoin, salicylates, anticoagulants; always mix powders as directed by manufacturer; unprocessed bran can be mixed with food
Granules Periden Plain Serutan		
Miscellaneous Naturacil (soft chewable pieces) Fiber Med Crackers		

Hyperosmotic

Rectal

Glycerin (solution or suppository)

Cause local rectal irritation

May produce rectal discomfort, irritation, burning

Oral or rectal

Sorbitol (solution or powder)

Lubricant

Oral

Mineral oil

Lubricant and emulsifier; augments fecal bulk and softens stool; acts in 6 to 8 hr after oral or rectal administration

Plain mineral oil should be given on empty stomach at bedtime to avoid reflux aspiration; emulsions may be given at mealtimes; helpful in clients who should avoid straining; seepage from rectum may occur with either oral or rectal route; should not be given to elderly clients or those with impaired gag reflex because aspiration can occur with subsequent lipid pneumonia; do not give with stool softeners

Emulsion

Agoral Plain (sugar free)
Zymenol (sugar free)
Kondremul Plain (sugar free)
Petrogalar Plain (sugar free)

Rectal

Fleet Mineral Oil Enema
Saf-Tip Oil Retention Enema

Data from Carnevali DL, Patrick MP, editors: *Nursing management for the elderly*, Philadelphia, 1979, Lippincott; Iseminger M, Hardy P: *Geriatr Nurs* 3:402, 1982; Nivatvongs S, Hooks VH: *Postgrad Med* 74:313, 1983; *Nursing 85 drug handbook*, Springhouse, Pa, 1985, Springhouse.
*This is not an all-inclusive list but rather highlights the most commonly used laxatives. In addition, combination laxatives were not addressed to avoid a cumbersome and confusing table. Please refer to a pharmacology text for such agents.

Continued.

Laxatives and Suppositories—cont'd

Laxatives—cont'd

Category examples	Actions/uses	Nursing considerations
Saline		
Oral		
Phillips Milk of Magnesia	Salts contained in these agents have osmotic attraction for water; absorbed water produces laxation; should be used infrequently and in single doses; oral doses produce watery stool in 3 to 6 hr or less, whereas rectal enemas cause evacuation in 2 to 5 min	For short-term therapy, should not be used for more than 1 wk; magnesium retention possible in clients with poor renal function which can cause CNS depression; dehydration possible with hypertonic solutions of sodium
Haley's M-O		
Fleet Phospho-Soda (sodium biphosphate, sodium phosphate, potassium phosphate)		
Evac-Q Mag		
Lactulose		
Rectal		
Evac-Q-Sert		
Fleet Enema		
Phosphate Enema		
Stimulants		
Oral		
Prune juice	Causes local irritation of mucosa or selective action on nerve plexi, which causes increased motility oral bisacodyl agents act	For short-term therapy, should not be used for more than 1 wk; stimulant laxatives are ones most often abused and are habit forming
Cascara sagrada		

Modane Liquid
Dorbane
Senokot (granules or tablets)
Castor oil
Bisco-Lax
Dulcolax
Feen-A-Mint
Ex-Lax
Evac-U-Lax

Rectal
Senokot
Bisco-Lax
Dulcolax

in 6 to 8 hr and within 15 to 60 min when given rectally; cascara sagrada and senna agents act in 6 to 24 hr

Stool softeners

Oral
Surfax
Colace
Doxinate
Bu-Lax
Laxinate
Modane Soft

Act as detergents and allow water to enter feces; only soften stool and have no effect on peristaltic movements; usually given in combination with stimulant laxative; usually begin to act in 1 to 3 days

Should not be given with mineral oil agents; should be given to prevent constipation and not to resolve existing constipation

Continued.

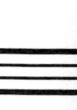

Laxatives and Suppositories—cont'd

Suppositories

Suppository (strength)	Action	Time when results expected	Disadvantages
Glycerin (mild/moderate)	Softens stool by irritating bowel, which responds by secreting fluid; irritation stimulates reflex peristalsis	Approximately 30 min	Irritant property may cause injury to mucous membrane with prolonged use
Vacuetts (mild/moderate)	Activated in water before insertion; suppository releases carbon dioxide which distends bowel and intiates reflex peristalsis	Varies	Use of petroleum lubricants negates effectiveness of suppository
Bisacodyl (Dulcolax) (strong)	Contact suppository that stimulates sensory nerve endings in colon and results in reflex peristalsis	15 to 20 min	Abdominal cramping possible

From Dittmar S: *Rehabilitation nursing: process and application*, St Louis, 1989, Mosby.

Suppositories and Medications Used for Bowel Programs in Clients with Spinal Cord Injury

Product	Action	Considerations
Laxatives		
Stimulant (contact laxative) Glycerine Bisacodyl	Acts on colonic mucosa to produce normal peristalsis through parasympathetic reflexes.	Very effective for initial bowel regulation for upper motor neuron lesion (reflex bowel); can be irritating to persons with rectal sensation.
Carbon dioxide evacuant	Acts by releasing carbon dioxide into rectum, stimulating peristalsis.	Expensive; may cause autonomic dysreflexia.
Medications		
Stool softeners Colace Surfax	Wetting agents that promote absorption of water and emulsifying fats.	Works well initially with Dulcolax suppository for clients with upper motor neuron lesion (reflex bowel).
Peristaltic stimulators Pericolace Doxidan Senekot (stimulator only)	Most are stool softeners and mild irritants that stimulate peristalsis.	Indicated initially for those with delayed response to bowel program.
Bulk formers Metamucil Fibermed	Dietary fibers that aid in absorbing water from intestinal contents and provide bulk.	Ensure adequate fluid intake. Effective with clients who have recurring problem of loose or semiformed stools and who are unable to get bulk from foods (i.e., on tube feedings).
Lactinex Yogurt	Assist in reinstating normal gastrointestinal flora.	Indicated for persons with prolonged loose stools associated with antibiotic therapy.

From Matthews PJ, Carlson CE, Holt NB: *Spinal cord injury: a guide to rehabilitation nursing*, Rockville, Md, 1987, Aspen. Copyright 1987 by Aspen Publishers, Inc.

Tricyclic and Tetracyclic Antidepressants: Side Effects/Adverse Reactions

Drug(s)	Side effects*	Adverse reactions†
Tricyclic	Most frequent: dizziness, dry mouth, headache, increased consumption of sweets, nausea, weakness, weight gain, unpleasant taste Less frequent: sweating, diarrhea, gas, insomnia, vomiting	Most frequent: not reported Less frequent: confusion, constipation (especially in geriatric clients), hypotension, dysrhythmia, nervousness, tremors, insomnia, tachycardia or bradycardia, visual pain or blurred vision
Amoxapine only		Less frequent: impairment of sexual functioning, extrapyramidal side effects (trouble speaking or swallowing, shuffle walk, slow movements, trembling, stiffness of arms and legs, loss of balance); tardive dyskinesia (abnormal chewing movements, lip smacking)
Tetracyclic Maprotiline	Most frequent: dizziness, blurred vision, dry mouth, pruritus, rash, insomnia, weakness, headache	Less frequent: severe constipation that may lead to impaction or paralytic ileus, nausea or vomiting, convulsions, tremors, increased excitement
Triazolopyridine Trazodone	Most frequent: sedation, dry mouth, nausea, vomiting, headache, dizziness, blurred vision Less frequent/rare: diarrhea, constipation, increased weakness, muscle pain or aches	Less frequent: muscle tremors, confusion Rare: hypotension, bradycardia or tachycardia, priapism, rash, excitement

Bicyclic

Fluoxetine

Most frequent: anorexia, weight loss, nausea, increased nervousness, anxiety, insomnia, increased sweating

Less frequent: tremors, dry mouth, visual disturbance, cough, chest pain

Less frequent: fever, rash, respiratory difficulties, muscle aches

Rare: convulsions

Phenylaminoketone

Bupropion

Most frequent: anorexia, dry mouth, light-headedness, nausea, vomiting, tremors, constipation, weight loss

Less frequent: chills, fever, increased weakness, sedation, bad dreams, inability to concentrate

Most frequent: increased anxiety, agitation, confusion, tachycardia, headache, convulsions with high doses

Less frequent: rash

From McKenry L, Salerno E: *Mosby's pharmacology in nursing*, ed 19, St Louis, 1995, Mosby.

*If side effects continue, increase, or disturb the client, inform the physician.

†If adverse reactions occur, contact physician, since medical intervention may be necessary.

Pharmacokinetic Overview: Benzodiazepines

Name	Duration of action*	Time to peak plasma concentration (hr) (oral)	Half-life (hr)	Active metabolites (half-life in hr)
Alprazolam (Xanax)	S-I	1-2	12-15	Alpha-hydroxy alprazolam (12-15)
Chlordiazepoxide (Librium, Libritab Medilium)	L	0.5-4	5-30	Desmethylchlordiazepoxide (18) Demoxepam (14-95) Desmethyldiazepam (30-100) Oxazepam (5-15)
Clonazepam (Klonopin, Rivotril)	S-I	1-2 (some clients from 4-8 hr)	18-50	None
Clorazepate (Tranxene, Novoclopate)	L	0.5-2	Parent drug not active	Desmethyldiazepam (30-100) Oxazepam (5-15)
Diazepam (Valium, Apo-Diazepam)	L	0.5-2	20-70	Desmethyldiazepam (30-100) Temazepam (9.5-12.4) Oxazepam (5-15)
Estazolam (Prosom)	L	2	10-24	Two identified metabolites, not believed to be active
Flurazepam (Dalmane, Apo-Flurazepam)	L	0.5-1	2.3	Desalkylflurazepam (30-100) N-1-hydroxyethylflurazepam (24)
Halazepam (Paxipam)	L	1-3	14	Desmethyldiazepam (30-100)

Drug	Classification*		Half-life	Active Metabolites (half-life)
Lorazepam (Ativan, Apo-Lorazepam)	S-I	1-6	10-20	None
Midazolam HCl (Versed)	S-I	0.5-1	2.5	1-Hydroxymethyl and 4-hydroxy midazolam
Oxazepam (Serax, Ox-pam)	S-I	1-4	5-15	None
Prazepam (Centrax)	L	2.5-6 hr for metabolite desmethyldiazepam (single dose)	Parent drug not active	Desmethyldiazepam (30-100) Oxazepam (5-15)
Quazepam (Doral)	L	2	39	Desalkylflurazepam (30-100) 2-Oxoquazepam (39)
Temazepam (Restoril)	S-I	2-3	9.5-12.4	None
Triazolam (Halcion)	S-I	Within 2	1.6-5.5	None

From McKenry L, Salerno E: *Mosby's pharmacology in nursing*, ed 19, St Louis, 1995, Mosby.
*S-I, short to intermediate acting; L, long acting.

Benzodiazepine Overdose

In conscious clients, administer an emetic followed by activated charcoal to adsorb the benzodiazepine. For unconscious clients, a gastric lavage with a cuffed endotracheal tube may be used.

Ensure maintenance of an adequate airway, closely monitor vital signs, administer oxygen for depressed respirations, and promote diuresis by the administration of intravenous fluids.

Medications that may be used include IV administration of flumazenil as a benzodiazepine antagonist and vasopressors such as norepinephrine, metaraminol, or dopamine to treat hypotension. Do not use barbiturates to treat excitation effects because they may exacerbate the condition.

Dialysis is of limited value in treating a benzodiazepine overdose.

Notes

From McKenry L, Salerno E: *Mosby's pharmacology in nursing,* ed 19, St Louis, 1995, Mosby.

Lithium Dosage and Administration

	Adults	Elderly	Children
Lithium carbonate tablets/capsules/syrup	Acute mania: 300 to 600 mg orally 3 times daily; adjust dosage as necessary according to client's response and development of side effects/adverse reactions. Maintenance: 300 mg 3 or 4 times daily, adjusted as necessary. Maximum: 2.4 g/day	Usually require a lower dosage	Children up to 12 yr, 15 to 20 mg/kg of lithium per body weight daily, divided into 2 or 3 doses. Adjust dosage weekly as necessary
Lithium carbonate extended-release tablets	450 to 900 mg orally twice a day or 300 to 600 mg orally 3 times a day; adjust dosage as necessary. Maintenance: 450 mg orally twice daily or 300 mg 3 times daily; adjust dosage as necessary. Maximum daily dose: 2.4 g/day	Usually require a lower dosage	Children less than 12 yr, not established

From McKenry L, Salerno E: *Mosby's pharmacology in nursing,* ed 19, St Louis, 1995, Mosby.

Factors Affecting Lithium Serum Levels

	Excretion:
Increased by:	
Diarrhea	
Diuretics or dehydration	
Low-salt diets	} Decreased
High fevers or strenuous exercise	
Decreased by:	
High salt intake	
High intake of sodium bicarbonate	} Increased
Pregnancy	

Characteristics of Insulin Preparations after Subcutaneous Administration

Insulins*	Onset (hours)	Peak effect (hours)	Duration of action (hours)
Rapid acting			
Insulin injection (Retular Insulin)[†]	½-1	2-4	5-7
Prompt insulin zinc suspension (Semilente)	1-3	2-8	12-16
Intermediate acting			
Insulin zinc suspension (Lente Insulin)	1-3	8-12	18-28
Isophane insulin suspension (NPH Insulin)	3-4	6-12	18-28
Isophane insulin suspension (70%) plus insulin injection (30%) (Mixtard, Novolin 70/30)	½	4-8	24
Long acting			
Extended insulin zinc suspension (Ultralente)	4-6	18-24	36
Protamine zinc insulin suspension (PZI)	4-6	14-24	36

From McKenry L, Salerno E: *Mosby's pharmacology in nursing,* ed 19, St Louis, 1995, Mosby.

*All above insulins, with the exception of Mixtard, Novolin combinations, are available in 100 unit strengths. Beef, pork, beef-pork, and human insulins are available in rapid-acting insulins and the three insulins listed under intermediate acting.

[†]This is the only insulin for intravenous use. Intravenously, the onset of action is within ⅙ to ½ hour, peak effect within ¼ to ½ hour, and duration of action within ½ to 1 hour.

Oral Hypoglycemic Agents: Pharmacokinetics

Drug	Absorption orally	Half-life (hours)	Peak effect (hours)	Duration of action (hours)	Metabolism (in liver)	Excretion
Acetohexamide	Good	6-8 (metabolite)	1-3	12-24	To active metabolite	Kidneys: bile
Chlorpropamide	Good	36	2-4	24-48 or more	80% metabolized; metabolites unknown	Kidneys
Glipizide	Good	2-4	1-3	12-24	To inactive metabolites	Kidneys
Glyburide	Good	10	4	24	To inactive metabolites	Kidneys: bile
Tolazamide	Fair (slow)	7	3-4	10	To slightly active metabolites	Kidneys
Tolbutamide	Good	5	3-4	6-12	To inactive metabolite	Kidneys: bile

From McKenry L, Salerno E: *Mosby's pharmacology in nursing*, ed 19, St Louis, 1995, Mosby.

Hypoglycemic Oral Agents:
Side Effects/Adverse Reactions

Side effects*	Adverse reactions[†]
Most frequent: diarrhea or constipation, dizziness, gas, anorexia, headache, nausea, vomiting, abdominal distress	Less frequent: chlorpropamide only—respiratory difficulties (CHF in persons with cardiac problems). Sedation; cramping of muscles; convulsions; edema of face, hands, or ankles; comatose, increased weakness (antidiuretic effect)
Less frequent/rare: photosensitivity, rash	Rare: pruritus, jaundice, light-colored stools, dark urine (impairment of liver function). Increased fatigue, sore throat, increased temperature, increased bleeding or bruising (blood dyscrasias)
	Overdosage: symptoms of hypoglycemia (see Diabetic Emergencies on p. 430)

From McKenry L, Salerno E: *Mosby's pharmacology in nursing,* ed 19, St Louis, 1995, Mosby.
*If side effects continue, increase, or disturb the client, inform the physician.
[†]If adverse reactions occur, contact the physician because medical intervention may be necessary.

Drugs with the Potential to
Cause Intellectual Impairment

Alcohol	Cimetidine
Analgesics	Digitalis
Anticholinergics	Diuretics
Antidepressants	Hypnotics
Antipsychotics	Sedatives
Antihistamines	Sudden withdrawal of benzodiazepines
Antiparkinsonism agents	

From Ebersole P, Hess P: *Toward healthy aging: human needs and nursing response,* ed 4, St Louis, 1994, Mosby.
Data compiled from Nolan L, O'Malley K: Prescribing for the elderly: part I, sensitivity of the elderly to adverse drug reactions, *Am Geriatr Soc* 3(2):142, 1988; Lamy PP: Drug interactions and the elderly, *J Geriatr Nurs* 12(2), 1986b; Lamy PP: Adverse drug effects, *Clin Geriatr Med* 6(2):293-307, 1990.

Some Preventable Drug Interactions through Proper Administration

Drug	Take with food, milk, meals	Do not take with milk or its products	May impair nutrient and electrolyte uptake and use	Do not take with alcohol	Do not take with fruit juice	Take on empty stomach
Alcohol			X			
Aminophylline and derivatives	X					
Ampicillin					X	
Antacids						X
Antihistamines				X		
Antiinfectives			X	X		
Atropine			X			
Belladonna and associated alkaloids						X
Benzathine penicillin G					X	X
Bisacodyl (Dulcolax)		X	X	X		

From Ebersole P, Hess P: *Toward healthy aging: human needs and nursing response,* ed 4, St Louis, 1994, Mosby.
Data from Knoben JE, Anderson PO: *Handbook of clinical data,* ed 6, Hamilton, Ill, 1988, Drug Intelligence Publications; Long JW: *Essential guide to prescription drugs,* New York, 1991, Harper-Collins.

Continued.

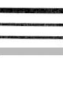

Some Preventable Drug Interactions through Proper Administration—cont'd

Drug	Take with food, milk, meals	Do not take with milk or its products	May impair nutrient and electrolyte uptake and use	Do not take with alcohol	Do not take with fruit juice	Take on empty stomach
Chloral hydrate				X		
Chlorpropamide (Diabinese)				X		
Cholestyramine (Questran)			X			
Clinamycin (Cleocin)			X			
Clofibrate (Atromid-S)			X			
Cloxacillin					X	X
Corticosteroids (oral)	X					
Diocytl sodium sulfosuccinate (Colace, Surfak)			X			
Diphenoxylate (Lomotil)			X			
Diuretics	X		X			
Donnatal						X

Erythromycin (oral)					X	X
Folic acid inhibitors			X			
Ibuprofen (Motrin)	X					
Indomethacin (Indocin)	X					
Iron salts						X
Monoamine oxidase inhibitors				X		
Methotrexate			X			
Methylphenidate (Ritalin)				X		X
Metronidazole (Flagyl)	X		X	X		
Mineral oil			X			
Narcotics				X		
Neomycin			X			
Nitrofurantoin (Furadantin)	X					

Continued.

Some Preventable Drug Interactions through Proper Administration—cont'd

Drug	Take with food, milk, meals	Do not take with milk or its products	May impair nutrient and electrolyte uptake and use	Do not take with alcohol	Do not take with fruit juice	Take on empty stomach
Nitrofurantoin macrocystals (Macrodantin)	X					
Penicillin (oral)						X
Phenazopyridine (Pyridium)						X
Phenylbutazone (Butazolidin)	X					
Phenytoin	X					
Potassium chloride solutions		X				
Rauwolfia derivatives	X			X		
Tetracyclines	X	X				
Tolbutamide (Orinase)				X		
Trimeprazine (Temaril)	X			X		

Effects of Systemic Drugs on Vision

Drug	Effect
Furosemide (Lasix)	Blurred vision, decreased tolerance to contact lenses, photophobia, allergic reactions to eyelids and conjunctivae
Propranolol (Inderal)	Transient blurred vision with diplopia, decreased accommodation
Dimetapp (antihistamine and anticholinergic effect)	Mydriasis (contraindicated in angle closure glaucoma), blurred vision, intolerance to contact lenses
Diazepam (Valium)	Allergic conjunctivitis
Digoxin (Lanoxin)	Diplopia, blurred vision, changes in color perception (warnings of toxicity)

From Ebersole P, Hess P: *Toward healthy aging: human needs and nursing response,* ed 4, St Louis, 1994, Mosby; modified from Osis M: Drugs and vision, *Gerontion* 1(5):15, 1986.

Notes

General Physiological System Characteristics of Drug Toxicity

Cardiovascular

Arrhythmias
Tachycardias
Palpitations
Hypotension
Congestive heart failure
Hypertension
Bone marrow depression
  Leukopenia
  Thrombocytopenia
  Anemia
  Agranulocytosis

Central nervous system

Confusion
Gait changes
Insomnia
Drowsiness
Blurred vision or visual changes
Slurred speech
Ototoxicity
Tremors
Irritability
Problems with temperature control
Anticholinergic effects
Seizures

Hepatic changes

Jaundice
Clotting problems
Decreased liver function

Gastrointestinal

Anorexia
Nausea and vomiting
Diarrhea
GI bleeding
Pancreatitis

Renal

Electrolyte imbalance
Polyuria
Urinary retenion
Fluid retention

Respiratory

Dyspnea
Asthmatic reactions

Skin

Rash
Urticaria
Pruritis
Photosensitivity

From Ebersole P, Hess P: *Toward healthy aging: human needs and nursing response,* ed 4, St Louis, 1994, Mosby.

Common Useful Over-the-Counter Preparations*

Medication (examples)	Use
Analgesic balm or ointment (Banalg, Ben-Gay)	Minor muscle aches and pain
Analgesic tablets (aspirin, acetaminophen)	Headaches, minor aches, pain, and fever
Antacids (Mylanta, Maalox)	Indigestion, upset stomach
Antidiarrheal (Kaopectate, Pepto Bismol)	Mild, uncomplicated diarrhea
Antihistamines (Benadryl, Chlortrimeton)	Allergies, allergic rhinitis
Antiseptics, liquid (hydrogen peroxide, isopropyl alcohol)	Hydrogen peroxide—minor cuts, scrapes and wounds; alcohol—sprains or muscle strain
Mouthwash (Gly-Oxide)	Oral wound cleansing product for minor dental inflammation or irritations
Throat lozenges (Cepacol)	Minor sore throat
Skin lotion (calamine lotion)	Insect bites, minor itching, poison ivy
Contraceptives (spermicides, condoms)	Prevention of pregnancy and sexually transmitted diseases
Ipecac syrup	Accidental poison treatment
Laxatives, mild (Milk of Magnesia)	Constipation
Motion or travel sickness preparations (Bonine, transdermal scopolamine)	Prevention of dizziness, nausea, vomiting

From Myers J: *Quick medication administration reference,* ed 2, St Louis, 1995, Mosby.

*The client should read the container label carefully, if there are any questions, the advice of the pharmacist or health care provider should be sought.

Considerations for the Elderly

Medications that Should and Should Not Be Used by Older Adults

Category	Do not use	Limited use	Okay
Cardiovascular	Aldomet Catapres Serpasil Persantine Cyclospasmol Pavabid Trental	Capoten Diazide Minipress Lasix	Inderal Lopressor Tenormin Lanoxin Nitrobid Coumadin K-Lor
Tranquilizers and hypnotics	Ativan Dalmane Halcion Librium Nembutal Restoril Valium Xanax	Serax	
Antidepressants	Elavil Triavil		
Antipsychotics		Desyrel Sinequan Tofranil Haldol Mellaril Navane Prolixin Stelazine Thorazine	Norpramine Aventyl Pamelor Lithium
Medication	Bufferin Feldene Darvocet Darvon Talwin Wygesic	Clinoril	Advil Aspirin Ecotrin Empirin Tylenol Demerol Dilaudid Percodan Vicodin

From Ebersole P, Hess P: *Toward healthy aging: human needs and nursing response,* ed 4, St Louis, 1994, Mosby. Compiled from Wolfe SM, Fugate L, Hulstrand EP et al: *Worst pills best pills,* Washington, DC, 1988, Public Citizen Health Research Group.

Category	Do not use	Limited use	Okay
Gastrointestinal	Mylanta Tigan Colace Dialose Plus Doxidan	Antivert Compazine Phenergan Reglan Milk of Magnesia	Tagamet Zantac Maalox Metamucil
Antiinfectives	Furadantin	Achromycin	Bactrim Gantrisin Keflex Penicillin Septra Vibramycin
Neurological	Artane Cogentin	Hydergine	Sinemet Dilantin Tegretol
Nutritional supplements	Vitamin E		Calcium Feosol Fergon Niacin Vitamins
Others	Norflex	Premarin	Synthroid

Special Drug Considerations for the Elderly

Drug	Special considerations
Analgesic agents	
Acetaminophen (APAP) (Tylenol, Datril)	Acetaminophen is the preferred analgesic agent with noninflammatory pain and is as effective as propoxyphene and codeine. Chronic daily ingestion of more than 4 to 5 g can lead to liver damage.
Aspirin (ASA)	Aspirin is the least expensive and is preferred over acetaminophen in inflammatory pain. It is as effective as propoxyphene and codeine. Gastrointestinal blood loss occurs in three fourths who take it and is of concern to clients with borderline anemia; concomitant liquid antacid minimizes. Antiplatelet effect may be of benefit in prevention of recurrent myocardial infarction and transient ischemic attack.
Propoxyphene and propoxyphene combinations (Darvocet-N 100 and Darvon compounds)	Single-ingredient propoxyphene is not as effective as aspirin or acetaminophen alone, but a combination is as effective as aspirin or acetaminophen. Confusional reactions are increased. Avoid long-term full-dose use.
Codeine and codeine combinations (Tylenol No. 1–4)	Codeine has equal potency with aspirin and acetaminophen. Combination has greater potency. Nausea, vomiting, and constipation are more common.
Pentazocine (Talwin)	Pentazocine is less effective than aspirin and is prone to causing confusional reactions.
Phenacetin	Never use phenacetin chronically because both prescription and OTC medications will lead to analgesic nephropathy, especially in combination analgesics.
Meperidine (Demerol), morphine, hydromorphone (Dilaudid)	Use one third to one half usual adult dose, since much more potent. No side effect differences in equal analgesic doses, but incidence increases with age.

Antiinflammatory analgesic agents

Phenylbutazone (Azolid, Buta-zolidin) and oxyphenbutazone (Tandearil)

Both have longer half-life and higher incidence of gastrointestinal upset and severe toxic reactions in older clients; therefore, give with meals or liquid antacid to minimize gastrointestinal effect. These are not recommended in those over 60 years of age by some authorities. Phenylbutazone and oxyphenylbutazone cause fluid retention, blood dyscrasias, and increased oral anticoagulant effect. Do not give full dose for more than 7 to 14 days.

Tolmetin (Tolectin), fenoprofen (Nalfon), sulindac (Clinoril), ibuprofen (Motrin), naproxen (Naprosyn)

All nonsteroidal antiinflammatory analgesics are less effective than aspirin in inflammatory disease but lower incidence of gastrointestinal side effects. These are much more expensive than aspirin.

Antidiabetic agents

Weight reduction and dietary measures control up to 70% of maturity-onset diabetes. Oral agents may increase cardiovascular morbidity. Hypoglycemic signs of tremor, sweating, and tachycardia are not as readily discernible. Chlorpropamide (Diabenese) and acetohexamide (Dymelor) have active metabolite and prolonged half-lives.

Cardiovascular drugs

Digitalis preparations

Digoxin (Lanoxin) is the preferred glycoside. Avoid digitoxin and digitalis leaf (long hepatic and renal half-lives). Although beneficial in low output failure and atrial fibrillation, digitalis preparations are successfully withdrawn in up to three fourths of clients. Subacute toxicity of anorexia with weight loss is more common than initial signs of gastrointestinal or cardiovascular effects. Baseline and follow-up electrocardiograms are essential. Dose is based on lean body weight and creatinine clearance with attention to electrolyte and thyroid status. One third to one half of clients are noncompliant.

From Ebersole P, Hess P: *Toward healthy aging: human needs and nursing response*, ed 4, St Louis, 1994 Mosby; modified from Deverau MO, Andrus L, Scott C: *Elder care*, New York, 1981, Grune & Stratton.

Continued.

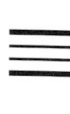

Special Drug Considerations for the Elderly—cont'd

Drug	Special considerations
Cardiovascular drugs—cont'd	
Quinidine	Quinidine has higher serum levels if used concurrently with both drugs and digoxin. Half-life is prolonged. Cinchonism (gastrointestinal effects, light-headedness, tinnitus) occurrence is more common with low body weight. Decrease loading dose by one third in clients with significant heart failure.
Propranolol (Inderal)	Toxic effects are more common, as is reduced beta-blocking responsiveness in older clients. Propranolol aggravates bronchospastic tendency in chronic obstructive pulmonary disease and can precipitate heart failure. Propranolol also affects diabetic control at higher doses, and there is increased tendency of "cold limb" effect in lower extremities in those with peripheral vascular or vasospastic diseases.
Nitroglycerin tablets (Nitrostat)	Nitrostat is the most stable form. Client must sit down before sublingual dose placement. Beware of orthostatic effect of all vasodilators.
Nitroglycerin ointment (Nitrol)	Never rub into skin. Headache may be relieved with aspirin or acetaminophen.
Long-acting nitrates (isosorbide [Isordil, Sorbitrate] and penta-erythritol tetranitrate [Peritrate])	Long-acting nitrates are variably effective. Be careful about blood pressure–lowering effect.
Antihypertensive agents	
Diuretics	All diuretics increase incontinence.
Thiazides (many; no significant difference; use hydrochloriazide generic)	Start with lowest possible dose. Clients must drink sufficient liquids. Watch volume, serum electrolyte, urate, and glucose effect.

Furosemide (Lasix)	Furosemide is most potent diuretic and should be held until thiazides no longer effective. It promotes calcium excretion and profoundly depletes sodium, potassium, and chloride. Cautious use of potassium supplements and salt substitutes is necessary because the elderly tend to have lower total body potassium with decreased muscle mass.
Spironolactone (Aldactone)	Spironolactone is a potassium-sparing diuretic often used in combination with thiazide (Aldactazide). Special caution is necessary if concurrent potassium supplement or salt substitute is used. Fatal hyperkalemia has been reported.
Triemterene (Dyrenium)	Triamterene is a potassium-sparing diuretic most often used in combination with thiazide (Dyazide) with similar precaution as spironolactone.
Sympatholytic antihypertensive agents	
Methyldopa (Aldomet)	Beware of continued blood pressure below 120/70, orthostatic effects, impaired male sexual function, and drowsiness or sedation. Reduce dosage when methyldopa is given in combination with thiazide (Aldoril). Sodium retention is seen when diuretic is not used. Daily dose at bedtime may take advantage of sedative effect, with therapeutic effect equivalent to multiple daily doses.
Propranolol (Inderal)	Propranolol is the only sympatholytic agent not requiring diuretic to prevent sodium retention. See cardiovascular section. If pulse is less than 50 to 60 beats per minute, drug is poorly tolerated.
Guanethidine (Ismelin)	Guanethidine is a profound sympatholytic agent with long second phase half-life. Use in small doses. Tricyclic antidepressants can interfere with antihypertensive effect.
Reserpine	Avoid giving reserpine to those with depression, sinusitis, peptic ulcer disease, and history of breast cancer.

Continued.

Special Drug Considerations for the Elderly—cont'd

Drug	Special considerations
Anticoagulant agents	
Heparin	Heparin increases risk of bleeding with age, especially in women over 60 years of age.
Warfarin (Coumadin)	Warfarin increases risk of bleeding with age because of altered sensitivity with genetic, nutritional, and liver factors. Carefully evaluate use, and do serial prothrombin times. Beware of risk of hemorrhage, especially with possible hemorrhagic stroke, peptic ulcer disease, hiatal hernia, and diverticulosis or any bleeding diathesis. Concurrent aspirin usage is not possible except with heart valve prostheses.
Sedative-hypnotics and minor tranquilizers	
Barbiturates (Butisol, Nembutal), phenobarbital, secobarbital (Seconal), amobarbital (Amytal)	With the exception of phenobarbital as an anticonvulsant, continued use of other barbiturates is irrational because of prolonged half-lives, paradoxic excitation in some, and tolerance and sleep pattern aberrations in all.
Benzodiazepines, chlordiazepoxide (Librium), diazepam (Valium), clorazepate (Tranxene), lorazepam (Ativan), oxazepam (Serax), and flurazepam (Dalmane)	Prolonged half-lives and cumulation of benzodiazepines have been reported with all except Ativan and Serax. Prolonged daily sedative (1 to 3 months) or hypnotic (7 to 14 days) use is not recommended because of depression of normal sleep pattern and resultant confusion, delirium, and psychological changes. Serax is best choice because of short half-life. No hypnotic should be used nightly longer than 14 days; instead skip to every third night.
Chloral hydrate (Noctec)	Chloral hydrate is an excellent hypnotic in clients with no liver disease.

Antihistamines

Diphenhydramine (Benadryl), hydroxyzine (Atarax, Visaril), phenylephrine (Dimetane), and chlorpheniramine (Chlor-Trimeton)

Antihistamines may be used for intercurrent use as needed for sedation and hypnotic effect. Beware of anticholinergic and tolerance effect with long-term use.

Nonbarbiturate hypnotic agents

Ethinamate (Valmid), methaqualone (Quaalude), methyprylon (Noludar), glutethimide (Doriden), and ethchlorvynol (Placidyl)

None of these are recommended because of same types of problems as in barbiturates.

Major tranquilizers—antipsychotic agents

Phenothiazines, thioridazone (Mellaril), trifluoperazine hydrochloride (Stelazine), triflupromazine (Vesprin), and fluphenazine (Prolixin)

Use lowest possible dose and titrate approximately. Increased incidence of extrapyramidal symptoms in elderly. Postural (orthostatic) hypotension is a problem. Temperature control and tardive dyskinesia are more common with higher doses.

Butyrophenone (Haldol) and thioxanthene (Navane)

Highest incidence of extrapyramidal symptoms occur with these drugs. These are potent antipsychotic agents with low order of side effects and create episodes of amnesia and confusion.

Continued.

Special Drug Considerations for the Elderly—cont'd

Drug	Special considerations
Antidepressant agents Amitriptyline (Elavil), nortriptyline (Aventyl), imipramine (Tofranil), desipramine (Pertofrane), protriptyline (Vivactil), and doxepin (Sinequan)	Antidepressants are useful only in endogenous depression in up to one half usual dosage. These drugs can exacerbate tremors, psychosis, constipation, postural hypotension, benign prostatic hypertrophy, delayed micturition, and arrhythmias. Because of prolonged half-life, use caution in full-dose bedtime use, especially with Elavil and Tofranil.
Antiparkinsonian agents Trihexyphenidyl (Artane), procyclidine (Kemadrin), benztropine (Cogentin), and diphenhydramine (Benadryl)	Prophylactic use with antipsychotic agents is generally not recommended. When extrapyramidal symptoms appear, 1 to 3 month use may be beneficial. Watch for constipation, tremors, and delirium resulting from prolonged use, especially with Cogentin.
Carbidopa-levodopa (Sinemet)	Carbidopa-levodopa is generally better tolerated than levodopa alone with less side effects (hypotension, syncope, anorexia, nausea, and emesis).

Side Effects of Drugs Used by the Elderly

Analgesic (mild)

ASA: gastric irritant, allergic rhinitis, anticoagulant, uric acid precipitation

Analgesic (strong)

Depress CNS, circulation, and respiration; some cause constipation, sedation

Antacids

Decrease nutrient absorption; interfere with absorption of some other drugs; decrease stomach acidity; decrease calcium metabolism and absorption

Antiarrhythmics

Procainamide may cause agranulocytosis, fever, chills, and hypersensitivity; lidocaine needs careful monitoring in persons with impaired liver function; quinidine can cause tinnitus, nausea, and arrhythmias; idiosyncrasies are common; propranolol (beta-adrenergic blocker), use cautiously with elderly

Antiarthritics

Phenylbutazone and oxyphenbutazone cause numerous side effects with high risk of severe or fatal toxic reactions; corticosteroids can cause gastrointestinal problems, depression, personality disturbance, irritability, and toxic psychoses

Anticholinergics

Blurred vision, dry mouth, urinary retention, intraocular pressure

Anticoagulants

Necessary to titrate to avoid internal bleeding; antibiotics and mineral oil decrease vitamin K production and thus potentiate anticoagulant effects

Anticonvulsants

Decrease folic acid activity, hypersensitivity; inhibit metabolism; primidone can cause anemia and visual hallucinations

Antidepressants

Imipramine, desipramine, amitryptyline, and nortriptyline all possess anticholinergic properties and must be used with caution in clients with glaucoma

Antihistamines

Drowsiness, blurred vision, and CNS depression, which is potentiated by alcohol

Antihypertensives

Thiazides and furosemide deplete potassium; triamterene or spironolactone may cause hyperkalemia; guanethidine and rauwolfia derivatives should be used together cautiously because they may cause excessive postural hypotension, bradycardia, and mental depression; hydralazine causes headaches, angina, and an arthritis-like syndrome

Antiinfectives

Hypersensitivity, gastrointestinal disturbance, pruritus, deafness, hepatic dysfunction, aplastic anemia; effects vary with the particular drug

Antiparkinsonians

Levodopa may cause nausea, hypotension, dyskinesia, agitation, restlessness and insomnia, cardiac and gastrointestinal effects; use with caution in clients with bronchial asthma or emphysema

From Ebersole P, Hess P: *Toward healthy aging: human needs and nursing response,* ed 4, St Louis, 1994, Mosby.

Continued.

Side Effects of Drugs Used by the Elderly—cont'd

Antipsychotics

In various degrees depending on the drug, all phenothiazines can cause photosensitivity, blood dyscrasias, agranulocytosis, and extrapyramidal effects (seen in 90% of clients after 10 weeks of therapy); haloperidol causes lethargy, decreased thirst, and jaundice, dosage should be considerably reduced for geriatric client; lithium carbonate has toxic level close to therapeutic; side effects are diarrhea, vomiting, tremors, sodium depletion, and muscular weakness; adequate salt and water intake is essential

Cough and cold preparations

OTC cough and cold preparations contain antihistamines and adrenergic decongestants; drugs with anticholinergic effects can contribute to a variety of drug interactions when taken with prescription drugs

Digitalis

Therapeutic and toxic levels close; frequent toxicity producing nausea, arrhythmias, hazy, yellow vision, and weight loss; potassium depletion sensitizes myocardium to digitalis and may also prolong toxicity, resulting in confusion and hallucinations

Diuretics

Thiazides can cause photosensitivity, pancreatitis, sodium and potassium depletion, and precipitate uric acid; ethacrynic acid can cause potassium depletion, vertigo, gastrointestinal problems, and hearing impairment; furosemide has similar side effects and may also alter color vision; spironolactone is potassium sparing but may cause hyperkalemia and drowsiness

Estrogens

Titrate dosage; use for 3 weeks with 1-week rest

Hypnotics

Barbiturates cause daytime drowsiness and hangover, aggravate cerebral anoxia, hypotension, delirium, and depress respiratory function, may cause decrease in REM sleep and rebound on withdrawal; chloral hydrate causes gastrointestinal irritation; dalmane may cause an arthritic-like allergic reaction

Hypoglycemics

Action altered by other drugs; avoid alcohol; oral preparations have numerous adverse side effects; some persons allergic to pork or beef insulin

Laxatives

Phenolphthalein may cause cardiac and respiratory distress in susceptible individuals

Psychotropics

Antianxiety drugs cause CNS depression and ataxia and may be habit forming with a definite withdrawal syndrome; benzodiazepines cause drowsiness, vivid dreams, ataxia, and convulsions on withdrawal; alcohol should be avoided

Vitamins

Ascorbic acids in dose of 1 g/day can cause diarrhea and precipitation of oxalic and uric acid crystals; vitamin D in large doses produces hypercalcemia, weakness, fatigue, headache, nausea, vomiting, and diarrhea

How to Assess the "At-Risk" Geriatric Client

1. Interview client to obtain a complete drug history. Carefully question him or her about disease states, illnesses, current use of medications (prescribed, over-the-counter, home remedies, herbals, vitamins, etc.), drug allergies (obtain description of allergy, time it occurred, intervention used, outcome), and any troubling side or adverse effects.

2. Make list of name, strength, and directions of each medication (prescribed and OTC) the person takes. Include prn medications, especially if person reports taking them one or more times per week.

3. Identify all physicians prescribing for this client. This information may be obtained by client interview and should be verified by checking prescription labels.

4. Prescription bottles may also provide additional information to review, for example, check name(s) of pharmacy(ies) that have dispensed medications to the person. If more than one pharmacy is involved, determine the reason why.

5. Check all prescription and OTC drug containers for expiration dates. Ask the client for permission to destroy any expired medications because they have the potential of being ineffective or causing harm.

6. Question clients on their self-medication practices, that is, how do they remember to take their scheduled medications; do they ever forget to take a dose and if so, what do they do; have they ever deliberately stopped their medication—if yes, obtain an explanation why, etc. Such information will help in evaluating compliance (or noncompliance) and if the medications are being consumed safely, according to the prescribed schedule.

7. Discover whether the client has any limitations that may impair safe, self-administration of medication. Examples include physical impairment, memory loss, health or cultural beliefs, financial constraints, and lack of social support.

From McKenry L, Salerno E: *Mosby's pharmacology in nursing,* ed 19, St Louis, 1995, Mosby.

Drugs Most Commonly Prescribed for the Elderly

- Diuretics
- Potassium salts
- H$_2$ antagonists
- Nitroglycerin
- Insulin
- Digitalis preparations
- Beta blockers
- Antianxiety agents
- Antihypertensives

From McKenry L, Salerno E: *Mosby's pharmacology in nursing,* ed 19, St Louis, 1995, Mosby.

Selected Problem Medications in the Elderly

Medication	Elderly response
Digoxin, digitalis preparations	Visual disorders, nausea, diarrhea, cardiac arrhythmias, hallucinations
Anticholinergics (antispasmodics)	Blurred vision, dry mouth, constipation, confusion, urinary retention, tachycardia
Phenothiazines	Hypotension, tremors, extrapyramidal side effects, restlessness
Analgesics, opioid	Confusion, constipation, urinary retention, nausea, vomiting, respiratory depression, addiction
Analgesics, nonnarcotic (aspirin)	Tinnitus, gastric distress, GI bleeding
Anticoagulant (heparin, warfarin)	Bleeding episodes, hemorrhage
Thiazide diuretics	Electrolyte imbalance (hypokalemia), rashes, fatigue, leg cramps, dehydration
Hypnotic-sedatives	Confusion, daytime sedation and ataxia, lethargy, increased forgetfulness
Antihypertensives (e.g., methyldopa)	Nausea, hypotension, diarrhea, bradycardia, heart failure
Antiarthritics (e.g., ibuprofen)	Edema, nausea, abdominal distress, gastric ulceration or bleeding

From McKenry L, Salerno E: *Mosby's pharmacology in nursing,* ed 19, St Louis, 1995, Mosby.

Toxic Characteristics of Specific Drugs Prescribed for the Elderly

Drugs	Signs and symptoms

Benzodiazepines
  Diazepam (Valium)
  Flurazepam (Dalmane)
  Lorazepam (Atavan)
	Ataxia, restlessness, confusion, depression, anticholinergic effect

Cimetidine (Tagamet)	Confusion, depression
Digitalis	Confusion, headache, anorexia, vomiting, arrhythmias, blurred vision or other visual changes (halos, frost on objects, color blindness), paresthesia
Furosemide (Lasix)	Electrolyte imbalance, hepatic changes, pancreatitis, leukopenia, thrombocytopenia
Gentamycin (Garamycin)	Ototoxicity (impaired hearing or balance), nephrotoxicity
L-Dopa	Muscle and eye twitching, disorientation, asterixis, hallucinations, dyskinetic movements, grimacing, depression, delirium, ataxia
Lithium (Eskalith, Lithane)	Confusion, diarrhea, drowsiness, anorexia, slurred speech, tremors, blurred vision, unsteadiness, polyuria, seizures, muscle weakness
Methyldopa (Aldomet)	Hepatic changes, mental depression, fever, bradycardia, nightmares, tremors, edema
Nonsteroidal antiinflammatory agents (NSAIA) Ibuprofen (Advil, Motrin, Nuprin, Rufin)	Photosensitivity, fluid retention, anemia, nephrotoxicity, visual changes

Indomethacin (Indocin)
  Fenoprofen (Nalfon)
  Phenylbutazone (Butazolodin)
  Piroxicam (Feldene)
  Sulindac (Clinoril)
  Tolmetin (Tolectin)
	Confusion plus the above

From Ebersole P, Hess P: *Toward healthy aging: human needs and nursing response,* ed 4, St Louis, 1994, Mosby. Data compiled from Skidmore-Roth L: *Nursing drug reference,* St Louis, 1992, Mosby; *Physicians' desk reference,* Ordell, NJ, 1992, Medical Economics; Salzman C: Basic principles of psychotropic drug prescription for the elderly, *Hosp Comm Psychiatr* 33:133, 1982; Todd B: Identifying drug toxicity, *Geriatr Nurs* 4:231, 1985. *Continued.*

Toxic Characteristics of Specific Drugs Prescribed for the Elderly—cont'd

Drugs	Signs and symptoms
Phenothiazide tranquilizers	Tachycardia, arrhythmias, dyspnea, hyperthermia, postural hypotension, restlessness, anticholinergic effects
Phenytoin (Dilantin)	Ataxia, slurred speech, confusion, nystagmus, diplopia, nausea and vomiting
Procainamide (Pronestyl, Procan, Promine, Sub-Quin, Rhythin)	Arrhythmias, depression, hypotension, SLE syndrome, dyspnea, skin rash, nausea and vomiting
Ranitidine (Zantac)	Liver dysfunction, blood dyscrasias
Sulfonyurals—1st generation Chlorpropamide (Diabinese)	Hypoglycemia, hepatic changes, CHF
Tolbutamide (Orinase)	Bone marrow depression, jaundice
Theophylline (Bronkotabs, Elixophyllin, Quinibron)	Anorexia, nausea, vomiting, GI bleeding, tachycardia, arrhythmias, irritability, insomnia, seizures, muscle twitching
Tricyclic antidepressants Amitriptyline (Elavil, Endep, Amitril) Doxepin (Sinequan, Adapin) Imipramine (Tofranil)	Confusion, arrhythmias, seizures, agitation, tachycardia, jaundice, hallucinations, postural hypotension, anticholinergic effects

INDEX

Italic page numbers indicate figures;
page numbers followed by a *t* indicate
tables.